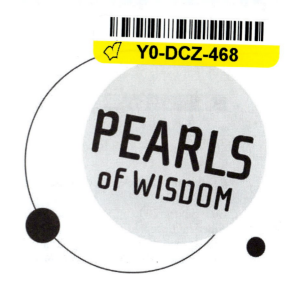

Pulmonary Medicine
REVIEW

Second Edition

Michael Zevitz
Richard Lenhardt

McGraw-Hill
Medical Publishing Division

New York Chicago San Francisco Lisbon London
Madrid Mexico City Milan New Delhi
San Juan Seoul Singapore
Sydney Toronto

Pulmonary Medicine Review, Second Edition

1 2 3 4 5 6 7 8 9 0   CUS/CUS   0 9 8 7 6 5

ISBN 0-07-146451-4

Notice

Medicine is an ever-changing science. As new research and clinical experience broaden our knowledge, changes in treatment and drug therapy are required. The authors and the publisher of this work have checked with sources believed to be reliable in their efforts to provide information that is complete and generally in accord with the standards accepted at the time of publication. However, in view of the possibility of human error or changes in medical sciences, neither the authors nor the publisher nor any other party who has been involved in the preparation or publication of this work warrants that the information contained herein is in every respect accurate or complete, and they disclaim all responsibility for any errors or omissions or for the results obtained from use of the information contained in this work. Readers are encouraged to confirm the information contained herein with other sources. For example and in particular, readers are advised to check the product information sheet included in the package of each drug they plan to administer to be certain that the information contained in this work is accurate and that changes have not been made in the recommended dose or in the contraindications for administration. This recommendation is of particular importance in connection with new or infrequently used drugs.

The editors were Catherine A. Johnson and Marsha Loeb.
The production supervisor was Phil Galea.
The cover designer was Handel Low.
Von Hoffmann Graphics was printer and binder.

This book is printed on acid-free paper.

Cataloging-in-Publication data for this title is on file at the Library of Congress.

INTERNATIONAL EDITION ISBN: 0-07-110892-0

DEDICATION

To my many mentors at Chicago Medical School.

Mike

To my Parents, for their constant love.

Richard

EDITORS-IN-CHIEF:

Mike Zevitz, M.D.
Assistant Professor
Chicago Medical School
Chicago, IL

Richard Lenhardt, M.D.
Havard Medical School
Boston, MA

CONTRIBUTING AUTHORS:

Bobby Abrams, M.D., FAAEM
Attending Physician
Macomb Hospital
Macomb, MI

Ishtiaq Ahmad, Ph.D., M.B.B.S.
Research Associate
Laboratory of Cellular and Molecular
Cerebral Ischemia
Departments of Neurology and Anatomy &
Cell Biology
Center of Molecular Medicine and Genetics
Center of Molecular and Cellular Toxicology
Wayne State University School of Medicine
Detroit, MI

James W. Albers, M.D., Ph.D.
Department of Neurology
University of Michigan
Ann Arbor, MI

W. Michael Alberts, M.D.
Professor and Associate Chair
Department of Internal Medicine
H. Lee Moffitt Cancer Center & Research
Institute
University of South Florida
Tampa, FL

Pranav Amin, M.D.
Department of Neurology
Duke University Medical Center
Durham, NC
Linda Anderson, M.D.
Department of Internal Medicine
Pulmonary and Critical Care Medicine
Section
University of Nebraska Medical Center
Omaha, NE

Michael L. Ault, M.D.
Instructor in Anesthesiology
Section of Critical Care Medicine
Department of Anesthesiology
Northwestern University Medical School
Chicago, IL

Howard Belzberg, M.D.
Los Angeles County and University of
Southern California Medical Center
Los Angeles, CA

Brian Bonanni, M.D.
Duke University Medical Center
Durham, NC

Jon M. Braverman, M.D.
Denver Health Medical Center
University of Colorado School of Medicine
Denver, CO

Gwenda Lyn Breckler, D.O.
Dept. of Surgery
Mt. Sinai Hospital
Chicago, IL

David F. M. Brown, M.D.
Instructor in Medicine
Harvard Medical School
Massachusetts General Hospital
Boston, MA

Edward Buckley, M.D.
Department of Neurology
Duke University Medical Center
Durham, NC

Leslie S. Carroll, M.D.
Assistant Professor
Chicago Medical School
Toxicology Director
Mt. Sinai Medical Center
Chicago, IL

Eduardo Castro, M.D.
Instructor in Medicine
Harvard Medical School
Massachusetts General Hospital
Boston, MA

Seemant Chatruvedi, M.D.
Assistant Professor of Neurology
Wayne State University School of medicine
Co-Director, Harper Hospital Acute Stroke
Unit
Detroit, MI

Willie Chen, M.D.
Louisville, KY

Ronald D. Chervin, M.D., MS
Sleep Disorders Center
Department of Neurology
University of Michigan Health System
Ann Arbor, MI

David Chiu, M.D.
Assistant Professor of Neurology
Director, Stroke Center
Baylor College of Medicine
The Methodist Hospital
Houston, TX

Charles H. Cook, M.D.
Assistant Professor of Surgery and Critical
Care
The Ohio State University Hospitals
Columbus, OH

Joseph T. Cooke, M.D., FACCP
Associate Professor of Clinical Medicine
Associate Director, Medical Critical Care
The New York Hospital-Cornell Medical
Center
New York, NY

William M. Coplin, M.D.
Assistant Professor
Neurology and Neurological Surgery
Wayne State University
Detroit, MI

C. James Corrall, M.D., MPH
Clinical Associate Professor of Pediatrics
Clinical Associate Professor of Emergency
Medicine
Indiana University School of Medicine
Indianapolis, IN

Douglas B. Coursin, M.D.
Professor of Anesthesiology and Internal
Medicine
Associate Director of the Trauma and
Life Support Center
University of Wisconsin School of Medicine
Madison, WI

Ruben Vargas-Cuba, M.D.
Instructor in Medicine
Chief Medical Resident
Department of Medicine
Tulane University School of Medicine
New Orleans, LA

G. Paul Dabrowski, M.D.
Assistant Professor of Surgery
University of Pennsylvania
Philadelphia, PA

Brian J. Daley, M.D.
Assistant Professor
Division of Trauma and Critical Care
The University of Tennessee Medical Center
Knoxville, TN

Carl W. Decker, M.D.
Madigan Army Medical Center
Fort Lewis, WA

Joshua De Leon, M.D.
Assistant Professor of Medicine
Mount Sinai School of Medicine
New York, NY
Director, Cardiac Catherization and Invasive
Cardiology
Elmhurst Hospital Center
Elmhurst, NY

Peter Emblad, M.D.
Boston City Hospital
Boston, MA

Phillip Fairweather, M.D.
Clinical Assistant Professor
Mount Sinai School of Medicine
New York, NY
Department of Emergency Medicine
Elmhurst Hospital Center
Elmhurst, NY

Craig Feied, M.D.
Clinical Associate Professor
George Washington University
Washington Hospital Center
Washington, D.C.

Eva L. Feldman, M.D., Ph.D.
Department of Neurology
University of Michigan
Ann Arbor, MI

Louis Flancbaum, M.D., FACS, FCCM,
FCCP
Associate Professor of Surgery,
Anesthesiology, and Human Nutrition
The Ohio State University Hospitals
Columbus, OH

Mark Franklin, M.D.
Department of Anesthesiology
Northwestern University Medical School
Chicago, IL

Rajesh R. Gandhi, M.D.
Critical Care/Trauma Fellow
University of Pennsylvania
Philadelphia, PA

Judith L. Geidebring, M.D.
Lecturer
University of Michigan
Ann Arbor, MI

Sheree Givre, M.D.
Clinical Assistant Professor
Department of Emergency Medicine
Mount Sinai School of Medicine
New York, NY
Associate Director
Department of Emergency Medicine
Elmhurst Hospital Center
Elmhurst, NY

Bill Gossman, M.D.
Chicago Medical School
Mt. Sinai Medical Center
Chicago, IL

Vicente H. Gracias, M.D.
Instructor of Surgery and Trauma
Surgical Critical Care Fellow
University of Pennsylvania
Philadelphia, PA

L. John Greenfield, Jr., M.D., Ph.D.
Assistant Professor
Department of Neurology
University of Michigan
Ann Arbor, MI

Rajan Gupta, M.D.
Instructor of Surgery and Trauma
Surgical Critical Care Fellow
University of Pennsylvania
Philadelphia, PA

Susan M. Harding, M.D.
Assistant Professor of Medicine
Pulmonary and Critical Care Medicine
University of Alabama
Birmingham, AL

Marilyn T. Haupt, M.D.
Professor, Department of Medicine
Wayne State University School of Medicine
Detroit, MI

Jeffrey W. Hawkins, M.D.
Co-Director, Pulmonary and Critical Care
Medicine
Norwood Clinic
Birmingham, AL

Thomas W. Hejkal, M.D.
Department of Ophthalmology
University of Nebraska Medical Center
Omaha, NE

James F. Holmes, M.D.
University of California, Davis
School of Medicine
Sacramento, CA

Eddie Hooker, M.D.
Assistant Professor
University of Louisville
Louisville, KY
Shyam Ivaturi, M.D.
Ridgeland, MS

Cameron Javid, M.D.
Department of Ophthalmology
Tulane University
New Orleans, LA

Mishith Joshi, M.D.
Stroke Fellow
Department of neurology
Wayne State University
Detroit, MI

Marc J. Kahn, M.D.
Assistant Professor of Medicine
Internal Medicine Residency Program
Director
Associate Director for Student Programs
Department of Medicine
Section of Hematology/Medical Oncology
Tulane University School of Medicine
New Orleans, LA

Henry J. Kaminski, M.D.
Case Western Reserve University School of
Medicine
Department of Veterans Affairs Medical
Center
University Hospitals of Cleveland
Cleveland, OH

Stuart Kessler, M.D.
Vice Chairman, Department of Emergency
Medicine
Mount Sinai School of Medicine
New York, NY
Director, Department of Emergency Medicine
Elmhurst Hospital Center
Elmhurst, NY

Ali M. Khorrami, M.D., Ph.D.
University Eye Institute
Syracuse, NY

Albert S. Khouri, M.D.
Kentucky Lions Eye Center
Louisville, KY

Lance W. Kreplick, M.D.
Assistant Professor
University of Illinois
EHS Christ Hospital
Oak Lawn, IL

Andrew Lee, M.D.
Department of Ophthalmology
Baylor College of Medicine
Houston, TX

Deborah Anne Lee, M.D., Ph.D.
Assistant Professor
Department of Psychiatry and Neurology
Section of Child Neurology
Clinical Assistant Professor
Department of Pediatrics
Director of the Child Neurology Training
Program
Tulane University Medical Center
New Orleans, LA

Kevin R. Lee, M.D.
Chief Resident
Neurological Surgery
Wayne State University
Detroit, MI

Klaus-Dieter K.L. Lessnau, M.D.
New York, NY

Gillian Lewke, P.A., CMA
Physician Assistant
Rockford Memorial Hospital
Rockford, IL

Joseph Lieber, M.D.
Associate Attending in Medicine
Chief, Medical Consult Service
Elmhurst Hospital Center
Elmhurst, NY
Clinical Associate Professor of Medicine
Mount Sinai School of Medicine
New York, NY

Mary W. Lieh-Lai, M.D.
Director, ICU
Associate Professor, Department of Pediatrics
Children's Hospital of Michigan
Wayne State University School of Medicine
Detroit, MI

Marijana Ljubanovic, M.D.
Fellow in Critical Care Medicine
Section of Critical Care Medicine
Department of Anesthesiology
Northwestern University Medical School
Chicago, IL

Bernard Lopez, M.D.
Assistant Professor
Thomas Jefferson Medical College
Thomas Jefferson University Hospital
Philadelphia, PA

Kenneth Maiese, M.D.
Associate Professor
Laboratory of Cellular and Molecular
Cerebral Ischemia
Departments of Neurology and Anatomy &
Cell Biology
Center of Molecular Medicine and Genetics
Center of Molecular and Cellular Toxicology
Wayne State University School of Medicine
Detroit, MI

John T. Malcynski, M.D.
Instructor of Surgery and Trauma
Surgical Critical Care Fellow
University of Pennsylvania
Philadelphia, PA

Mary Nan S. Mallory, M.D.
Instructor
University of Louisville
Louisville, KY

Sanjeev Maniar, M.D.
Department of Neurology
Wayne State University
Detroit, MI

Gregory P. Marelich, M.D., FACP, FCCP
Assistant Professor of Clinical Internal
Medicine
Division of Pulmonary and Critical Care
Medicine
University of California Davis Medical Center
Sacramento, CA

Joseph Masci, M.D.
Associate Director of Medicine
Mount Sinai Services
Elmhurst Hospital Center
Elmhurst, NY
Associate Professor of Medicine
Mount Sinai School of Medicine
New York, NY

Terence McGarry, M.D.
Pulmonary and Critical Care Medicine
Elmhurst Hospital Center
Elmhurst, NY
Assistant Professor of Medicine
Mount Sinai School of Medicine
New York, NY

Luis Mejico, M.D.
Department of Neurology
Georgetown University Medical Center
Washington, DC

Kevin Miller, M.D.
Jules Stein Eye Institute
Los Angeles, CA

David Morgan, M.D.
University of Texas
Southwestern Medical Center
Parkland Memorial Hospital
Dallas, TX

Gholam K. Motamedi, M.D.
Department of Neurology
Baylor College of Medicine
Houston, TX

Debasish Mridha, M.D.
Department of Neurology
Wayne State University School of Medicine
Detroit, MI

Anthony M. Murro, M.D.
Associate Professor of Neurology
Department of Neurology
Medical College of Georgia
Augusta, GA

Debra Myers, M.D.
Pulmonary/Critical Care Division
Sleep Disorders Medicine
Assistant Professor
Department of Internal medicine
Wayne State University School of Medicine
Detroit, MI

Sarah T. Nath, M.D.
Sleep Disorders Center
Department of Neurology
University of Michigan Health System
Ann Arbor, MI

Kurt M. Nellhaus, M.D., FCCP
Pulmonary Service, Department of Medicine
Lakes Region General Hospital
Laconia, NH

N. K. Nikhar, M.D., MRCP
Chief Resident
Department of Neurology
University Health Center
Detroit, MI

Scott Olitsky, M.D.
Children's Hospital of Buffalo
Buffalo, NY

Lavi Oud, M.D.
Department of Critical Care Medicine
Wayne State University School of Medicine
Detroit, MI

Igor Ougorets, M.D.
Chief Resident
Department of Neurology
Department of Veterans Affairs Medical
Center
University Hospitals of Cleveland
Cleveland, OH

Edward A. Panacek, M.D.
Associate Professor
University of California, Davis
School of Medicine
Sacramento, CA

Deric M. Park, M.D.
Department of Neurology
The University of Chicago
Chicago, IL
Professor and Chairman
Department of Anesthesiology
Fletcher Allen Health Care
University of Vermont College of Medicine
Burlington, VT

Anthony T. Reder, M.D.
Associate Professor of Neurology
Department of Neurology
The University of Chicago
Chicago, IL

Juan Carlos Restrepo, M.D.
Diplomat of the American Board of
Anesthesiology
Board Certified in Critical Care Medicine
VA Medical Center – Jackson Memorial
Hospital
University of Miami
Miami, FL

Perry Richardson, M.D.
Department of Neurology
George Washington University Medical
Center
Washington, DC

Karen Rhodes, M.D.
University of Chicago Medical Center
Chicago, IL

Luis R. Rodriquez, M.D., F.A.A.P.
Assistant Professor of Pediatrics
Mount Sinai School of Medicine
New York, NY
Elmhurst Hospital Center
Elmhurst, NY

Lisa Rogers, D.O.
Associate Professor of Neurology
Wayne State University School of Medicine
Detroit, MI

Carlo Rosen, M.D.
Instructor in Medicine
Harvard Medical School
Massachusetts General Hospital
Boston, MA

Jeffrey Rosenfeld, Ph.D., M.D.
Director Neuromuscular Program
Carolinas Medical Center-Internal Medicine
Charlotte, NC

James A. Rowley, M.D.
Assistant Professor of Medicine
Division of Pulmonary/Critical Care Medicine
Wayne State University School of Medicine
Medical Director
Harper Hospital Sleep Disorders Center
Detroit, MI

Bruce K. Rubin, M.D.
Professor of Pediatrics, Physiology and
Pharmacology
Brenner Children's Hospital
Winston-Salem, NC

David Rubenstein, M.D.
Division of Cardiology
Elmhurst Hospital Center
Elmhurst, NY

Robert L. Ruff, M.D., Ph.D.
Departments of Neurology and Neurosciences
Case Western Reserve University School of
Medicine
Department of Veterans Affairs Medical
Center
University Hospitals of Cleveland
Cleveland, OH

James W. Russell, M.D.
Department of Neurology
University of Michigan
Ann Arbor, MI

Nelson R. Sabates, M.D.
Eye Foundation of Kansas City
University of Missouri, Kansas City School of Medicine
Kansas City, MO

Carla Siegfried, M.D.
Department of Ophthalmology and Visual Sciences
Washington University
St. Louis, MO

Harvey M. Shanies, Ph.D., M.D.
Clinical Associate Professor of Medicine
Mount Sinai School of Medicine
New York, NY
Associate Director of Medicine for Clinical and Academic Pulmonary and Critical Care Medicine
Elmhurst Hospital Center
Elmhurst, NY

Arunabh Sharma, M.D.
Fellow in Pulmonary and Critical Care Medicine
Brigham and Women's Hospital
Havard Medical School
Boston, MA

Anders A.F. Sima, M.D., Ph.D.
Professor of Pathology and Neurology
Wayne State University School of Medicine
Detroit, MI
Visiting Professor of Pathology
University of Michigan
Ann Arbor, MI
Staff Neuropathologist
Harper Hospital and Detroit Medical Center
Detroit, MI

Sabine Sobek, M.D.
Department of Critical Care Medicine
Wayne State University School of Medicine
Detroit, MI

Dana Stearns, M.D.
Instructor in Medicine
Harvard Medical School
Massachusetts General Hospital

Girish D. Sharma, M.D., FCCP
Assistant Professor of Pediatrics
Section of Pediatric Pulmonology
The University of Chicago Children's Hospital
Chicago, IL

Jack Stump, M.D.
Attending Physician
Rogue Valley Medical Center
Medford, OR

Joan Surdukowski, M.D.
Assistant Professor
Chicago Medical School
Mt. Sinai Hospital
Chicago, IL

Michael J. Taravella, M.D.
University of Colorado
Denver, CO

William O. Tatum, IV, M.D.
Clinical Assistant Professor
Tampa General Hospital Epilepsy Center
Tampa, FL

Menno Terriet, M.D.
Department of Anesthesia
Veterans Affairs Medical Center
Miami, FL

Carlo Tornatore, M.D.
Assistant Professor of Neurology
Department of Neurology
Georgetown University Medical Center
Washington, DC

R. Scott Turner, M.D., Ph.D.
Assistant Professor Department of Neurology
University of Michigan
Ann Arbor, MI

Mythili Venkataraman, M.D.
Attending, Pulmonary Medicine
Director, Bronchology and Invasive Procedures
Elmhurst Hospital Center
Elmhurst, NY
Assistant Professor of Medicine
Mount Sinai School of Medicine
New York, NY

Mladen Vidovich, M.D.
Department of Anesthesiology
Northwestern University Medical School
Chicago, IL

John J. Wald, M.D.
Department of Neurology
University of Michigan
Ann Arbor, MI

Martin Warshawsky, M.D., FACP, FCCP
Director, Respiratory Intensive Care Unit
Elmhurst Hospital Center
Elmhurst, NY
Assistant Professor of Medicine
Mount Sinai School of Medicine
New York, NY

Thais Weibel, M.D.
Department of Neurology
George Washington University Medical
Center
Washington, DC

Maria-Carmen B. Wilson, M.D.
Assistant Professor
Department of Neurology
Director, Headache and Pain Program
University of South Florida
School of Medicine
Tampa, FL
Assistant Professor of Medicine
Director of the Trauma and Life Support
Center
University of Wisconsin School of Medicine
Madison, WI

A. Zacharias, M.D.
Department of Neurology
Emory University School of Medicine
Atlanta, GA

Jingwu Zhang, M.D., Ph.D.
Associate Professor of Neurology
Department of Neurology
Baylor College of Medicine
Houston, TX

Kristin Zeller, M.D.
Norfolk, VA

INTRODUCTION

Congratulations! *Pulmonary Medicine Review: Pearls of Wisdom* will help you learn about pulmonary medicine as well as prepare for the pulmonary board examination.

This book is structured in a question and answer format. Such a format is most useful in certain situations. It is useful to enable one to assess strengths and weakness in a particular area before starting a rotation in pulmonary medicine or a board exam review. This permits the reader to concentrate on areas of interest or weakness. Some readers will find answering questions the preferred way to study for a board exam, as by going through the problems while having a textbook open. After completing a *Pulmonary Medicine Review* chapter, these readers are encouraged to examine the corresponding textbook chapter entirely, for comprehensiveness.

Most readers will probably use this book in a post-textbook review mode. One such method would involve reading a chapter in a textbook then proceeding to answer the questions posed in this book. Other readers will prefer to comprehensively study the contents of pulmonary medicine entirely and use this book afterwards. The purpose of the last two methods is to permit the reader to uncover areas of weakness and to become familiarized with the process of answering questions. Answering questions during a board exam is a cognitive task which requires different faculties than reading a textbook.

It must be emphasized that a question and answer book is most useful as a learning tool when used in conjunction with a textbook of pulmonary medicine. This is because the question/answer format is an active learning process that is optimized when the questioning process continues further along than ending with answering the *Pulmonary Medicine Review* question. The more active the learning process, the better the understanding. When the reader approaches a question that he/she cannot recall the answer to or uncovers a topic of interest (heard of a patient with such a condition, etc.), he/she is encouraged to read in the textbook at hand.

Most of the questions are short with short answers. This is to facilitate moving through a large body of knowledge. Some of the questions have longer answers. In these situations, the question posed could not be tersely answered. The questions were not altered because of the clinically interesting question posed.

The chapters are organized to include all aspects of pulmonary medicine. The questions within each chapter are randomly presented, to simulate board exams and the way questions arise in real life. The entirety of this book is not directed at one group of physicians. Some chapters have minimal bearing to certain readers. For example, the chapter on pediatric pulmonology has more utility to a pediatric pulmonologist than the chapter does to an adult pulmonologist. The chapter on airway management, likewise, is more useful to those who work on the anesthesiology/surgical side than the internal medicine side of the hospital.

Each question is preceded by a hollow bullet, to permit the reader to check off areas of interest, weakness, or simply noting that it has been read. This allows for re-reading without having uncertainty of what was reviewed earlier.

Great effort has been made to verify that the questions and answers are accurate. Some answers may not be the answer you would prefer. Most often this is attributable to variance between original sources. Please make us aware of any errors you find. We hope to make continuous improvements and would greatly appreciate any input with regard to format, organization, content, presentation, or about specific questions.

Study hard and good luck!

TABLE OF CONTENTS

AIRWAY MANAGEMENT

"The king shall drink to Hamlet's better breath"
Hamlet, Shakespeare

O **Speaking of RSI, discuss some agents that may be used to induce unconsciousness.**

Agent	Trade name	Class	Onset	Duration	Dose
Thiopental	Pentothal	Barbiturate	~ 30 seconds	2 to 30 minutes, depending on source	2.0 to 5.0 mg/kg at 40 mg/minute
Methohexital	Brevital	Barbiturate	Fast	Very short	5 to 12 ml of 1% solution at 1 ml/5 seconds
Fentanyl	Sublimaze	Opiate	2 minutes	~ 20 minutes	20 to 100 mcg/kg
Midazolam	Versed	Benzodiazepine	~ 5 minutes	~ 30 minutes	0.1 mg/kg
Etomidate	Amidate	Benzoderiv.	1 minutes	3 to 12 minutes	0.2 to 0.4 mg/kg

O **In a trauma patient with multiple fractures, internal injuries and an unstable airway, emergent endotracheal intubation in the emergency department is considered prior to definitive surgical therapy. What are the most likely hemodynamic consequences of intubation and initiation of mechanical ventilation in this subject?**

Hypotension may occur during and/or following endotracheal intubation and the institution of positive-pressure ventilation. This cardiovascular collapse is due to a decrease in venous return associated with both the use of sympatholytic agents for induction and the positive-pressure induced increase in intrathoracic pressure.

O **What is the average distance from the external nares to the carina in males and females?**

32 cm and 27 cm, respectively.

O **How many cartilages are included in the structure of the larynx?**

9. Three single (epiglottic, thyroid and cricoid) and three paired (arytenoid, corniculate and cuneiform) cartilages.

O **The involvement of which laryngeal joint produces hoarseness in rheumatoid arthritis?**

The cricoarytenoid synovial joint.

O **Which of the physiologic functions involving the larynx can occur even in the absence of the epiglottis?**

Phonation and deglutition.

O **What is the only abductor muscle of the vocal cords?**

The posterior cricoarytenoid muscle.

O **What is the only muscle of the larynx supplied by the superior laryngeal nerve?**

The cricothyroid muscle.

O   **At what thoracic vertebral level is the carina situated during full inspiration and full expiration?**

At the sixth and fourth thoracic vertebral level, respectively.

O   **What is the effective dose of intravenous lidocaine able to partially blunt the cardiovascular response to intubation?**

1.5 mg/kg.

O   **How long does it take for preoxygenation to achieve a 96% denitrogenation (a level which enables apnea for 5-6 minutes without hypoxemia)?**

7 minutes.

O   **What is the oxygen store of the lungs at 96% denitrogenation?**

2.5 liters.

O   **What is the minimal time required for preoxygenation before induction of general anesthesia?**

3 minutes.

O   **What is the mean average rise of carbon dioxide in apneic oxygenation?**

3 mmHg.

O   **What are the optimal angles of flexion of the neck and extension of the atlanto-occipital joint to achieve axial alignments before intubation ("sniffing" position)?**

30° and 15°, respectively.

O   **What is the mortality rate of epiglottitis with a conservative treatment approach (no preventive endotracheal intubation)?**

6.1%.

O   **How difficult is conventional endotracheal intubation in a patient with rheumatoid arthritis who presents with a stiff neck and limited mouth opening?**

Impossible.

O   **What is the reason for elective preoperative tracheostomy in some acromegalic patients?**

Bilateral recurrent laryngeal nerve palsy.

O   **What is the reported failure rate at first attempt and the final failure rate with blind nasal intubation?**

70% and 20%, respectively.

O   **In which clinical situation are retrograde and lightwand intubation considered better choices than fiberoptic assisted intubation?**

Bleeding in the oral cavity.

○ **What is the maximum safe dose of lidocaine for topical anesthesia of the airway?**

3 mg/kg.

○ **What is the maximum safe dose of cocaine for topical anesthesia of the airway?**

1.5 mg/kg.

○ **What is the toxic limit of the serum level of lidocaine?**

5 micrograms per milliliter of serum.

○ **In a scenario of failed intubation and impossible mask ventilation, is the use of a laryngeal mask airway contraindicated in a patient with an increased risk for aspiration of gastric contents (i.e. hiatus hernia)?**

No, it is not contraindicated. In fact the use of LMA in this situation may be life saving. Hypoxemia and not aspiration kills most patients after failed intubation and ventilation.

○ **What are the three most frequent causes of failure of fiberoptic laryngoscopy?**

Lack of training, "red out" and "white out" of the view and inadequate topical anesthesia.

○ **Which are the only "fail safe" signs of the correct placement of an endotracheal tube?**

Visualization of the tube passing through the cords and fiberoptic confirmation.

○ **What is the safest technique of intubation for children suffering from epiglottitis?**

Intubation in the OR after induction of anesthesia with an inhaled anesthetic (halothane or sevoflurane) in the semi-sitting position.

○ **Are there any differences between endotracheal intubation and Combitube with regard to oxygenation and ventilation?**

Yes. The $PaCO_2$ is higher with the Combitube. The PaO_2 is also higher due to the physiologic PEEP maintained by the vocal cords.

○ **What is the reported incidence of laryngeal injuries after endotracheal intubation?**

6.2%.

○ **What is the incidence of failed intubation in the general surgical population?**

1 in 2230 anesthetics.

○ **What is the incidence of impossible mask ventilation?**

1 in 5000 anesthetics.

○ **What should be done immediately after a failed intubation and impossible mask ventilation?**

A laryngeal mask airway should be inserted.

❍   **What is the most effective external laryngeal manipulation to achieve a better laryngoscopic view?**

BURP. Backward, upward and rightward pressure on the cricoid cartilage.

❍   **What is the incidence of malposition of double lumen tubes revealed by fiberoptic bronchoscopy?**

40% to 48%.

❍   **At what peak inspiratory pressure should an air leak be detected in pediatric patients intubated with an appropriate sized endotracheal tube?**

25 - 30 cm H_2O.

❍   **What are the initial ATLS steps of resuscitation?**

A - Airway maintenance with cervical spine control
B - Breathing and ventilation
C - Circulation with hemorrhage control
D - Disability: neurologic status
E - Exposure/Environmental Control: completely undress the patient, but prevent hypothermia

❍   **In what circumstances should the above order be modified?**

When a patient in a monitored setting arrests with sudden pulseless ventricular fibrillation. This requires immediate defibrillation.

❍   **What is the most common cause of upper airway obstruction?**

The tongue occluding the posterior oropharynx.

❍   **Name some important adjuncts often needed to help establish basic airway control.**

Suction equipment to remove secretions from mouth and throat, chin lift-jaw thrust maneuver, oral/nasal airway and bag-valve-mask device and mouth-to-mask ventilation device.

❍   **What are some advanced techniques for airway management?**

Orotracheal intubation, nasotracheal intubation, esophageal obturator airway (EOA), esophageal gastric tube airway (EGTA), pharyngotracheal airway, combination esophageal-tracheal tube, cricothryoidotomy and tracheostomy.

❍   **What are some indications for intubation?**

Apnea, burns, acute airway obstruction, expanding neck hematomas, hemodynamic instability, severe head injuries, poor oxygenation, poor ventilation, prevention of aspiration, inability to maintain a patent airway and impending or potential compromise of the airway.

❍   **What must be kept in mind when performing endotracheal intubation in a trauma patient?**

The potential for cervical spine injury.

❍   **What is a potential problem with bag-valve-mask ventilation?**

Air can enter the stomach via the esophagus causing gastric distention and aspiration.

❍   **How many people does it take to effectively ventilate a patient via the bag-valve-mask technique?**

Two. One to hold the mask securely to the face and a second to squeeze the bag with two hands.

○   **Does tracheal intubation prevent aspiration?**

No. Microaspiration can still occur.

○   **What characteristic of gastric contents causes the greatest harm following aspiration?**

Although the particulate matter can clog the airways leading to atelectasis, it is the acidity of the gastric contents that leads to the greatest airway injury.

○   **Name some factors that place a patient at risk for aspiration.**

Full stomach, trauma, intra-abdominal pathology (obstruction, inflammation, gastric paresis), esophageal disease (symptomatic reflux, motility disorders), pregnancy, obesity and uncertainty about intake of food or drink.

○   **Are esophageal, combination esophageal-tracheal tube or pharyngotracheal airways better than orotracheal intubation?**

No. These are substitutes when no trained personnel are available for orotracheal intubation.

○   **What properties of succinylcholine make it particularly useful as an aid for intubation?**

Succinylcholine, a depolarizing paralytic agent, has a brief duration of action (3 to 5 minutes) and a rapid onset of action (within 60 seconds).

○   **T/F: Succinylcholine has sedative and amnestic effects as well as muscle relaxant properties.**

False.

○   **What is the usual dose for succinylcholine?**

1 to 1.5 mg/kg.

○   **What are the possible deleterious effects of succinylcholine?**

Increased intragastric, intraocular and intracranial pressure.
Hyperkalemia, particularly in neurologic and burn injuries.
Increased duration of action in the rare patient with pseudocholinesterase deficiency.

○   **What maneuver should be performed during any tracheal intubation?**

The Sellick maneuver (occlusion of the esophagus by pressure on the cricoid cartilage). It can help prevent aspiration during tracheal intubation.

○   **What equipment is needed to assist with endotracheal intubation?**

Suction for the mouth and pharynx, bag-valve-mask system for oxygenation, functioning laryngoscope, stylets and endotracheal tubes.

○   **What type of endotracheal tube is used in children?**

Uncuffed.

○   **Why are uncuffed tubes used in children?**

Young children have a narrow subglottic area. Uncuffed tubes help avoid subglottic edema and ulceration.

○   **What is the correct tube size for the typical adult male and female?**

Male 8.0 mm ± 1.0 and female 7.0 mm ± 1.0.

○   **T/F: Female patients have larger airways compared to males but actually need smaller sized tubes.**

False. Female patients have smaller airways necessitating smaller tubes.

○   **What three axes should be aligned when attempting to perform endotracheal intubation on a patient when motion of the cervical spine is not contraindicated?**

Pharyngeal, oral and laryngeal.

○   **Where is the tip of the curved blade placed during orotracheal intubation?**

Into the vallecula just anterior to the epiglottis.

○   **Where is the tip of the straight blade placed during orotracheal intubation?**

Beneath the epiglottis to directly lift the epiglottis anteriorly.

○   **T/F: To use the laryngoscope correctly, the back of the blade is placed against the upper front teeth and the handle is rotated posteriorly, thus lifting the epiglottis anteriorly.**

False. Once positioned correctly, the handle and blade are lifted anteriorly without rotation to lift the epiglottis and expose the cords.

○   **In the typical male patient, what length of ET tube should lie distal to the lips?**

23 cm.

○   **In the typical female patient, what length of ET tube should lie distal to the lips?**

21 cm.

○   **What is the consequence of an ET tube placed too far distally?**

Respiratory insufficiency secondary to right mainstem bronchus intubation.

○   **How is right mainstem intubation diagnosed?**

Decreased breath sounds on the left that corrects with repositioning of the ET tube.

○   **What type of endotracheal tube cuff is presently used?**

High-volume, low pressure cuffs. (Pressure = 20 to 25 mmHg.)

○   **What type of endotracheal cuff was formerly used?**

Low volume, high pressure cuffs. (Pressure = up to 180 to 250 mmHg.)

○   **When does tracheal ischemia occur?**

When the transmitted pressure equals or exceeds capillary perfusion pressure (typically 25 to 35 mmHg).

○ **Immediately after inserting an ET tube, what is the next most appropriate step?**

Confirm tube placement.

○ **How is proper endotracheal tube placement confirmed?**

Symmetric chest expansion, breath sounds in axillae but not over epigastrum, tube fogs with respirations, end-tidal CO_2, monitoring of oxygen saturation and visualizing the tube passing through the vocal cords all assist with confirming proper positioning of the ET tube.

○ **Does a chest x-ray guarantee correct endotracheal tube placement?**

No. Clinical signs (see last question) are needed for confirmation of endotracheal tube placement.

○ **What is the correct position of the tip of the endotracheal tube?**

Approximately 4 cm above the carina.

○ **What are two contraindications to nasotracheal intubation?**

Maxillofacial trauma (with suspected fracture of the cribiform plate) and apnea.

○ **What is the most common complication of nasotracheal intubation?**

Epistaxis.

○ **How is transtracheal needle jet insufflation performed?**

A #12 or #14 gauge plastic cannula can be placed through the cricothyroid membrane into the trachea. The cannula should be connected to oxygen at 15 liter/minute (40 to 50 psi) and be given intermittently, one second on and four seconds off.

○ **How long can a patient be adequately temporized with needle jet insufflation?**

Approximately 45 to 60 minutes.

○ **What limits this form of surgical airway?**

Hypercapnia, due to inadequate ventilation.

○ **When is an emergent cricothyroidotomy indicated?**

When a patient cannot adequately oxygenate or ventilate and standard intubation and bag ventilation cannot be performed.

○ **T/F: Cricothyroidotomy is generally contraindicated in children.**

True. Needle jet insufflation is considered a better choice to avoid injuring the cricoid cartilage

○ **Why is emergent tracheostomy usually not recommended?**

The trachea lies deeper in the neck than the cricothyroid membrane. The trachea is surrounded by a number of veins and the isthmus of the thyroid gland. Complications such as recurrent laryngeal nerve injury, pneumothorax and esophageal perforation can occur.

❍   **When may emergent tracheostomy be performed instead of emergent cricothryoidotomy?**

In pediatric patients. Cricothyroidotomy is generally contraindicated in the pediatric population. Because of the smaller size and greater soft-tissue compliance of the pediatric airway the cricoid cartilage plays a major role in maintaining patency of the tracheal lumen. An injury to this structure could be disastrous.

❍   **The three divisions of the airway are:**

1.   Extrathoracic - nose to the trachea before it enters the thoracic inlet
2.   Intrathoracic, extrapulmonary - trachea at the thoracic inlet to the right and left mainstem bronchi before they enter the lungs
3.   Intrapulmonary - bronchi within the lungs

❍   **According to Poiseuille's law, if the airway radius of the conducting airway is reduced from 4 mm to 2 mm, how much will resistance to airflow increase?**

Sixteen-fold.

❍   **The funnel-shaped narrowing of the glottis and subglottic airway, commonly known as the "steeple sign" is observed in what type of extrathoracic airway obstruction?**

Croup or laryngotracheobronchitis.

❍   **What is the narrowest part of the adult airway?**

The glottic opening.

❍   **What is the most common offender in foreign body aspiration?**

Organic substances such as nuts and corn.

❍   **What great vessel anomalies result in airway obstruction?**

1.   Right aortic arch with or without a left ligamentum arteriosum
2.   Double aortic arch
3.   Anomalous innominate or left carotid artery
4.   Aberrant right subclavian
5.   Anomalous left pulmonary artery

❍   **The total work of breathing is divided into what two parts?**

Overcoming lung and chest wall compliance and overcoming airway resistance.

ALTITUDE MEDICINE

"Thy turfy mountains, where live nibbling sheep"
The Tempest, Shakespeare

○ **At what altitude does acute mountain sickness typically develop?**

8000 feet.

○ **Do I really have to review Dalton's Law again?**

Yes. It states that the partial pressure of each gas in a mixture of gases is described by the following equation:

$P1 = F1 \times P$

Where P1 is the partial pressure of a gas in a mixture, F1 is the fractional concentration of that gas in the mixture and P is the total pressure at which the mixture exists.

○ **SO?**

So, as altitude increases, total ambient pressure decreases. At all levels of the atmosphere, oxygen represents about 20% of the molecules present in air. Thus, the partial pressure of oxygen at any altitude is equal to 20% of the ambient atmospheric pressure.

○ **What is the partial pressure of oxygen in air at sea level?**

20% of 760 torr, or approximately 150 torr.

○ **How rapidly does atmospheric pressure decrease with ascent?**

It's not a linear relationship. The following table gives you a feel for the logarithmic changes.

Altitude (m)	atmospheric pressure (torr)	partial pressure of 02 (torr)
0 (sea level)	760	152
30	733	147
1000	674	135
3000	525	105
5000	405	81
10,000	199	40

○ **What are the effects of acute exposure to altitude on ventilation?**

Decreased partial pressures of oxygen stimulate ventilation. The threshold for increased ventilation appears at about 1500 meters breathing air. These changes are very small until an altitude of about 3500 meters is achieved, at which there is approximately a 10% increase in ventilation. At 5500 meters, the increase in minute ventilation is approximately 30%. At 6700 meters minute ventilation ordinarily has almost doubled.

○ **How is the effect of progressive hypoxemia on human performance measured?**

Effective performance time (EPT) is the length of time one can perform useful cognitive and physical activities while breathing a decreased partial pressure of oxygen. The EPT is indefinite below 3000 meters. The table below shows the limitations in human performance breathing air at altitude.

Altitude (meters)	Effective Performance Time (minutes)
3000 and less	Indefinite
6700	10
8500	2.5
10,000	1

○ **So, if an aviator breathes 100% oxygen, is ascent to extreme altitude possible?**

The table below shows the alveolar total pressure and arterial partial pressure of oxygen at various altitudes breathing air or 100% oxygen. You can see that, even breathing 100% oxygen, the arterial PO_2 falls below 60 at altitudes greater than 12,000 meters (39,000 ft.). Please do not open windows or doors on commercial jet aircraft at their usual cruising altitudes of approximately 35,000 feet!

Altitude (ft)	Total Pressure (mmHg)	Arterial PO_2 (mmHg)	
		Breathing Air	100%
0	760	94	580
5,000	630	74	540
10,000	525	55	435
15,000	430	40	340
20,000	350	29	260
25,000	280	25	190
30,000	220	X	125
35,000	180	X	85
40,000	140	X	52

○ **So, why do we not breathe extra oxygen when flying on a commercial jet aircraft?**

One <u>does</u> need additional oxygen at cabin altitudes exceeding approximately 12,000 ft. Commercial airliners solve this problem, however, by increasing the total pressure within the cabin (Dalton's Law helps out again – as total pressure within the cabin increases, the partial pressure of oxygen increases). A commercial airliner is typically pressurized to a cabin altitude of approximately 2,500 meters (7500 ft).

○ **What is the clinical significance of this?**

Patients with borderline or overt respiratory insufficiency at sea level may be seriously challenged or injured at altitude. At a cabin altitude of 7000-8000 ft., commonly encountered in a Boeing 737 or 747, the arterial partial pressure of oxygen is 70 torr in a healthy individual (down from the sea level normal of approximately 100 torr). For a patient with a sea level room air PO_2 of 65 or 70, this will result in an arterial PO_2 of approximately 35 torr!

○ **How does decompression sickness fit in with all of this?**

Decompression sickness occurs when ambient pressure decreases too rapidly and dissolved gases in the blood and tissue (nitrogen for ordinary people doing ordinary things) come out of solution too rapidly. When this occurs, micro or even macro bubbles develop which cause tissue injury, ischemia and symptoms of pain and/or organ system dysfunction. In the context of altitude physiology and flight, the incidence of decompression sickness is vanishingly low unless the cabin altitude suddenly reaches at least 8000 meters. Such an event may occur with unplanned decompression of the cabin at altitudes exceeding that level.

○ **How could sudden decompression occur?**

A structural element could fail (spontaneous failure of a window seal with loss of the window), a bird could break a windshield, or you could be unlucky enough for your plane to be hit by a meteorite.

○ **How is decompression sickness treated?**

Primarily by re-exposing the victim to a pressure similar to or greater to that experienced prior to the onset of symptoms. Usually this is done in a hyperbaric chamber and involves breathing 100% oxygen. Treatment duration and pressure are a matter of clinical judgment and protocol and depend greatly on the pressure to which the victim was exposed prior to onset of symptoms.

○ **Besides aviators and their passengers, who else has medical problems with ascent to altitude?**

Climbers, adventurers and tourists visiting a variety of high altitude locations.

○ **How long does it take for the human body to acclimate to altitude?**

Tolerance to hypoxemia appears with widely varying speed (a few days to several weeks) depending on poorly understood individual differences.

○ **How is the increase in ventilation associated with hypoxemia mediated?**

The carotid body senses decreased arterial partial pressures of oxygen and sends afferent signals to the medullary respiratory center, which increases minute ventilation.

○ **What factors limit the ventilatory response to hypoxemia?**

The hypocapnia produced causes an alkalosis that blunts the output of the respiratory center, limiting further increases in minute ventilation.

Secondarily (24-48 hours), renal compensation returns the pH to a level at which ventilation may increase again.

○ **What else does the body do to acclimate and adjust?**

Hemoglobin levels increase in all mammals exposed chronically to high elevations. Erythropoietin is secreted in increased amounts within two hours of ascent and immature red blood cells can be found in the peripheral circulation within 48 hours.

○ **Can the hematocrit "overcompensate" or go dangerously high?**

Hematocrits in excess of 60-65% do occur with chronic exposure to altitude. This is associated with "sludging" in the cerebral circulation.

○ **What are the acute clinical effects of ascent to altitude?**

Dyspnea on exertion, a sense of breathlessness at rest, easy fatigability and sleep disturbance. Periodic breathing is common.

○ **What illness may occur as a result of exposure to altitude?**

Acute mountain sickness is an illness attributed directly to hypobaric hypoxemia.

○ **What are the symptoms of acute mountain sickness?**

The syndrome covers a spectrum from mild headache and fatigue to life threatening cerebral and pulmonary edema. Headache is throbbing, worse at night and early after awakening and is made worse by lowering the head or performing a Valsalva maneuver. Loss of appetite is common and nausea is frequent

○ **What behavioral symptoms are associated with acute mountain sickness?**

Irritability and apathy resembling an acute depressive reaction are very common.

○   **What are the physical findings of acute mountain sickness?**

There are no pathognomonic signs in acute mountain sickness. Rales may be present with the onset of mild pulmonary edema. When present they should be taken seriously, since overt pulmonary edema can occur.

○   **What is the differential diagnosis of acute mountain sickness?**

It is commonly misdiagnosed as a viral influenza like illness, dehydration, mere physical exhaustion or alcohol-associated hangover. A key diagnostic point is that mountain sickness is not associated with fever or myalgia. Exhaustion may cause the same symptoms as mountain sickness but should not cause rales. Dehydration may cause most of the symptoms of acute mountain sickness but responds to fluid administration, while acute mountain sickness does not. Carbon monoxide poisoning, which is a danger in tents with cooking flames at altitude, should be considered in the differential diagnosis as well.

○   **What causes pulmonary and cerebral edema in acute mountain sickness?**

The mechanism is not certain but is generally accepted to be a cytotoxic injury as a direct result of the hypoxemia.

○   **How does one treat acute mountain sickness?**

Avoid further ascent. The presence of neurologic problems or symptoms or signs of pulmonary edema dictate immediate descent. Stable generalized symptoms without suggestion of pulmonary or cerebral edema can be observed without ascent for 24 hours. Acclimatization will take place within 12 hours to 3 days.

○   **Is any drug therapy indicated?**

Acetazolamide produces a central stimulation of respiration and enhances renal excretion of bicarbonate. Symptomatic improvement may be dramatic. When available, oxygen usually provides prompt improvement in symptoms but may not be available where the problems exists (on the side of a mountain). Dexamethasone is associated with improvement.

○   **Is it possible to prevent mountain sickness?**

Gradual ascent is the best prevention. Persons living below 1000 meters ought to avoid overnight ascents to greater than 3000 meters and ought to spend at least 48 hours near 3000 meters before going higher. Daytime trips to higher altitude with nighttime return to lower altitude for sleep seems to help in acclimatization.

○   **Is there such an entity as chronic mountain sickness?**

Chronic mountain polycythemia or sickness is characterized by headache, sleep disturbance, fatigue and polycythemia greater than anticipated even for the altitude of chronic residence. Males are at much greater risk (perhaps tenfold) than women, for unknown reasons. These symptoms are similar to those of acute mountain sickness, but they do not resolve with chronic exposure. Descent to and living at a lower altitude solves the problem. Supplemental oxygen and phlebotomy to a hematocrit less than 60% are helpful.

○   **Is there a quick and easy way to predict which of COPD patient will be at risk while flying on a commercial airliner?**

Yes. Researchers have found that a resting room air arterial PO_2 greater than or equal to 72 identifies 90% of subject who will have an arterial PO_2 of greater than 55 at a cabin altitude of 7500 ft. Patients with a resting room air PO_2 lower than 72 will almost always have a PO_2 less than 55 and arterial oxygen saturation less than 90% at usual cabin altitudes.

ACUTE RESPIRATORY DISTRESS SYNDROME (ARDS)

"Thy life's a miracle"
King Lear, Shakespeare

○ **What is the American-European Consensus Conference definition for the diagnosis of ARDS?**

PaO2/FIO2 ratio < 200, bilateral infiltrates and wedge pressure < 18.

○ **What is the cause of hypoxemia in ARDS?**

An increase in alveolar fluid that causes a reduction in the diffusion of oxygen into the capillaries, increasing the shunt.

○ **What is the mortality of ARDS?**

40 to 60%.

○ **What are the major risk factors for ARDS?**

Sepsis, trauma, aspiration, multiple transfusions, shock and pulmonary contusions. Many other systemic and local insults may trigger ARDS.

○ **Why is the pulmonary artery wedge pressure an important feature in the diagnosis of ARDS?**

The presence of a significantly elevated wedge pressure implies that the pulmonary edema may be hydrostatic and, therefore, due to left ventricular dysfunction rather than alveolar dysfunction.

○ **Does PEEP improve ARDS?**

PEEP commonly improves oxygenation. However, it does not reduce the amount of total lung water

○ **What is the distribution of pulmonary edema in ARDS?**

Routine chest x-ray appears to show a diffuse distribution. However, CT scan studies reveal an increased involvement in the dependent portions of the lung fields.

○ **What are the x-ray findings in ARDS?**

Commonly, patchy bilateral peripheral infiltrates. Cardiogenic pulmonary edema typically demonstrates an enlarged heart, pleural effusions and peribronchial cuffing with septal lines.

○ **What complications are associated with ARDS?**

Pneumothorax, pulmonary infection, pulmonary hypertension and multisystem organ failure.

○ **What is the advantage of pressure controlled ventilation in ARDS?**

It often allows for higher mean airway pressures and, therefore, better oxygenation with relatively lower peak airway pressures.

○   **Has the strategy of minimizing plateau pressures been demonstrated to improve outcome in ARDS?**

This strategy is commonly employed. It is controversid as to whether such a strategy improves the clinical outcome.

○   **What is the theory behind the strategy to minimize plateau pressures for ARDS?**

Decreasing plateau pressures decreases the propensity for alveolar overdistention. Animal studies have demonstrated that alveolar overdistention will result in the same pathological changes as ARDS. The most practical way to currently estimate alveolar overdistention is by measuring plateau pressure.

○   **Is surfactant therapy helpful in ARDS?**

While there is some evidence that exogenous surfactant is helpful in some pediatric cases, the studies in adults have failed to show a benefit.

○   **What are the three phases of ARDS?**

Acute or exudative (up to 6 days), proliferative (4 to 10 days) and fibrotic phase (after 7 days).

○   **What is the role of PEEP in ARDS?**

To maintain alveolar inflation and functional residual capacity. This optimizes V/Q matching and improves oxygenation.

○   **What is compliance and how is it calculated?**

Compliance measures the elasticity of the lungs. It is calculated by measuring the change in volume for a given change in pressure.

○   **What are the changes in compliance in ARDS?**

The compliance is decreased due to increased fluid and debris in the alveoli.

○   **What are the negative effects of PEEP on cardiac output?**

PEEP may reduce cardiac output by reducing venous return, by increasing pulmonary vascular resistance and by shifting the interventricular septum to the left, thus reducing the left ventricular end diastolic volume.

○   **What are the ways that the optimal level of PEEP can be determined?**

Compliance, oxygenation, calculation of oxygen delivery and elucidation of the lower inflection point on the volume-pressure curve.

○   **What is the role of corticosteriods in ARDS?**

Steroids have not been shown effective in the early phase of ARDS. In the later stages of ARDS, steroids may have a role by reducing lung fibrosis.

○   **What interventions have been shown to reduce the mortality of ARDS?**

There never has been a clinically useful interventional study completed in adults that has clearly demonstrated an improved mortality in ARDS.

○ **Which drugs can cause ARDS?**

Opiates, salicylates, cocaine, protamine and certain chemotherapeutic agents.

○ **How long after an initial insult does ARDS usually occur?**

12 to 72 hours.

○ **What does ARDS stand for?**

Acute Respiratory Distress Syndrome is a better term than Adult Respiratory Distress Syndrome as this syndrome occurs in children.

○ **What is the characteristic histologic change in the alveoli in ARDS?**

Pathologists call this diffuse alveolar damage. It is characterized by a process of diffuse lung inflammation that progresses to fibrosis. Interestingly, the number of inflammatory cells observed is not large. There is heterogeneity both in time and space as to which alveoli are in the inflammatory phase and which are in the fibrotic phase. Another name for ARDS is hyaline membrane disease, which refers to the hyaline membranes seen histopathologically. These are collections of sloughed type 1 pneumocytes and other cellular debris.

○ **In patients diagnosed with ARDS, what are the most common causes of death?**

Multisytem organ failure or sepsis syndrome, not respiratory failure.

○ **T/F: Any cause of shock can cause ARDS.**

True.

○ **T/F: Too much oxygen can cause ARDS.**

True.

○ **T/F: A patient with ARDS can have a fever without having a source of infection.**

True.

○ **What is in the differential diagnosis of ARDS?**

Broadly three categories - cardiogenic pulmonary edema, pneumonia (PCP, fungi, bacteria, legionella, miliary TB) and inflammatory lung conditions (drug reaction, collagen vascular disease, BOOP, acute eosinophilic pneumonia).

○ **What is the optimal fluid management strategy in ARDS?**

No such strategy has been clearly demonstrated as the preferred strategy. However, current thinking is to avoid hypervolemia and, at the same time, maintain enough intravascular volume to optimize oxygen transport to peripheral organs.

○ **How does the pressure-volume curve appear in a patient with ARDS?**

Generally, with pressure on the horizontal axis and volume on the vertical axis, the curve has three components. Initially, the curve is relative flat, until shifting to a steeper rising curve. The changeover is called the lower inflection point and is thought to reflect the opening of atelectatic alveoli in the dependent portions of the lungs. The curve continues to rise until it flatness again. This second change is called the upper inflection point and is thought to reflect the overdistention of alveoli.

○   **What is the current ventilator strategy in ARDS utilizing the lower and upper inflection points?**

To give enough PEEP to exceed the lower inflection point, thereby minimizing sheer forces on alveoli that results from the atelectatic alveoli being excessively opened and closed. This has an additional benefit of optimizing oxygenation by keeping the atelectatic alveoli open. The second component is to minimize the lung volume by keep the peak pressure below the upper inflection point, thereby avoiding overdistention of the alveoli.

This strategy makes pathophysiological sense but has not been clinically demonstrated to be clearly advantageous. Clinical trials are underway.

○   **Does nitric oxide improve oxygenation in ARDS?**

Yes, but outcome studies have not been completed.

○   **T/F: ECMO improves the mortality in ARDS.**

False.

○   **What is permissive hypercapnia?**

The ventilator strategy of protecting the lungs from alveolar overdistention by reducing lung volumes and accepting, as a cost, the rise in pCO_2 and fall in pH. This is a controversial strategy, although two consensus conferences suggested that this strategy be utilized when plateau pressures are elevated. Studies are underway which will hopefully resolve the controversy.

○   **What is the plateau pressure? What is the peak airway pressure?**

The plateau pressure is the static pressure that exists when, at end inspiration, the airway is occluded. Occlusion of the airway creates a static column of air from the endotracheal tube to the alveoli. Because a static column of air is in pressure equilibrium, the pressure measured at the endotracheal tube is the same as that in the alveoli. The plateau pressure is a method to measure the alveolar distending pressure. An excessive elevation of this pressure is thought to reflect alveolar overdistention.

Peak airway pressure is the maximal excursion of the airway pressure gauge during the inspiratory and expiratory cycle.

○   **Does inverse ratio ventilation improve oxygenation in ARDS? Does it improve mortality?**

Inverse ratio ventilation is the strategy to reverse the normal 1:2 inspiration to expiration ratio in spontaneous breathing. This has been shown to improve oxygenation by increasing mean airway pressure at lower peak pressure. The controversy is whether it has any beneficial effect over simply increasing PEEP. It is unknown if this strategy improves mortality.

○   **What is the effect of PEEP on right ventricular preload and afterload? How about on left ventricular preload and afterload?**

PEEP decreases preload to both ventricles, increases RV afterload and decreases LV afterload.

○   **What is the long term lung function in ARDS survivors?**

Mild reduction of DLCO and mild restrictive ventilatory defect. Some have normal lung function.

○   **T/F: Patients with ARDS do not develop auto-PEEP.**

False.

○   **Why does PEEP improve oxygen exchange in ARDS?**

PEEP reverses atelectasis and redistributes lung water from the alveoli to the interstitium.

○   **How does prone positioning improve oxygenation in ARDS?**

Prone positioning recruits dorsal lung units and improves V/Q matching.

○   **Are there any side effects noted with prone positioning?**

Yes. Although unusual, hypotension, desaturation and arrhythmias have occurred after prone positioning.

○   **What level is suggested as the maximal transalveolar pressure that will avoid barotrauma in a patient with ARDS?**

35 cm H2O is commonly suggested in the literature. A recent editorial suggested that higher levels may be acceptable. Randomized trials using a pressure-targeted goal in conjunction with permissive hypercapnia are ongoing.

ASPIRATION SYNDROMES, NEAR-DROWNING AND HEMOPTYSIS

"Lord, Lord! Methought, what pain it was to drown!"
King Richard III, Shakespeare

O **What 4 physical examination findings would make posterior epistaxis more likely than anterior epistaxis?**

1. Inability to see the site of bleeding. Anterior nosebleeds usually originate at Kiesselbach's plexus and are easily visualized on the nasal septum.
2. Blood from both sides of the nose. In a posterior nosebleed the blood can more easily pass to the other side because of the proximity of the choanae.
3. Blood trickling down the oropharynx.
4. Inability to control bleeding by direct pressure.

O **What is the best initial method for localizing hemoptysis in a patient who is actively bleeding?**

Bronchoscopy.

O **What is the location for aspiration pneumonias?**

In the supine patient, it is in the posterior segment of the upper lobe and in the superior segment of the lower lobe. In the upright patient, it is in the basilar segments of the lower lobes. The right lung is favored over the left because of the straighter takeoff of the right mainstem bronchus.

O **What are the common directly toxic (non-infected) respiratory tract aspirates?**

Gastric contents, alcohol, hydrocarbons, mineral oil, animal and vegetable fats. All of these produce an inflammatory response and pneumonia. Gastric contents are the most common offender.

O **What are the consequences of aspirating acid?**

The response is rapid, with near immediate bronchitis, bronchiolitis, atelectasis, shunting and hypoxemia. Pulmonary edema may occur within 4 hours. The clinical manifestations are dyspnea, wheezing, cough, cyanosis, fever and shock.

O **What is the antibiotic of choice for gastric acid aspiration?**

None.

O **What is the role of corticosteroids in gastric acid aspiration?**

None.

O **What is the main priority in treating gastric acid aspiration?**

Maintenance of oxygenation. Intubation, ventilation and PEEP (positive end expiratory pressure) may be required.

○   **What are the radiographic manifestations of acid aspiration?**

Varied. There may be bilateral diffuse infiltrates, irregular "patchy" infiltrates or lobar infiltrates.

○   **What outcomes occur in patients who do not rapidly resolve gastric acid aspiration pneumonitis?**

ARDS (adult respiratory distress syndrome), progressive respiratory failure and bacterial superinfection.

○   **Under what circumstances are antibiotics used in aspiration?**

Aspiration of infected material, intestinal obstruction, immunocompromised host and evidence of bacterial superinfection after a non-infected aspirate (new fever, infiltrates, or purulence after the initial 2 to 3 days).

○   **What is the usual source of infected aspirated material?**

The oropharynx.

○   **What pleuripulmonary infections may occur after aspirating infected oropharyngeal material?**

Necrotizing pneumonia, lung abscess, "typical" pneumonia and empyema.

○   **What is the predominant oropharyngeal flora in outpatients?**

Anaerobes. Community acquired aspiration is usually anaerobic. The most common aerobes involved are streptococcus species.

○   **What is the antibiotic of choice for outpatient acquired infectious aspiration pneumonia?**

Clindamycin.

○   **What is the bacteriology of inpatient acquired infectious aspiration pneumonia?**

Mixed aerobic and anaerobic organisms. Unlike outpatients, Staphylococcus aureus, Escherichia coli, Pseudomonas aeruginosa and Proteus species are common.

○   **What antibiotics treat inpatient acquired infectious aspiration pneumonia?**

Beta-lactamase resistant penicillins, cephalosprins, or imipenem.

○   **How long after aspiration is a lung abscess usually detected?**

Two weeks or more.

○   **What is the duration of treatment for lung abscess?**

Until radiographic resolution or stabilization with a small residual scar or cyst. This may take 6 weeks or more.

○   **What are the clinical consequences of aspiration of liquid gastric contents with a pH less than 2.5?**

Hypoxemia, bronchospasm and atelectasis may develop, but usually resolve within 24 hours.

○   **What is the annual U.S. mortality from drowning?**

9000.

○   **What is the preferred antibiotic for near drowning in polluted (high coliform count) water?**

None.

○   **What is the priority in treatment of near drowning?**

Maintenance of airway and oxygenation.

○   **What are the indications for intubation and ventilation after near drowning?**

Apnea, pulselessness, altered mental status, severe hypoxemia and respiratory acidosis.

○   **What is the frequency of ARDS (adult respiratory distress syndrome) after near drowning?**

40%.

○   **What are the major causes of massive hemoptysis?**

Tuberculosis, bronchiectasis and lung cancer.

○   **What causes hemoptysis in patients with tuberculosis (either active or healed)?**

Pulmonary artery (Rasmussen's) aneurysm, bronchiolar ulceration and necrosis, bronchiectasis, broncholithiasis, lung cancer and mycetoma (fungus ball).

○   **What is the purpose of bronchoscopy in hemoptysis?**

Localization and diagnosis.

○   **What are the invasive therapies for massive hemoptysis?**

Thoracotomy, embolization, balloon tamponade (via bronchoscopy), double-lumen tube for lung separation and independent ventilation and laser bronchoscopy.

○   **What is the most feared complication of bronchial artery embolization?**

Anterior spinal artery embolization.

○   **When is surgery indicated for massive hemoptysis?**

Localized massive hemoptysis unresponsive to other therapy, or electively, after stabilization, for long term control of localized bleeding.

○   **What is the most common cause of hemoptysis in the United States?**

Bronchitis.

○   **What percentage of patients with an endobronchial neoplasm and a normal chest x-ray present with hemoptysis?**

15%.

○   **What metastatic tumors can produce hemoptysis?**

Breast, colon, kidney and malignant melanomas.

❍   **What tumor other than squamous cell, adeno-, large cell, or small cell carcinoma is likely to cause hemoptysis?**

Bronchial carcinoid.

❍   **What is the most common cause of hemoptysis in patients with leukemia?**

Fungal infections, often aspergillus.

❍   **Which bacterial pneumonias frequently cause frank hemoptysis?**

Pseudomonas aeruginosa, Klebsiella pneumoniae and Staphylococcus aureus.

❍   **What are the major cardiovascular causes of hemoptysis?**

Mitral stenosis, pulmonary hypertension and Eisenmenger's complex.

❍   **How does pulmonary artery catheterization produce hemoptysis?**

By pulmonary artery rupture, aneurysm formation, or pulmonary infarction.

❍   **What is the frequency of hemoptysis in pulmonary embolization?**

20%.

❍   **What is a common definition for massive hemoptysis?**

Coughing of more than 600 ml of blood in 24 hours.

❍   **What are the most common causes of hemoptysis in non-hospitalized patients?**

Bronchitis, bronchogenic carcinoma and idiopathic.

❍   **What systemic illnesses cause hemoptysis?**

Amyloidosis, CHF, mitral stenosis, sarcoidosis, SLE, vasculitis, coagulation disorders and pulmonary-renal syndromes.

❍   **When should life threatening hemoptysis be suspected?**

When there is a large volume of blood, the appearance of a fungus ball in a pulmonary cavity on chest x-ray and hypoxemia.

❍   **How can aspiration be prevented when intubating?**

By avoiding unnecessary increase in intragastric pressure from overzealous bag-valve-mask ventilation and by applying cricoid pressure during intubation.

❍   **When is aspiration most likely to occur during surgery?**

During the induction of anesthesia.

❍   **In a sitting patient, where does aspiration generally occur as revealed by chest x-ray?**

The basilar segments of the right lower lobe.

○   **What is the pH of aspirated fluid that suggests a poor prognosis?**

PH < 2.5.

○   **What is the clinical significance of fixed, dilated pupils in a near-drowning victim?**

Don't give up the ship! Ten to twenty percent of patients presenting with coma and fixed, dilated pupils recover completely. Asymptomatic patients should be observed for a minimum of 4 to 6 hours.

○   **What are the expected blood gas findings of a near-drowning victim?**

Metabolic acidosis from poor perfusion and hypoxia.

○   **Describe the airway defenses during swallowing.**

The soft palate is pulled up, preventing reflux into the nose, the epiglottis covers the glottis and the respiratory center in the medulla is inhibited.

○   **Liquids pass from stomach to duodenum in 2 hours. Solids pass from stomach to duodenum in _____.**

4 to 6 hours

○   **What may delay gastric emptying?**

Anxiety, pain, drugs, diabetes mellitus, gastric outlet obstruction and pregnancy.

○   **Where is the vomiting center is located?**

In the medulla.

○   **Under what circumstances is aspiration of vomitus, oral secretions or foreign material likely?**

Anything resulting in an altered level of consciousness (e.g. alcohol, overdose, general anesthesia and stroke), impaired swallowing, abnormal gastrointestinal motility, or disruption of esophageal sphincter function predisposes to aspiration.

○   **T/F: Nasogastric and gastric tubes increase the risk of aspiration.**
True.

○   **T/F: Healthy people may aspirate small amounts of oral contents without developing clinical complications.**

True.

○   **What determines the likelihood of pulmonary complications from aspiration?**

The frequency of aspiration, volume of aspirate and character of the aspirate.

○   **What factors characterize an aspiration?**

Solid or liquid, size if solid, pH and infected or non-infected.

○   **Is foreign body aspiration more common in children or adults?**

Children. In adults it is more common from the fourth decade onwards. It is more likely in adults when food is poorly chewed and when alcohol or sedative drugs are taken.

○   **What are the signs of a large obstructing foreign body in the larynx or trachea?**

Respiratory distress, stridor, inability to speak, cyanosis and loss of consciousnes.

○   **What are the symptoms of a smaller (distally lodged) foreign body?**

Cough, dyspnea, wheezing, chest pain and fever.

○   **(T/F): Adults are more likely to aspirate into the right side.**

True. Up to the age of 15, aspiration is equally likely to either side.

○   **Complete upper airway obstruction by a foreign body is treated by the _____ maneuver.**

Heimlich.

○   **What are the complications of the Heimlich maneuver?**

Rib fractures, ruptured viscera, pneumomediastinum, regurgitation (and aspiration) and retinal detachment

○   **What is the procedure of choice for foreign body removal?**

Rigid bronchoscopy. Fiberoptic bronchoscopy is an alternate procedure in adults, not in children.

○   **What are the common radiographic findings in foreign body aspiration?**

Normal film, atelectasis, pneumonia, contralateral mediastinal shift (more marked during expiration) and visualization of the foreign body

○   **(T/F): Aspiration of fluids with a pH less than 5 produces chemical pneumonitis.**

False. Aspirate pH less than 2.5 produces chemical injury.

○   **The chemical pneumonitis produced by aspirated gastric acid is called _____ _____.**

Mendelson's syndrome.

○   **T/F: Aspiration of liquid gastric contents with a pH greater than 2.5 produces no clinical consequences.**

False. Hypoxemia, bronchospasm and atelectasis may develop but usually resolve within 24 hours.

○   **What are the consequences of aspirating small (non-obstructing) food particles?**

Inflammation and hypoxemia that may result in chronic bronchiolitis or granulomatosis.

O   **Name the commonly aspirated hydrocarbons.**

Gasoline, kerosene, furniture polish and lighter fluid

O   **What are the effects of hydrocarbon aspiration?**

Hypoxemia, intrapulmonary shunting, pulmonary edema, hemoptysis and respiratory failure.

O   **What is the role of emesis induction or gastric lavage in hydrocarbon ingestion?**

These maneuvers are not recommended as the patient may aspirate during regurgitation.

O   **Lipoid pneumonia is associated with chronic aspiration of _____ _____ _____.**

Mineral, animal, or vegetable oils (as oil-based nose drops).

O   **What is the definition of drowning?**

Death due to suffocation by submersion in water

O   **Can drowning occur without aspiration of water?**

Yes. 10% of victims die from intense laryngospasm.

O   **How much fluid can be drained from the lungs after drowning in fresh water?**

Little, as hypotonic fresh water is rapidly absorbed from the lung, unlike salt water which is hypertonic and is retained. There is no difference in outcome.

O   **When is the Heimlich maneuver applied after near drowning?**

It is not applied unless foreign body aspiration is suspected

O   **Is the prognosis of hemoptysis better in a patient with active or with healed tuberculosis?**

Active, which is more amenable to treatment.

O   **What is the cause of death in hemoptysis?**

Asphyxiation, not exsanguination

O   **What is the flaw of prognosis based on volume of hemoptysis alone?**

Lethal bleeding may occur with little or no hemoptysis in patients with impaired cough.

O   **May sedation and cough suppression be used in hemoptysis?**

Yes. Mild sedation and mild cough suppression to prevent excessive anxiety and cough may be used. High levels should be avoided.

O   **Why is rigid bronchoscopy preferred in massive hemoptysis?**

Better suctioning ability, vision and airway control and ability to pack the airway.

O   **What are the advantages of fiberoptic bronchoscopy?**

Less invasive, better access to upper lobes and ability to visualize to fifth or sixth generation bronchi.

○   **What non-invasive bedside maneuver may assist management of massive hemoptysis?**

Positioning the bleeding lung in a dependent position

○   **What are the invasive therapies for massive hemoptysis?**

Thoracotomy, embolization, balloon tamponade (via bronchoscopy), double lumen tube for lung separation and independent ventilation and laser bronchoscopy.

○   **What is the major complication of a double lumen tube for independent lung ventilation?**

The tube may slip distally, such that no ventilation is provided to one lung, or proximally, so that separation of the 2 sides is lost.

○   **How does blood retained in the lung alter pulmonary function other than volume restriction?**

It increases the diffusion capacity.

○   **How does hemoptysis differ from hematemesis?**

Blood in hemoptysis is often frothy and bright red. Alveolar macrophages may be seen on microscopy. Hematemesis is often acidic with a pH less than 2.5

○   **What is the most common cause of hemoptysis in the Far East?**

Paragonimus westermani.

○   **What other parasites may produce hemoptysis?**

Schistosomes, echinococcus, amebiasis, strongyloides, trichinosis, ascaris and ancylostoma.

○   **What factors are considered in evaluating the differential diagnosis of hemoptysis?**

Associated symptoms, co-existent disease, clubbing, patient population, travel, smoking history, duration and quantity of blood expectorated and history of bleeding disorders.

○   **What is the etiology of hemoptysis associated with menses?**

Catamenial hemoptysis, caused by endometrial tissue in the lung.

ASTHMA, OCCUPATIONAL ASTHMA AND COPD

"When all around the wind doth blow
And coughing drowns the parson's saw"
Love's Labour's Lost, Shakespeare

○ **What is the Reid Index?**

The ratio of airway mucus gland depth (thickness) to epithelial depth (wall thickness) in cartilaginous airways. This is increased in chronic inflammatory pulmonary diseases like chronic bronchitis.

○ **Name some processes that cause the work of breathing to increase markedly in patients with COPD.**

Increased dead space ventilation requiring a higher minute ventilation, decreased respiratory muscle efficiency due to hyperinflation and increased airway resistance.

○ **A patient has severe status asthmatics associated with 20 mmHg of pulsus paradoxus. After another half-hour the degree of pulsus paradoxus decreases to 5 mmHg and the degree of wheezing heard over the chest diminishes. What two exactly opposite ventilatory conditions can produce this identical picture?**

The bronchospasm may be resolving, such that the swings in intrathoracic pressure that caused the pulsus paradoxus decrease along with the intensity of wheezing. The swings in intrathoracic pressure could also decrease if the patient were tiring, such that the respiratory efforts decrease as the patient slipped into a hypercarbic acidosis.

○ **What local complication can result from prolonged use of inhaled steroids?**

Oral candidiasis. Patients should rinse their mouth after each treatment.

○ **What term is used to describe the over expansion of a pulmonary lobe that may be a cause of respiratory distress in infants?**

Lobar emphysema.

○ **What conditions or commonly used medications result in an increase in serum theophylline concentration?**

Cimetidine, macrolides, quinolones, verapamil, congestive heart failure and liver failure.

○ **What conditions or commonly used medications result in a decrease in serum theophylline concentration?**

Barbiturates, phenytoin, carbamazepine, rifampin, smoking and barbecued or smoked food consumption.

○ **How is chronic bronchitis defined?**

Daily expectoration of sputum for a minimum of three months in a year for at least two years in a patient without other underlying pulmonary disease.

○ **What spirometric test best discriminates COPD from restrictive lung disease?**

FEV_1/FVC.

○ **What parameters should make you consider initiating home oxygen therapy for a patient with COPD?**

If the patient has a resting pO_2 less than 55 mmHg, or a pO_2 of less than 60 mmHg with evidence of tissue hypoxia. O_2 desaturation with exercise may also require home O_2.

○ **What percentage of cigarette smokers develop chronic bronchitis?**

10 to 15%. Chronic bronchitis generally develops after 10 to 12 years of smoking.

○ **Other than smoking, what are the risk factors for COPD?**

Environmental pollutants, recurrent URI (especially in infancy), eosinophilia or increased serum IgE, bronchial hyperresponsiveness, a family history of COPD and protease deficiencies.

○ **Is there any hope for patients with COPD who quit smoking?**

Yes. Symptomatically speaking, coughing stops in up to 80% of these patients. Fifty-four percent of COPD patients find relief from coughing within a month of quitting.

○ **If a patient with chronic bronchitis suffers an acute exacerbation of his illness, such as dyspnea, cough, or purulent sputum, what type of O_2 therapy should be initiated?**

Patients with COPD are no longer prompted to breathe by hypercarbia, but by hypoxia alone. However, in the case of an acute exacerbation of bronchitis, oxygen therapy should be guided by pO_2 levels. Adequate oxygen must be maintained to a pO_2 above 60 mmHg. This should be accomplished with the minimal amount of oxygen necessary. The pO_2 must be kept above 60 mmHg even if the patient loses the drive to breathe.

○ **Which pulmonary function test shows an increase in COPD?**

Residual volume and total lung capacity. All other tests (FEV_1, FEV_1/FVC and $FEV_{25-75\%}$, DLCO) decrease.

○ **Which part of the lung is affected by emphysema? By chronic bronchitis?**

Emphysema: respiratory bronchioles.
Chronic bronchitis: bronchi and membranous bronchioles.

○ **What is the risk of placing a patient with COPD on a high FIO2?**

Suppression of the hypoxic ventilatory drive.

○ **What is a blue bloater?**

An overweight patient with chronic bronchitis and central cyanosis. These individuals have normal lung capacity and are hypoxic.

○ **What is a pink puffer?**

A patient with emphysema. These patients are generally thin and non-cyanotic. They have an increased total lung capacity and a decreased FEV_1.

○ **In treating a patient with a common cold, you prescribe an oral decongestant. Is it necessary to add an antitussant?**

No. Most coughs, arising from a common cold, are caused by the irritation of the tracheobronchial receptors in the posterior pharynx as a result of postnasal drip. Postnasal drip can be relieved with decongestant therapy, thus eliminating the need for cough suppressant therapy.

○   **What drugs can induce a chronic cough?**

ACE inhibitors cause chronic cough as a result of the accumulation of prostaglandins, kinins, or substances that excite the cough receptors. Beta-blockers evoke bronchoconstriction and coughing by blocking beta-2 receptors. Never give beta-blockers to asthmatics or other patients with an airway disease.

○   **Which beta-adrenergic receptors primarily control bronchiolar and arterial smooth muscle tone?**

Beta-2 adrenergic receptors.

○   **Is theophylline useful in the emergency management of a severely asthmatic patient?**

No. It has not been shown to affect further bronchodilatation in patients fully treated with beta-adrenergic agents.

○   **What effect does pre-existing acidosis have on the efficacy of treatment with beta-adrenergic agonists?**

Decreased efficacy.

○   **If mechanical ventilation is required for a patient with status asthmaticus, what is an appropriate setting for the initial tidal volume?**

10 ml/kg.

○   **A 29 year-old triathlete develops wheezing when exercising. What would be a reasonable treatment program?**

A sodium cromoglycate (cromolyn sodium) inhaler. Sodium cromoglycate stabilizes mast cells that are involved in the early and late phase bronchoconstrictive reactions of asthma. Sodium cromoglycate is only a prophylactic treatment for exercise-induced asthma and is not effective once the attack has begun.

○   **What x-ray markings may be observed in a patient with a long history of bronchial asthma?**

Increased bronchial wall markings and flattening of the diaphragm. The bronchial wall markings are caused by inflammation and thickening of the bronchial walls.

○   **What is test is most useful to demonstrate airway caliber constriction in asthma?**

FEV_1/FVC. This test determines the amount of air exhaled in 1 second compared to the total amount of air in the lung that can be expressed. A ratio under 0.70% is consistent airway constriction seen in asthma. Peak flow monitors are helpful in monitoring asthma at home or during an acute exacerbation.

○   **Is wheezing an integral part of asthma?**

No. Thirty-three percent of children with asthma will only have the cough variant of asthma with no wheezing.

○   **Which is more effective for relieving an acute exacerbation of asthma in a conscious patient: nebulized albuterol or albuterol MDI administered via an aerosol chamber?**

They are both equally effective.

O   **Asthmatics will most likely have a family history of what?**

Asthma, allergies, or atopic dermatitis.

O   **What type of exercise usually triggers an asthmatic episode in patients with exercise-induced asthma?**

High intensity exercise for more than 5 to 6 minutes.

O   **What medications should be avoided for a pregnant patient with asthma?**

Epinephrine and parenteral beta-adrenergic agonists.

O   **What is a normal peak expiratory flow rate in adults?**

Males: 550 to 600 L/minute. Females: 450 to 500 L/minute. However, this varies somewhat with body size and age.

O   **Sympathomimetic agents are used to treat asthma. What enzyme do they activate?**

Adenylate cyclase.

O   **What reaction is catalyzed by adenyl cyclase?**

Adenyl cyclase catalyzes ATP to cyclic AMP.

O   **What effects do increased levels of c-AMP have on bronchial smooth muscle and the release of chemical mediators, such as histamine, proteases, platelet activation and chemotactic factors, from airway mast cells?**

Smooth muscles are relaxed and release of mediators is decreased. Recall that the effects of c-AMP are opposed by c-GMP. Thus, another treatment approach can be provided by decreasing the levels of cyclic GMP via the use of anticholinergic (antimuscarinic) agents, such as ipratropium bromide.

O   **What should be suspected if a very young, non-smoking patient has symptoms similar to those associated with emphysema?**

Alpha-1 antitrypsin deficiency. Without alpha-1 antitrypsin, excess elastase accumulates, resulting in lung damage. Treatment for this condition is the same as that for emphysema. An alpha-1 protease inhibitor may also be useful.

O   **Can theophylline be dialyzed?**

Yes.

O   **What may decrease theophylline metabolism and increase theophylline levels?**

Factors including age greater than 50, prematurity, liver and renal disease, pulmonary edema, CHF, pneumonia, obesity and viral illness in children. Drugs that increase theophylline levels include cimetidine, erythromycin, allopurinol, troleandomycin, oral contraceptives and quinolone antibiotics.

O   **What may decrease the theophylline level?**

In smokers, the theophylline half-life is decreased, which causes the levels of serum theophylline to decrease. Phenobarbital, phenytoin, rifampin, carbamazepine, marijuana smoking, exposure to environmental pollutants and the consumption of charcoal-broiled foods may decrease serum theophylline levels.

○   **What two diseases are usually seen in patients with COPD?**

Chronic bronchitis and emphysema.

○   **What is the only known genetic abnormality that leads to COPD?**

Alpha-1 antitrypsin deficiency

○   **When is a patient too old to benefit from smoking cessation?**

Smoking cessation improves prognosis regardless of age.

○   **What pathologic type of emphysema is associated with longstanding cigarette smoking?**

Centrilobular emphysma.

○   **What three pathogens are most often cultured from purulent sputum during an acute exacerbation of COPD?**

Streptococcus pneumoniae, Haemophilus influenzae and Moraxella catarrhalis.

○   **What is the most successful smoking cessation strategy?**

Quitting "cold turkey" is more likely to be successful than gradual withdrawal.

○   **What factor in cigarettes is responsible for the addiction of smoking?**

Nicotine is the ingredient in cigarettes primarily responsible.

○   **Should oxygen therapy be withheld in hypoxemic COPD to prevent hypercapnia?**

No. Hypercapnia is more often caused by ventilation-perfusion mismatching rather than respiratory center depression.

○   **Should oxygen therapy be used on an as needed basis in COPD patients?**

No. Oxygen therapy should be based on blood gas measurements and administered continuously in hypoxemic patients.

○   **Does transcutaneous pO2 allow accurate assessment of oxygenation in adults with COPD?**

No. In adults the skin surface characteristics and problems with local blood flow have limited the accuracy of such measurements.

○   **Has noninvasive pulse oximetry replaced ABG in the assessment of acid-base status in patients with COPD?**

No. Oximetry is useful for assessing SaO2 but it cannot determine PCO2 or acid base status.

○   **What are the absolute Medicare reimbursement guidelines for oxygen therapy?**

PaO2 less than or equal to 55 or SaO2 less than or equal to 88%.

○   **Does participation in pulmonary rehabilitation reduce health-care costs?**

Yes. After pulmonary rehabilitation hospitalization frequency and length of stay have been shown to decrease.

○   **Does participation in pulmonary rehabilitation increase survival?**

No. There have been no prospective randomized controlled studies that provide evidence of increased survival.

○   **What is "pursed-lips" breathing and what benefit does it have?**

Patients breathe in slowly and deeply through the nose, purse their lips (as if to whistle) and breathe out slowly through pursed lips, taking twice as long to exhale as to inhale. This decreases dyspnea.

○   **What serum theophylline level is appropriate when aminophylline is used to treat exacerbations of COPD?**

A level of 8 to 12 ug/ml is usually appropriate.

○   **Has chest physiotherapy with postural drainage been shown to improve mucus clearance in COPD?**

No. Trials have not shown improvement in sputum volume or pulmonary function.

○   **Which patients with COPD are most likely to benefit from chest physiotherapy?**

Patients with mucus plugging and lobar atelectasis.

○   **Is intermittent positive pressure breathing (IPPB) the best method for promoting clearance of airway secretions?**

No. IPPB has been abandoned in the care of patients with COPD.

○   **Does the inhalation of aerosolized saline help liquefy airway secretions?**

No. Sufficient volumes cannot be administered by jet nebulization to liquefy airway secretions.

○   **Does systemic over-hydration enhance mucous clearance in patients with exacerabation of COPD?**

No data support systemic hydration beyond euvolemia.

○   **Does nasotracheal suctioning of nonintubated patients with COPD improve respiratory function?**

No. It may impair ventilatory function.

○   **Does hypopnea in the setting of acute exacerbation of COPD require assisted ventilation?**

Not unless progressive worsening of respiratory acidosis and/or altered mental status develop.

○   **What is auto-PEEP?**

Intrinsic positive end-expiratory pressure.

○   **When does a patient require tracheostomy for prolonged mechanical ventilation due to COPD?**

No study confirms a time limit. Clinical judgment will determine when weaning appears difficult and benefits of surgery outweigh immediate and long-term risks of prolonged endotrachal intubation.

○   **What are the risks of positive pressure mechanical ventilation?**

Ventilator-associated pneumonia, pulmonary barotrauma and laryngotracheal complications.

○   **Has noninvasive positive pressure ventilation been shown to improve clinical outcome in acute exacerbation of COPD?**

Yes. Improved survival and hospital stay has been found in some studies examining certain subgroups of COPD patients.

○   **Is a patient with an acute COPD exacerbation and impaired mental status a good candidate for a trial of noninvasive ventilation?**

No. Impaired mental status makes success less likely with noninvasive ventilation.

○   **Does noninvasive ventilation decrease the staffing requirements for treatment of respiratory failure in COPD?**

No. Experience and extensive training of physicians, nurses and respiratory care practitioners is required to maintain the necessary supervision of patients managed with noninvasive positive pressure ventilation.

○   **Can patients with COPD be successfully extubated without a weaning period?**

Yes. Many patients with COPD who undergo mechanical ventilation for acute bronchospasm, fluid overload, oversedation or inadvertent hyperoxygenation may be successfully extubated without weaning.

○   **What are the currently available techniques for weaning patients with COPD from mechanical ventilation?**

Assist-control ventilation with T-piece trials, intermittent mandatory ventilation and pressure support ventilation.

○   **What is the approximate FI02 delivered via nasal cannula at 2 liters per minute?**

Fl02 = 21% + (2-4 x oxygen liter flow) = 25-29%.

○   **When should an ABG be sampled following a change in FIO2?**
20 to 30 minutes to achieve a steady state.

○   **What is lung volume reduction surgery?**

Resection of noncompressive emphysema intended to reduce hyperinflation and improve respiratory symptoms. Studies are underway to evaluate the role of this surgery.

○   **What is glomectomy?**

Surgical resection of the carotid body designed to blunt symptoms of dyspnea. The procedure was abandoned due to problems with patients who developed ventilatory failure because of insensitivity to hypoxia.

○   **Do patients with COPD need overnight sleep studies?**

Patients who have symptoms of coexistent obstructive sleep apnea, unexplained polycythemia or cor pulmonale should have overnight sleep study.

○   **Are physicians required to honor properly established advance directives by a patient with severe COPD to forego intubation and mechanical ventilation?**

Respect for patient autonomy requires a physician to honor such requests or transfer the patient's care to another physician who can honor the patient's directives.

O **Is there an ethical difference between withholding and withdrawing life-support measures in patients with acute respiratory failure?**

Ethical principles underlying the decision to withhold intubation and mechanical ventilation apply equally when patients or proxies request discontinuance of care for patients who have no hope for an acceptable and meaningful recovery.

O **What method of evaluation of a patient with COPD gives prognostic information and serves as a guide for therapy?**

Spirometry before and after bronchodilator.

O **Is unilateral lung transplantation a feasible option for patients with end-stage COPD?**

Multiple centers have confirmed the feasibility of single lung transplantation in patient with obstructive lung disease. Because of the large number of patients with COPD, it has overtaken fibrotic disease as the number one indication for single lung transplantation.

O **Which pulmonary function test is the best predictor of the severity of emphysema?**

The carbon monoxide diffusing capacity has consistently been the best predictor with correlation coefficients from 0.60 to 0.87.

O **After cessation of smoking, is lung function lost as a result of smoking regained?**

No. The rate of decline of lung function slows, but lung function is not regained.

O **Is anti-inflammatory therapy with corticosteroids required to slow the progression of COPD?**

No, unlike asthma COPD is not primarily a disorder of inflammation. Only 15-20% of stable COPD patients have objective improvement with corticosteroids.

O **What are the 3 major pathophysiological components of airway obstruction in asthma?**

Airway wall thickening from chronic inflammation and edema, mucus plugging and bronchoconstriction.

O **What are the common triggers of asthma in children?**

1. Respiratory viral infections (rhinovirus, RSV).
2. Air pollutants (ozone, cigarette smoke).
3. Allergens (house dust mite, cockroaches, molds, pollens).
4. Exercise.
5. Emotions.

O **What is the stepwise approach for managing asthma?**

It's a 4-step set of guidelines designed to assist clinicians in decision making. The idea is to gain control as quickly as possible and then decrease treatment to the least medication necessary to maintain control. Gaining control may be accomplished by either starting treatment at the step most appropriate to the initial severity of their condition, or by starting at a higher level of therapy. One of the basic concepts of this approach is that the use of short-acting beta-2 agonists on a daily basis indicates the need for additional long-term control therapy.

O **What is the estimated prevalence of asthma in the United States?**

Three to six percent of the population

O   **What is the estimated prevalence of occupational asthma among asthmatics?**

Conservatively, two to five percent of all asthmatics. However, in a survey of disability by the Social Security Administration in 1978, 15.4% of respondents attributed their self-reported diagnosis of asthma to their working conditions.

O   **What percentage of workers sufficiently exposed to toluene diisocyanate will develop occupational asthma?**

Approximately five percent.

O   **How many agents have been reported to cause asthma in exposed workers?**

Approximately 200 to 300.

O   **By what mechanism do high molecular weight (>50,000 daltons) substances cause occupational asthma?**

Immunologic response mediated by IgE. The pathogenesis is no different from that of the more common inhalant allergens, such as house dust mites or pollens.

O   **Is atopy a predisposing factor for the development of occupational asthma?**

Yes, for high molecular weight substances. No, for low molecular weight substances.

O   **By what mechanism do low molecular weight substances (<50,000 daltons) cause occupational asthma?**

They may elicit an IgE mediated immunologic response by serving as haptens with a native protein carrier molecule to form a complete allergen. In many circumstances, however, an IgE mediated response to low molecular weight substances has not been demonstrable. In such circumstances the mechanism remains to be elucidated.

O   **What is the asthma-like syndrome that may result from an exposure to irritant gases, fumes and vapors?**

Reactive Airways Dysfunction Syndrome (RADS).

O   **What type of exposure may result in RADS?**

A single episode of inhaling a high concentration of an irritant (or toxic) gas, fume, or vapor. Generally, the intensity of the exposure is such that the affected individual seeks immediate medical attention and may require hospitalization.

O   **What occupational airway disorder is caused by exposure to textile dusts, including cotton, flax and hemp?**

Byssinosis. A similar syndrome is caused by exposure to grain dust.

O   **What is the characteristic progression of symptoms during a typical work-week in a patient with byssinosis?**

Chest tightness, cough and dyspnea develop several hours after returning to work on Monday. The symptoms disappear later in the day. If symptoms develop on Tuesday, they are milder. Later in the week, the worker becomes asymptomatic.

O   **What is the causative agent in the development of Western Red Cedar asthma?**

Plicatic acid.

O   **What is colophony?**

A solid material left after turpentine has been distilled from pine tree resins. Asthma among soldering workers in the electronics industry has been associated with exposure to colophony contained in soldering fluxes.

O   **What is the most common cause of occupational asthma in North America?**

Toluene diisocyanate. Hexamethylene diisocyanate (HDI), diphenylmethane diisocyanate (MDI) and naphthalene diisocyanate (NDI) also cause asthma.

O   **Acid anhydrides are essential precursors of what substances?**

Epoxy resins. This substance has a wide range of applications in such products as reinforced plastics, adhesives, molding resins and surface coating. All of the common acid anhydrides, such as phthalic, tetrachlorophthalic, maleic and trimellitic anhydride (TMA) may cause respiratory disease. TMA is the best studied.

O   **Salts of which heavy metals have been commonly reported to cause occupational asthma?**

Nickel, chromium and platinum.

O   **Occupational asthma may, at first, present with atypical symptoms. Name three.**

Cough, chest discomfort and easy fatigability.

O   **In retrospect, what symptoms are commonly identified as the very first signs of development of occupational asthma?**

Rhinitis and ocular irritation are common where protein antigens are involved. A dry tickly cough is also a common presenting symptom.

O   **What is the first step in the diagnosis of occupational asthma?**

Confirm that the patient's complaints are due to asthma. The demonstration of bronchial hyperresponsiveness (either by methacholine/histamine challenge or a significant spirometric response to an inhaled bronchodilator) would confirm a clinical suspicion of asthma.

O   **If a diagnosis of asthma is confirmed, what is the next step in the diagnosis of occupational asthma?**

Establishing an association between symptoms and exposure at the workplace. The key here is the history.

O   **In obtaining a history from a patient with possible occupational asthma, what two questions will identify the majority of patients with occupational asthma?**

1.   Are your symptoms improved on your days off?
2.   Are your symptoms improved while on vacation?
The latter question may be especially important in those with more severe disease. In this case, symptoms may not improve over a one or two day weekend but might disappear with an extended period of 10 - 14 days.

O   **A patient with pre-existing asthma develops cough, shortness of breath and wheezing after an exposure to an irritating gas at the worksite. Is this occupational asthma?**

No. Occupational asthma generally refers to a situation whereby the asthmatic condition is caused by exposure at the worksite. The patient in question has suffered a non-specific temporary exacerbation of symptoms due to his pre-existing bronchial hyperresponsiveness.

O   **A patient without a history of pre-existing asthma develops cough, shortness of breath and wheezing after an exposure at the worksite on his first day of work. Is this occupational asthma?**

No. With the exception of RADS, occupational asthma does not develop immediately upon first exposure to a sensitizer. Sensitization occurs during a latent period. The latent period is variable and may range from weeks to months to years.

O   **What is the average latent period in a patient who develops TDI asthma?**

Two years.

O   **What are the immediate and late responses in asthma?**

An "immediate response" occurs within minutes of exposure, is maximal within 10 - 15 minutes, will reverse with bronchodilator, will abate without treatment in one hour, may be prevented by pre-treatment with a beta-agonist and is not followed by an increase in non-specific bronchial responsiveness.

A "late response" develops within several hours of exposure, is maximal within 4 - 8 hours, may be more severe, will resolve within 12 - 36 hours, may prove more difficult to treat, may be prevented by corticosteroids and is followed by an increase in non-specific bronchial responsiveness.

Patients may demonstrate an immediate, a late, or dual responses. Atypical patterns, however, may occur in up to 22% of patients.

O   **In what percentage of patients, felt to have occupational asthma by history alone, will the diagnosis be confirmed by objective testing?**

Approximately 60%. A recent study found that of 162 patients with a history suggestive of occupational asthma, only 66 (63%) actually had the disorder based on objective testing. The diagnosis of occupational asthma may be inferred from the history but must be confirmed objectively.

O   **What test is commonly used to confirm an association between symptoms and workplace exposures?**

A "stop-resume" work test with serial measurement of peak expiratory airflow rate (PEFR). The patient measures his/her PEFR at least four times daily for a period of 2 - 3 weeks while at work and at least 10 days away from work. Criteria for interpreting the test have not been firmly established. An "eyeball" test of a graph of serial measurements is commonly employed.

O   **What is a "MSDS"?**

Material safety data sheet. Employers are required to have information on substances and materials used in the workplace available for review. The worker may request these reports for use in the diagnosis and management of exposure related health problems

O   **Of what value is skin testing and serologic testing in the diagnosis of occupational asthma?**

In a few circumstances, appropriate extracts are available for specific skin testing. For example, skin testing with flour and wheat is useful in the diagnosis of Baker's Asthma. For a few substances, such as the anhydrides and platinum salts, antibodies may be detected and measured by RAST and ELISA techniques. Positive tests only document exposure and sensitization and do not confirm a cause-and-effect relationship.

O   **Why are specific bronchial challenge tests infrequently performed?**

These tests are time consuming and not without risk. Testing should be done by experienced personnel and usually in a hospital setting. As a result, these studies are not widely available and should not be pursued in most clinical settings. In some circumstances, however, the specific challenge may be the only way to establish the diagnosis.

O   **How does the treatment of occupational asthma differ from that of common asthma?**

In general, the treatment of occupational asthma is no different from any other type of asthma. With occupational asthma, however, an emphasis is placed on environmental control, particularly cessation of exposure.

O   **Will improved ventilation of the work area and the use of personal protective equipment allow the patient with occupational asthma to return to the worksite?**

In general, no. Improved ventilation and respiratory protection may decrease the incidence of new sensitization in co-workers but are not adequate to prevent symptoms in most sensitized individuals.

O   **Will patients with RADS be able to return to the worksite?**

Yes. If the level of exposure to irritants does not exceed the symptom threshold for that individual, he/she may return to the worksite. The patient with RADS is no more sensitive to the substance that caused the problem than is any other asthmatic with a similar degree of non-specific bronchial hyperresponsiveness.

O   **What strategies have proven beneficial in preventing occupational asthma?**

Persuading workers to stop smoking, keeping concentrations of possible occupational agents low, avoiding spills, use of personal respiratory protective devices, engineering controls, industrial hygiene surveys, product formulation changes, medical surveillance and screening and worker education.

O   **What is the natural history of occupational asthma after cessation of exposure?**

Signs and symptoms may completely resolve. The disorder may persist as a chronic asthmatic condition associated with permanent non-specific bronchial hyperresponsiveness. In a study of patients with Western Red Cedar asthma, 60% did not recover during a 4 year follow-up.

O   **What factors influence whether symptoms resolve after exposure cessation?**

The total duration of exposure, the duration of exposure after the onset of symptoms and the severity of the asthma at the time of diagnosis.

O   **By what mechanism do many pesticides induce bronchoconstriction?**

Exposure, primarily inhalational, to organophosphate pesticides may result in bronchoconstriction. The toxicological mechanism is competitive inhibition of acetylcholinesterase, the enzymatic deactivator of the neurotransmitter acetylcholine.

O   **In what way are the physical examination and chest roentgenogram helpful in the diagnosis of occupational asthma?**

Only in the negative sense of excluding other causes of the presenting symptom complex. There are neither characteristic physical findings nor chest x-ray changes of occupational asthma.

O   After cessation of exposure, how long may skin testing and RAST findings be expected to remain positive?

In general, when positive, they may be expected to remain positive for up to 6 to 12 months.

O   What is the main sensitizer in laboratory animal allergy?

Protein in the urine of the animal, rather than dander, is the main cause of sensitization. The important urinary proteins seem to be an alpha 2 globulin in the rat and a prealbumin in the mouse.

O   What is the estimated prevalence of laboratory animal allergy?

Varies between 15% to 30% of exposed workers.

O   What feature separates the two types of occupational asthma?

Two types of occupational asthma are recognized, depending on whether or not they develop after a latency period. Occupational asthma with a latency period is characterized by a variable time during which "sensitization" takes place. Occupational asthma without a latency period may be termed "irritant-induced asthma," an example of which is RADS.

O   What is the "healthy worker effect"?

Many workers who experience respiratory symptoms at the worksite will merely leave the workplace and change occupations. Therefore, in cross-sectional studies of working populations, those who experience no ill effects from the workplace will tend to be overrepresented.

O   What is the most common high molecular weight agent that causes occupational asthma in North America?

Flour.

O   What is the reported sensitivity and specificity of serial PEFR monitoring as compared to the "gold standard" specific inhalation challenge studies?

They vary from 72% to 89%, depending on the study.

O   What is the main pitfall in using serial PEFR monitoring in the diagnosis of occupational asthma?

Patient compliance and honesty.

O   What four separate clinical syndromes caused by exposure to trimellitic anhydride have been identified?

1. Toxic airway irritation.
2. IgE mediated immediate rhinitis and asthma.
3. IgG mediated late asthma with systemic symptoms ("TMA flu").
4. Pulmonary hemorrhage with hemolytic anemia syndrome.

O   What four respiratory reactions to inhaled diisocyanates have been reported?

1. Inhalation of toxic concentrations may result in the RADS.
2. Occupational asthma with a latent period.
3. An accelerated decline in FEV1 among exposed workers.

4. Hypersensitivity pneumonitis.

○   **What causes occupational asthma in bakery workers?**

Although grain contaminants such as mites and molds have been suggested as causes, current evidence implicates cereal flour proteins as the most important cause. Asthma in bakers may also be caused by exposure to an enzyme (alpha-amylase) used in bread making.

○   **What are the side effects of selective beta-2 adrenergic agonists?**

Tachycardia, tremor secondary to skeletal muscle stimulation and hypokalemia.

○   **What is the mechanism of action of theophylline?**

Unknown! It is no longer considered to mediate its effects through inhibition of c-AMP phosphodiesterase.

○   **What are the pharmacological effects of theophylline?**

Bronchodilation, increased endogenous catecholamine, enhanced contractility of diaphragm and inhibition of the immediate and late phase asthmatic responses.

○   **What are the signs and symptoms of theophylline toxicity?**

Nausea, insomnia, irritability, tremors, headache, seizure, tachycardia, cardiac rhythm disturbances, hypotension, ataxia, hallucinations, hypokalemia and hyperglycemia.

○   **How do you treat theophylline toxicity?**

For gut decontamination, multi-dose activated charcoal is used. The method of choice for serum removal is charcoal hemoperfusion.

○   **What side effects can be observed in high doses of terfenadine or astemizole?**

Cardiac arrest secondary to QT prolongation and ventricular tachycardia (Torsades de Pointes).

○   **Two hours after receiving corticosteroids, what occurs in the peripheral blood count?**

A fall in peripheral eosinophils and lymphocytes.

○   **What effects of corticosteroids are likely after six to eight hours?**

An improvement in pulmonary function in asthmatics and hyperglycemia.

○   **What are the clinical effects of phenobarbital and phenytoin on corticosteroids?**

Increased steroid clearance and decreased plasma concentration.

○   **What are some possible adverse effects of chronic steroid use?**

1. Posterior subcapsular cataract
2. Osteoporosis
3. Hypertension
4. Diabetes mellitus
5. Cushingoid body habitus
6. Infections
7. Pancreatitis

8.   Gastritis
9.   Myopathy

O   **What constitutes triad asthma?**

The syndrome of nasal polyps, asthma and aspirin intolerance.

O   **What is the most effective treatment of allergic rhinitis?**

Topical use of corticosteroids, such as beclomethasone nasal spray.

O   **What are the major risk factors of asthma?**

1.   Poverty
2.   African-American ancestry
3.   Maternal age <20 years old
4.   Birth weight < 2,500 grams
5.   Maternal smoking
6.   Small home size
7.   Intense allergic exposure (dust mite)
8.   Large family size
9.   Frequent respiratory infection

O   **Is cor pulmonale, resulting from sustained pulmonary hypertension, a common complication of asthma?**

No.

O   **What is extrinsic asthma?**

Asthmatic exacerbation following environmental exposure to allergens such as dust, pollens and dander.

O   **What is intrinsic asthma?**

Asthmatic exacerbation not associated with an increase in IgE or a positive skin reaction.

O   **Is clubbing a feature of severe asthma?**

It is rarely observed in either mild or severe asthma.

O   **Why are acute asthmatic exacerbations more common at night?**

Patency of the airway decreases at night, which precipitates an acute attack.

O   **A 20 year-old male who appears pale and alert, presents to the ER with shortness of breath. He can only speak in short phrases, his respiratory rate is 28/min, he has audible inspiratory and expiratory wheezing and obvious intercostal retractions and chest hyperinflation are noted on exam. A blood gas demonstrates oxygen saturation of 90-95% and carbon dioxide of 39. What is the estimated asthma severity?**

Moderate.

O   **When administering epinephrine in the treatment of asthma, how might the side effects of epinephrine be minimized?**

Side effects, such as pallor, tremor, anxiety, palpitations and headache, can be minimized if doses of no more than 0.3 ml are given.

○   **What are the historical risk factors for status asthmaticus?**

1.   Chronic steroid-dependent asthma
2.   Prior ICU admission
3.   Prior intubation
4.   Recurrent ER visits in past 48 hours
5.   Sudden onset of severe respiratory distress
6.   Poor therapy compliance
7.   Poor clinical recognition of attack severity
8.   Hypoxic seizures

○   **What should be reserved for refractory status asthmaticus after the patient has been intubated?**

Halothane anesthesia produces prompt bronchodilation, but is difficult to administer and is reserved for the most severe cases.

○   **A 20 year-old asthmatic has had a poor response to treatment in the ER despite nebulizers and steroids. His PEFR is still 40% below baseline, his oxygen saturation is 91% and he now exhibits pulsus paradoxus on physical exam. What is your next step in management?**

Hospitalize.

○   **What are the criteria for ICU admission in a severe asthma case?**

1.   PEFR <30% baseline
2.   PCO2 >40 mmHg
3. O_2 saturation <90%
4.   Severe obstruction with evidence of decreased air movement
5.   Pulsus paradoxus >15 mmHg.

○   **What is the mortality rate of asthma?**

In the United States, the mortality rate is 2.0/100,000.

○   **T/F: Dynamic hyperinflation in obstructive airway disease can cause hypotension.**

True.

○   **T/F: Briefly disconnecting the endotracheal tube from the ventilator tubing is a way to correct the hypotension associated with dynamic hyperinflation.**

True. Be careful to avoid oxygen desaturation.

○   **T/F: Complications in patients with obstructive airway disease that are mechanically ventilated have been shown to correlate with the degree of hyperinflation, as measured by the volume of gas exhaled after disconnecting the patient from the ventilator for 40 to 60 seconds.**

True.

○   **T/F: The complications mentioned above include barotrauma (as pneumothorax) and hypotension.**

True.

BRONCHIECTASIS AND CYSTIC FIBROSIS

"After life's fitful fever he sleeps well"
Macbeth, Shakespeare

○ **A chest x-ray shows honeycombing, atelectasis and increased bronchial markings.**

What is the most likely diagnosis?

Bronchiectasis, an irreversible dilation of the bronchi that is generally associated with infection. Bronchography shows dilatation of the bronchial tree but this method of diagnosis is not recommended for routine use.

○ **Bronchiectasis occurs most frequently in patients with what conditions?**

Cystic fibrosis, immunodeficiencies, consequent to lung infections, or foreign body aspirations.

○ **What is bronchiectasis?**

An abnormal dilatation of the proximal medium sized bronchi greater than 2 mm in diameter. It is due to the destruction of the muscular and elastic components of their walls, usually associated with chronic bacterial infection.

○ **Is bronchiectasis always associated with purulent expectoration?**

No. Tuberculosis induced bronchiectasis is not.

○ **How do you classify bronchiectasis?**

The most widely used system is the Reid classification, which classifies bronchiectasis as:

Cylindrical bronchiectasis: sections of the bronchi are consistently widened. It is the mildest form of bronchiectasis.

Varicose bronchiectasis: local constrictions in cylindrical bronchiectatic areas cause irregularities of the bronchial wall outline resembling varicose veins.

Saccular or cystic bronchiectasis: dilatation increases towards the lung periphery causing the bronchi to terminate as balloon like cystic structures measuring several centimeters in diameter. It is the most severe form of bronchiectasis.

○ **What is the advantage of the Reid classification system?**

Since the Reid classification is based on a pathologic - bronchographic correlation, it helps in the roentgenographic description of the process.

○ **What are the disadvantages of the Reid classification system?**

Little clinical, epidemiological or pathologic difference has been demonstrated between the three types of bronchiectasis. As the Reid system is based on light microscopic analysis, it does not benefit from the recent advances in the understanding of bronchiectasis attained by electron microscopy.

○ **What is the major mechanism in the pathogenesis of bronchiectasis?**

Inflammation mediated by elastase from neutrophils and cytokines from monocytes that are recruited into the lung.

○   **Describe the pathogenesis of bronchiectasis.**

Injury/Inflammation

Recruitment of neutrophils and monocytes

Release of elastase from neutrophils and cytokines from monocytes

Inflammation of the bronchial walls

Destruction of the elastic and muscular components of the wall

Contractile force by the surrounding undamaged lung tissue

Expansion of the bronchi by the pull, creating the characteristic dilatation on radiographs

○   **Which lung segments are most frequently involved in bronchiectasis?**

The posterior basal segments of the left or right lower lobes.

○   **Describe the lobar distribution of bronchiectasis?**

Unilateral involvement is seen in left or right lungs with equal frequency.
50% with left lower lobe bronchiectasis have involvement of the lingular segment.
Right middle lobe is more commonly affected than the right upper lobe.
Upper lobe bronchiectasis usually involves the posterior and apical segments.

○   **What are the most common causes of upper lobe bronchiectasis?**

Tuberculous bronchitis and allergic bronchopulmonary aspergillosis (ABPA).

○   **What is the most important functional impairment of the bronchiectatic airway?**

Impaired tracheobronchial clearance that predisposes to airway colonization and infection with pathogenic organisms.

○   **What physiologic and anatomic alterations have been described in patients with bronchiectasis?**

1.   Impaired tracheobronchial clearance.
2,   Enlargement of the bronchial arteries and extensive anastamosis between these vessels and the pulmonary arteries.
3.   Diminished total pulmonary arterial blood flow.
4,   Functional decrease in the cross sectional area of the pulmonary vasculature with hypoxia.
5.   Left to right intrapulmonary shunting.
6.   Decreased ventilation of bronchographically abnormal areas.

○   **Which population group in the U.S. has the highest incidence of postinfectious bronchiectasis?**

Native Americans in Alaska.

○   **What are the major pulmonary function abnormalities in bronchiectasis?**

Most patients have some amount of airflow obstruction. Restriction may be noted in patients with bronchiectasis associated with restrictive lung diseases.

○ **Is cor pulmonale a common feature of bronchiectasis?**

No. The hypoxia is usually mild.

○ **What are the symptoms of bronchiectasis?**

1. Chronic cough
2. Purulent sputum
3. Fever
4. Weakness
5. Weight loss
6. Dyspnea in some patients
7. Hemoptysis: generally mild, originates from bronchial arteries, and not a common cause of death (< 10% of deaths attributed to hemoptysis)

○ **How do you grade the severity of bronchiectasis based on sputum production?**

Mild bronchiectasis: < 10 ml/ 24 hrs
Moderate bronchiectasis: 10 - 150 ml/ 24 hrs
Severe bronchiectasis: > 150 ml/ 24 hrs

○ **What are the most common complications of bronchiectasis?**

Recurrent attacks of pneumonia, empyema, pneumothorax and lung abscess.

○ **What are the less common complications that can be seen in bronchiectasis?**

Brain abscess, amyloidosis and cor pulmonale.

○ **Describe the sputum in bronchiectasis?**

On allowing to stand, the sputum settles into three layers:
1. Upper frothy and watery layer
2. Middle turbid, mucopurulent layer
3. Bottom purulent layer containing white or yellow particles known as Dittrich's granules.

○ **Describe the radiographic findings in bronchiectasis?**

May be normal.
Cylindrical bronchiectasis: tram tracking - thin parallel linear radiolucencies radiating from the hila.
Varicose bronchiectasis: thick parallel shadows.
Cystic bronchiectasis: isolated or clustered cystic spaces with air fluid levels.

○ **What is reversible bronchiectasis?**

Bronchial dilatation occurring in association with acute pneumonia, developing as a result of retained secretions and atelectasis. With resolution of the pneumonia, the dilatation gradually resolves over a period of 3 to 4 months.

○ **What is the primary indication for bronchography?**

For presurgical evaluation of patients with focal bronchiectasis. It has been supplanted by high resolution CT.

○ **What precautions should be followed prior to bronchography?**

The procedure should be withheld during an exacerbation and should be deferred in bronchospastic patients. It should be postponed by several months (4 - 6 months) after an infection, as reversible changes in airway dimensions may occur. Bronchography should be performed in only one lung at a time.

○   **What is the specificity of CT scan in detecting bronchiectasis?**

At least 85%.

○   **What laboratory investigations aid in the evaluation of idiopathic bronchiectasis?**

1. Serum protein electrophoresis to rule out alpha-1 antitrypsin deficiency.
2. Ig levels with IgG subclass.
3. Pilocarpine iontophoresis sweat test.
4. Serum precipitins for Aspergillus.
5. Electron microscopy of sperm or respiratory epithelium for primary ciliary dyskinesia (PCD).

○   **What is the mainstay of treatment of bronchiectasis?**

Antibiotics.

○   **How should the choice of antibiotic treatment be guided?**

Sputum culture for aerobes and mycobacteria.

○   **What is an acceptable cost-effective choice of empirical antibiotic in bronchiectasis with mixed flora?**

Amoxicillin with clavulanic acid or trimethoprim/sulfamethoxazole.

○   **What are the adjunctive treatment measures that may be beneficial in patients with bronchiectasis?**

1. Chest physiotherapy.
2. Nutritional support.
3. Bronchodilators.
4. Supplemental oxygen.
5. Immunoglobulin administration for Ig deficiency.
6. Replacement treatment for patients with alpha-1 antitrypsin deficiency.
7. Recombinant DNase to reduce sputum viscosity in patients with cystic fibrosis (CF).

○   **What are the indications for surgery in bronchiectasis?**

1. Patients with focal bronchiectasis who fail medical management.
2. Patients who are non-compliant with medical management.
3. Patients with massive, life threatening hemoptysis.

○   **What are the treatment options for massive, life threatening hemoptysis?**

1. Endobronchial bronchoscopic tamponade with a Fogarty balloon catheter.
2. Bronchial arteriography and embolization - may cause serious neurologic deficits from inadvertent obstruction of the spinal arteries.
3. Surgical resection of the involved lobe.

○   **What is middle lobe syndrome?**

Bronchiectasis and chronic recurrent pneumonia of the right middle lobe.

○   **What are the causes of middle lobe syndrome?**

Angulation at the origin of the right middle lobe bronchus.
Extrinsic compression of the right middle lobe bronchus by enlarged lymph nodes combined with an absence of collateral ventilation.

○   **What is Kartagener's syndrome?**

Triad of: situs inversus, bronchiectasis and nasal polyps or recurrent sinusitis.

○   **What is primary ciliary dyskinesia (PCD)?**

Previously known as immotile cilia syndrome, this is an autosomal recessive disorder affecting 1 in 20,000 to 40,000 people, causing recurrent sinopulmonary infections and bronchiectasis due to uncoordinated movement of the cilia. 50% of patients also have situs inversus.

○   **What are the diagnostic criteria for PCD?**

1.   Chronic or recurrent sinopulmonary infections from childhood.
2.   Situs inversus.
3.   Living but immotile spermatozoa with a normal appearance.
4.   Absent or near absent tracheobronchial clearance.
5.   Nasal or bronchial biopsy specimen demonstrating cilia with the ultrastructural defects typical of this syndrome.

○   **What proteins in the cilia interact to produce ciliary beating (bending)?**

Dynein and tubulin.

○   **What is the most common abnormality that causes primary ciliary dyskinesia?**

Dynein arm defects or dynein arm absence.

○   **What are the most common clinical presentations of primary ciliary dyskinesia?**

Sinusitis, recurrent otitis media, bronchiectasis and male infertility. Because sperm flagella have the same ultrastructure as respiratory cilia, spermatozoa are also dyskinetic.

○   **What percentage of patients with primary ciliary dyskinesia have situs inversus?**

50%. Normal ciliary activity appears to regulate visceral situs. In the absence of ciliary activity, visceral situs orientation is random.

○   **What percentage of patients with primary ciliary dyskinesia have digital clubbing?**

About 30%. Clubbing appears to be associated with saccular bronchiectasis.

○   **What is the prevalence of primary ciliary dyskinesia?**

This is thought to be approximately 1 in 20 to 25,000.

○   **What does it mean when megacilia (fusion cilia) are seen on a transmission electron micrograph of the airway epithelium?**

Megacilia represent airway inflammation and is a nonspecific finding not associated with primary ciliary dyskinesia.

○   **What are the different ciliary ultrastructural defects described in patients with PCD?**

1.   Absence of outer dynein arms.

2.   Absent or defective inner dynein arms.
3.   Deficient central sheath.
4.   Absent or short radial spokes.
5.   Absent central microtubules.
6.   Transposition of the peripheral microtubules.
7.   Supernumerary microtubules.

○   **What are the radiographic features of PCD?**

1.   Bronchial wall thickening.
2.   Hyperinflation.
3.   Segmental atelectasis.
4.   Consolidation.
5.   Bronchiectasis.

○   **What are the major diagnostic criteria for allergic bronchopulmonary aspergillosis (ABPA)?**

1.   History of asthma.
2.   Increased IgE levels.
3.   Peripheral blood eosinophilia.
4.   Precipitating antibodies against Aspergillus.
5.   Central bronchiectasis.

○   **What is the most characteristic pattern of bronchiectasis in ABPA?**

Saccular proximal bronchiectasis of the upper lobes.

○   **What is the cause of bronchiectasis in ABPA?**

Airway plugging by viscid secretions containing aspergillus hyphae.

○   **What has been shown to be associated with bronchiectasis?**

Abnormal B-lymphocyte function.
Congenital or acquired hypogammaglobulinemia with decreased circulating IgG levels.
IgG subclass deficiency in the presence of normal total IgG levels.

○   **What is the most common immunoglobulin (Ig) deficiency?**

Selective IgA deficiency, which affects 1 in 800 individuals. It is usually associated with IgG subclass deficiency (most often IgG2 or IgG4) and presents with recurrent sinopulmonary infections.

○   **What is Young's syndrome?**

Also known as obstructive azoospermia, it is a primary male infertility with normal spermatozoa in the testes, but none in the ejaculate, due to defective mucociliary activity.

○   **A 6 year old male child, born to Jewish parents, is brought to the clinic with recurrent episodes of fever, cough with purulent expectoration and shortness of breath. On physical exam, the patient has a temperature of 101F, orthostatic hypotension and rales in the right mid zone with bronchial breath sounds. Chest X-ray shows a bronchopneumonia pattern in the mid zone of the right lung. What is the most likely diagnosis?**

Familial dysautonomia. It is an autosomal recessive condition seen exclusively in Jews, manifested by dysfunction of the autonomic nervous system leading to hypersecretion of mucous glands, obstruction of the bronchial tree, recurrent sinopulmonary infections and bronchiectasis.

○ **What are the possible manifestations of alpha-1 antitrypsin deficiency?**

Panlobular emphysema, bronchiectasis and hepatic cirrhosis.

○ **What is a unilateral hyperlucent lung?**

Also known as Swyer-James syndrome (MacLeod syndrome in the UK). This is a unilateral hyperlucency of one lung related to recurrent bronchopulmonary infections in infancy causing hypoplasia of the lung parenchyma and pulmonary artery on the involved side.

○ **What are the mean dimensions of the airway in normal adults?**

Trachea = 20 mm
Right main stem bronchus = 16 mm
Left main stem bronchus = 15 mm

○ **What is tracheobronchomegaly?**

Also known as Mounier-Kuhn syndrome, it is described when the mean dimensions of the airways are increased as follows:
Trachea > 31 mm
Right main stem bronchus > 24 mm
Left main stem bronchus > 23 mm

○ **What is yellow nail syndrome?**

Association of yellow discoloration of fingernails, lymphedema, bilateral pleural effusions and bronchiectasis. All four features need not be present in the same patient.

○ **What is cystic fibrosis (CF)?**

CF is a multisystem disorder affecting children and young adults, characterized by chronic obstruction and infection of the airways and exocrine pancreatic insufficiency.

○ **What is the incidence of CF?**

1 in 2500 live births among whites and 1 in 17,000 live births among blacks.

○ **What is the inheritance pattern of CF?**

Autosomal recessive.

○ **What is the site of mutation in CF?**

At a single gene locus on the long arm of chromosome 7. This locus codes for a large protein (cystic fibrosis transmembrane regulator - CFTR protein) that has several transmembrane domains, phosphorylation sites and two cytoplasmic ATP binding sites.

○ **What is the chance of having a child with CF, when one parent is a carrier and the other is heterozygous for the CF gene?**

25%.

○ **Pathology in CF is confined predominantly to what part of the lung?**

Mucous obstruction and infection in the lungs are confined mostly to the conducting airways.

O   **Why is a pneumothorax more common in advanced CF?**

Subpleural cysts often occur on the mediastinal surfaces of the upper lobes and are thought to contribute to pneumothorax in patients with advanced disease.

O   **What is the most common site of non-pulmonary pathology in CF?**

The GI tract, with striking changes seen in the exocrine pancreas. The islets of Langerhans are spared.

O   **What are the reproductive abnormalities in CF?**

In males: The vas deferens, tail and body of the epididymis and the seminal vesicles are either absent or rudimentary.
In females: Uterine cervical glands are distended with mucous and the cervical canal is plugged with tenacious mucoid secretions. Endocervicitis also seen.

O   **What are the most frequent respiratory pathogens in patients with CF?**

Staphylococcus aureus and Pseudomonas aeruginosa.

O   **What are the immunological defects in CF?**

CF patients have low levels of serum IgG in the first decade of life, which increase dramatically once chronic infection is established. T-lymphocyte numbers are adequate. With advancing severity of pulmonary disease, lymphocytes of CF patients proliferate less briskly in response to P. aeruginosa and other gram-negative organisms. Deficient opsonic activity of alveolar macrophages is seen in patients with established P. aeruginosa infection.

O   **T/F: Patients with CF have a higher incidence of atopy and asthma when compared to the general population.**

False. The presence of atopy or asthma does not affect the severity, natural course or prognosis compared to non-atopic or non-asthmatic patients with CF.

O   **What is the earliest manifestation of CF lung disease?**

Cough, later associated with greenish, tenacious, purulent sputum, reflecting Pseudomonas aeruginosa infection.

O   **What are the respiratory symptoms of CF?**

Cough with greenish sputum and wheezing.

O   **What are the earliest organisms to be detected in airway of patients with CF?**

S. aureus and H. influenza. P. aeruginosa is typically cultured from respiratory secretions months to years later.

O   **What is the most common organism to be detected from the airways of patients with advanced CF?**

Pseudomonas aeruginosa.

O   **T/F: The recovery of P. aeruginosa, particularly the mucoid form, from the lower respiratory tract of a child or young adult with chronic lung symptoms is virtually diagnostic of CF.**

True.

○   **What other organisms have been found to colonize the respiratory tract of patients with CF?**

Pseudomonas cepacia, Escherichia coli, Xanthomonas maltophilia, klebsiella, proteus and anaerobes.

○   **What is the earliest radiographic change seen in CF?**

Hyperinflation of the lung, reflecting obstruction of small airways.

○   **What are the initial lung function abnormalities in CF?**

1.   Small airway obstruction as evidenced by decreased maximum mid expiratory flow.
2.   Reduced flow at low lung volumes.
3.   Elevation of RV/TLC ratio.
4.   Decreased diffusion capacity.

○   **What are the various radiographic manifestations of CF?**

1.   Hyperinflation.
2.   Peribronchial cuffing.
3.   Mucous impaction in airways seen as branching finger like shadows.
4.   Bronchiectasis.
5.   Subpleural blebs, most prominent along the mediastinal border.
6.   Prominent pulmonary artery segments with advanced disease.

○   **What tests are most often used to follow the course of pulmonary function in patients with CF?**

Spirometry, lung volume measurements and measurements of oxygenation.

○   **What are the features of pneumothorax in CF?**

1.   More common than atelectasis.
2.   Incidence increases with age.
3.   Incidence equal in both sexes.
4.   More frequent on the right side.

○   **Hemoptysis in CF correlates best with what radiographic manifestation?**

Bronchiectasis.

○   **What is the clinical significance of hemoptysis?**

The occurrence of both small and large volume hemoptysis correlates strongly with exacerbation of lung infection.

○   **What is the immediate mortality with massive hemoptysis?**

~ 10%.

○   **Does the severity of digital clubbing correlate with that of the lung disease present in CF?**

Yes.

○   **What is the relation of hypertrophic pulmonary osteoarthropathy (HPO) with that of the pulmonary disease?**

Symptoms of HPO frequently correlate with exacerbation of pulmonary disease activity.

○   **What is the most common cause of rectal prolapse in children in the U.S.?**

CF.

○   **What is the incidence of exocrine pancreatic insufficiency in CF?**

90 to 95%.

○   **What is the incidence of symptomatic biliary cirrhosis in patients with CF?**

2 to 5%.

○   **What is the most characteristic pattern of hepatobiliary disease in CF?**

Focal biliary cirrhosis.

○   **What are the diagnostic criteria for CF?**

Primary:
Characteristic pulmonary manifestations and/or,
Characteristic gastrointestinal manifestations and/or,
A family history of CF
PLUS
Sweat Cl concentration > 60 mEq/L [repeat measurement if sweat Cl is 50 - 60 mEq/L].

Secondary Criteria:
Documentation of dual CFTR mutations and evidence of one or more characteristic manifestations.

○   **What conditions are associated with an elevated sweat chloride?**

CF, hypothyroidism, pseudohypoaldosteronism, hypoparathyroidism, nephrogenic diabetes insipidus, type I glycogen storage disease, mucopolysaccharidosis, malnutrition, hypogammaglobulinemia and pancreatitis.

○   **What is the test recognized by the CF foundation to be the definitive diagnostic test for CF?**

Collection of sweat (at least 50 mg in a 45 minute period) by pilocarpine iontophoresis, coupled with chemical determination of the chloride concentration (> 60 mEq/L in children, >80 mEq/L in adults).

○   **What is the sensitivity and specificity of pilocarpine iontophoresis sweat test in detecting CF?**

Sensitivity = close to 100%
Specificity > 90%

○   **What are the advantages of chest physical therapy in CF?**

Clears secretions and improves flow rates and lung function.

○   **What is the effect of nutritional supplementation on CF?**

Patients with adequate nutrition experience a slower rate of decline of lung function.

○   **What is the 2-year survival after a double lung transplant?**

> 50%.

○   **How do you manage pulmonary complications of CF?**

PULMONARY COMPLICATION	MANAGEMENT
Right heart failure	Improve oxygenation through intensive pulmonary therapy.
Respiratory failure	Vigorous medical therapy of the underlying lung disease and infection.
Atelectasis	Frequent chest physiotherapy.
Pneumothorax	Conservative if < 10% and patient asymptomatic. Pleurodesis to avoid recurrence.
Small volume hemoptysis	Aggressive treatment of lung infection.
Persistent massive hemoptysis	Bronchial artery embolization along with aggressive treatment of the lung infection.

O   **What is the life expectancy in CF?**

50% patients survive to 28 - 30 years of age.

O   **What factors improve survival in CF?**

Better survival in patients living in northern climates.
Males.
African-American athnicity.
Patients followed at established care centers.
Patients with better pancreatic function.

O   **What are the 2 most important clinical manifestations of cystic fibrosis?**

1.   Respiratory: abnormal Cl transport --> thick airway mucus production -->airway obstruction and secondary infection --> bronchiectasis, pulmonary fibrosis --> respiratory failure and death.
2.   Gastrointestinal: abnormal Cl transport --> pancreatic insufficiency and abnormal viscid mucus secretions --> malabsorption, failure to thrive, meconium ileus (in neonates), meconium ileus equivalent (in older children).

O   **What are the main treatments for cystic fibrosis?**

1.   Respiratory: bronchodilators, antibiotics (inhaled, oral or IV), inhaled DNase and chest physiotherapy.
2.   Gastrointestinal: Pancreatic enzymes and vitamin (ADEK) supplementation, high calorie - high protein diet and H_2 receptor antagonists.

O   **What is the predominant type of gene mutation in CF?**

3 base pair deletion at position 508 (F508 mutation) of chromosome 7, which causes a loss of a single amino acid (phenylalanine) at position 508 on the CF gene.

O   **Does screening for the F508 mutation identify all cases of CF?**

No. F508 identifies < 75% of CF cases.

O   **What is the earliest macroscopic pathologic lesion in CF?**

Mucus obstruction of the bronchioles.

O   **Is the disease in the conducting airways acquired antenatally or postnatally?**

Postnatally. The airways of children with CF who have died within the first days of life display no obvious abnormality.

O   What pathologic changes can occur with progression of disease?

1. Submucosal gland hypertrophy.
2. Goblet cell hyperplasia.
3. Complete obstruction of small airways by secretions.
4. Bronchiolectasis.
5. Bronchiectasis (with upper lobe predominance).
6. Pneumonia.
7. Inflammatory edema of the nasal mucosa with pedunculation and polyp formation.

O   What is the chemical structure of the CFTR protein?

CFTR is a N-glycosylated single peptide chain with 1480 amino acids having a molecular weight of about 170 KD.

O   What are the functions of CFTR?

Serves as an anion channel and transports ATP molecules.

O   What is the diagnostic biophysical hallmark of CF in airway epithelia?

Raised transepithelial electric potential difference (PD).

O   What is transepithelial potential difference?

The product of the active ion transport rate and the ionic resistance of the epithelium (RT).

O   What is the dominant resting electric abnormality of the superficial epithelium in CF airways?

Studies with Amiloride, a Na^+ channel blocker, indicate that the elevated Na^+ absorption rate rather than the defective Cl conductance is the predominant resting electric abnormality.

O   What are the abnormalities of the superficial epithelial chloride transport in CF?

1. CF airway epithelial cells exhibit a conductive chloride permeability of the apical membranes.
2. CF airway and other affected epithelia, unlike normal airway epithelia, do not respond with chloride secretion to agents that raise cellular cAMP, e.g., alpha-adrenergic agonists.
3. CF airway epithelia unlike normal airway epithelia, do not respond with chloride secretion to activation of protein kinase C (PKC).
4. CF airway epithelial cells retain the capacity to secrete chloride in response to elevations in intracellular calcium.

O   What is the prognosis of CF, based on lung function?

Less than 50% of patients with an FEV1 less than 30% predicted, arterial pCO2 greater than 50 mmHg or arterial pO2 less than 55 mmHg live for 2 years.

O   What are the upper respiratory tract manifestations of CF?

1. Chronic rhinitis.
2. Increased volume of upper airway secretions.
3. Moderate airflow obstruction.
4. Nasal polyps in 15 to 20% patients.

❍ **What is the incidence of atelectasis in CF?**

Lobar and segmental atelectasis is uncommon, occurring in approximately 5% of patients, most prevalent in the first 5 years of life.

❍ **What is the most common site of atelectasis in CF?**

The right lung.

❍ **What is the incidence of massive hemoptysis in CF?**

~ 5%.

❍ **What is the incidence of meconium ileus in newborns with CF?**

5 to 15%. It is virtually diagnostic of CF if present in the newborn.

❍ **What is the incidence of a normal sweat chloride in patients with compatible clinical features of CF?**

1 to 2%

❍ **How do you diagnose such patients?**

Bioelectric potential differences across respiratory epithelia are elevated in patients with CF.
CF sweat glands do not produce sweat in response to alpha-adrenergic agonists.
DNA analysis techniques for detection of the CF gene.

❍ **What method can be used for newborn screening of CF?**

Assay of immunoreactive trypsin in dried blood spots collected on filter paper in the first several days of life.

❍ **What is the physiologic basis of postural drainage with chest percussion?**

This approach for clearance of mucus is based on the fact that cough clears the mucus from large airways and chest vibrations facilitate movement of secretions from the smaller airways to the larger airways.

❍ **What are the principles of antibiotic therapy in CF?**

1. Initiation of antibiotic guided by symptoms.
2. Choice of antibiotic guided by identification of pathogens in the lower respiratory tract.
3. Early, aggressive use of appropriate antibiotics may improve outcome.
4. Dosages of antibiotics should be higher and continued for a longer duration.

❍ **Are corticosteroids routinely indicated in CF?**

No. They may be used for specific indications such as allergic bronchopulmonary aspergillosis (ABPA).

❍ **Is exercise beneficial for patients with CF?**

Exercise is beneficial and should be encouraged for all but those with severe lung disease.

❍ **What are the physiologic effects of exercise?**

1. Increases exercise tolerance.
2. Improves cardiorespiratory fitness.
3. Improves respiratory muscle endurance.

4. Promotes deep breathing and effective coughing.
5. Does not improve pulmonary function.

○   What are the indications for hospitalization in CF?

1. Increased cough or wheezing.
2. Respiratory distress.
3. Decreased exercise tolerance.
4. Weight loss.
5. Deterioration in lung function.
6. Worsening hypoxemia.
7. Pulmonary complications of CF, e.g., atelectasis, pneumothorax, hemoptysis.

○   What is the most common surgical procedure performed in patients with CF?

Nasal polypectomy.

○   What is the most commonly performed transplant procedure to treat CF?

Double lung transplant.

○   What is the most common presentation of newborns with cystic fibrosis?

GI obstruction due to meconium ileus.

AIRWAY CONDITIONS OTHER THAN ASTHMA, BRONCHIECTASIS, COPD AND CYSTIC FIBROSIS

"How art thou out of breath, when thou hast breath
To say to me that thou are out of breath?"
Romeo and Juliet, Shakespeare

○   **What are the most common etiologies of a chronic cough not due to cigarette smoking?**

Postnasal drip (40%), asthma (25%) and gastroesophageal reflux (20%). Other etiologies include bronchitis, bronchiectasis, bronchogenic carcinoma, esophageal diverticuli, sarcoidosis, viruses and drugs.

○   Stridor is observed in what phase of respiration?

Inspiratory.

○   **What is the etiology of stridor?**

With extrathoracic airway obstruction, the pressure inside the extrathoracic part of the airway is much more negative relative to atmospheric pressure. This results in further narrowing of the airway during inspiration and therefore, stridor.

○   **Grunting is observed during what phase of respiration?**

Expiratory. It is an exhalation against a closed glottis.

○   **What is the etiology of retropharyngeal abscesses?**

Lymphatic spread of infections from the nasopharynx, oropharynx or external auditory canal.

○   **What is the preliminary test most helpful in establishing the presence of a vascular ring?**

Contrast esophagram.

○   **What is the time constant?**

The product of compliance and resistance.

○   **A 22-year-old with cerebral palsy and in a vegetative state was intubated for 10 days because of aspiration pneumonia. She was weaned from mechanical ventilation, extubated and one hour later, developed stridor and severe retractions. She is appropriately suctioned and given three aerosol treatments of racemic epinephrine. She has a pH of 7.20, PCO_2 of 80, and PO_2 of 80 on 100% oxygen. What should be done next?**

Intubation.

○   **A 17 year-old male complains of dysphagia and fever. Tonsillar exudates and anterior cervical adenitis are noted. What sign differentiates Group A Strep from other causes of pharyngitis?**

A sandpaper-like rash.

○   **A 24 year-old female presents with a high fever, sore throat, hoarseness and increased stridor of 3 hours duration. Examination reveals an ill appearing woman with a temperature of 40° C, inspiratory stridor, drooling and mild intercostal retractions. She prefers to sit up. What is the most likely diagnosis?**

Epiglottitis or supraglottitis.

○   **What is the predominant auscultatory finding in a patient with a foreign body lodged in the right mainstem bronchus?**

Expiratory wheezing.

○   **When a radiolucent foreign body is lodged in the right mainstem bronchus with resultant incomplete obstruction, inspiratory and expiratory films show air-trapping and increased lucency of the lung on the involved side. What is the cause of this phenomenon?**

Ball-valve air trapping. Air enters around the foreign body during inspiration and is trapped as the airway closes around the foreign body during expiration, preventing emptying of that side.

○   **What are the flow-volume characteristics of obstruction of the upper airways?**

Variable extrathoracic: decreased flow during inspiration, as with vocal cord paralysis.
Variable intrathoracic: decreased flow during expiration, as with tracheomalacia.
Fixed intra- or extrathoracic: decreased flow during both inspiration and expiration, as with scar tissue.

○   **What causes hereditary angioedema?**

Deficiency in the production or function of C1 esterase inhibitor.

○   **What screening test can obtained if hereditary angioedema is suspected?**

C4 complement level. It is low during and between attacks.

○   **What is type 1 and type 2 hereditary angioedema?**

Type 1 patients have low serum C1 esterase inhibitor levels. Type 2 patients have abnormal C1 esterase inhibitor function.

○   **What is the treatment for hereditary angioedema?**

C1 esterase inhibitor. Epinephrine, antihistamines and steroids are often used, although they have not been proven effective.

○   **What is functional asthma?**

A conversion disorder in which patients present with dyspnea and voluntary adduction of the vocal cords during expiration. Patients often have a psychiatric history. Fiberoptic laryngoscopy demonstrates paradoxical adduction of the vocal cords during inspiration.

○   **What is the treatment for angioneurotic edema due to ACE inhibitors?**

Epinephrine, antihistamines and corticosteroids.

❍ **How does inhalation of noxious fumes result in injury to the trachea?**

The initial insult results in severe tracheobronchitis that when severe enough can result in sloughing of the mucosa, granulation tissue formation and ultimately, scar and stenosis.

❍ **What is a double aortic arch?**

It is caused by persistence of the right and left fourth aortic arches. These remnants form a true vascular ring surrounding the trachea and esophagus. Stridor, dysphagia and aspiration are common symptoms.

❍ **What is tracheobronchomegaly (Mounier-Kuhn syndrome)?**

A disease with enlarged central airways resulting in pooling of secretions in redundant tissue. Complications include bronchiectasis, fibrosis and recurrent infections.

❍ **What are the characteristics of relapsing polychondritis?**

Episodic inflammation of the cartilaginous tissue throughout the body, including the laryngotracheobronchial tree. Inflammation of the airway cartilage may result in stenotic lesions.

❍ **What tumors cause endobronchial metastases?**

Renal cell, colonic, rectal, cervical and breast carcinoma, malignant melanoma and bronchogenic carcinoma.

❍ **What organisms cause mediastinal fibrosis and, possibly, airway obstruction?**

Histoplasmosis and tuberculosis.

❍ **Where do foreign bodies most frequently lodge?**

In the right mainstem bronchus.

❍ **What is broncholithiasis?**

The presence of a calcified tissue fragment in the airways. Any process that causes calcification of lung parenchyma or lymph nodes may lead to this. It is usually due to granulomatous infections such as histoplasmosis or tuberculosis.

❍ **What is bronchomalacia?**

The softening of the bronchial walls that may result in collapse of the bronchi during forced expiration.

❍ **What fungi cause tracheobronchitis?**

Aspirgillus, mucormycosis, cryptosporidiosis, blastomycosis and actinomycosis.

❍ **What is the most common type of congenital tracheoesophageal fistula?**

A blind ending esophagus with a more proximal connection to the trachea. The H-type of fistula is far less common.

❍ **What are the most common causes of acquired tracheoesophageal fistulas?**

Malignancy (bronchogenic or esophageal), instrument perforation, histoplasmosis and broncholithiasis.

○   **What is amyloidosis?**

The extracellular deposition of amyloid, a substance that has green birefringence when viewed with a polarized light after staining with Congo red. Lesions in the airway include polyp-type, submucosal masses and diffuse tracheobronchial involvement. Profuse bleeding after biopsy has been reported.

○   **What are the characteristics of bronchiolitis obliterans (obliterative bronchiolitis)?**

Stenosis of the bronchiolar lumen that results from chronic inflammation, scarring and smooth muscle hypertrophy.

○   **What are the most common causes of bronchiolitis obliterans?**

Toxic fume inhalation, viral, mycoplasma and legionella infection, bone marrow transplantation, lung transplantation (form of chronic rejection), rheumatoid arthritis, penicillamine, lupus, dermatomyositis and polymyositis.

○   **How does bronchiolitis obliterans (BO) differ from bronchiolitis obliterans with organizing pneumonia (BOOP)?**

BO is characterized by an obstructive ventilatory defect, while BOOP causes a restrictive ventilatory defect. In BOOP, the exudate and granulation tissue extend into the alveoli, whereas they do not in BO. The CXR is often patchy in BOOP whereas it can show miliary, diffuse nodular or reticulonodular infiltrates or be normal in BO. BOOP is generally more responsive to corticosteroids than BO.

○   **What is the source of airway mucus?**

Respiratory mucus is a mixture of submucous gland, goblet cell and epithelial cell secretions. Submucous glands are innervated by cholinergic, adrenergic and noncholinergic, nonadrenergic nerves.

○   **What is the purpose of airway mucus?**

Mucus is the first defense mechanism of the airway. It captures inhaled foreign particle so that these can be cleared, inhibits invading particles and organisms from reaching the airway epithelium and prevents dehydration of the airway surface

○   **What are the layers of the airway surface fluid?**

In the large airways, this is believed to consist of a gel layer on a low-viscosity, periciliary fluid layer that is approximately as deep as the standing height of a cilium.

○   **What is the daily volume of mucus produced in the airway?**

Between 10 and 100 ml/day.

○   **What is the normal ciliary beat frequency?**

Between 8 and 15 Hz.

○   **What effect do beta agonists have on ciliary beat frequency?**

Increased.

○   **What is a mucolytic agent?**

A medication that reduces the viscosity of secretions by disrupting the polymer networks of mucin or of DNA/F-actin.

❍   **What is the mechanism of action of the classic mucolytics?**

They sever disulfide bonds within the mucin polymer network. These agents generally contain thiol residues.

❍   **What is the major side effect associated with the inhalation of N-acetylcysteine?**

Cough and bronchospasm, most likely due to irritation by the low pH (2.2) of the aerosol solution.

❍   **What is the mechanism of action of peptide mucolytics?**

They disrupt the pathologic network of neutrophil-derived F-actin or DNA filaments. Dornase alfa (Pulmozyme) is the only peptide mucolytic approved for use in the United States.

❍   **What is the function of mucokinetic agents?**

Mucokinetics increase cough clearability either by increasing airflow or by decreasing mucus tenacity.

❍   **What are expectorants?**

These are agents thought to increase the hydration of secretions. There have been no studies that demonstrate a consistent clinical benefit when expectorants are used for the therapy of either acute or chronic lung disease.

❍   **What are mucoregulatory agents?**

Medications that reduce the volume of mucus secretion. This group of medications includes the anticholinergic agents, antiinflammatory agents (steroids and indomethacin) and macrolide antibiotics.

❍   **What is the primary use of chest percussion and postural drainage?**

Secretion clearance in patients with cystic fibrosis. Clearly beneficial effects have not been shown for other COPD.

❍   **What are the contraindications to the use of chest physical therapy?**

Gastroesophageal reflux can be exacerbated by postural drainage or by chest percussion.

❍   **What alternatives are there to chest percussion and postural drainage?**

Devices such as external high frequency oscillators (ThAIRpy vest) or positive expiratory pressure (PEP) breathing have been demonstrated to be an effective replacement for standard chest physical therapy in some patients with cystic fibrosis. There are no controlled trials that have demonstrated short or long term clinical benefits with other devices such as oral high frequency oscillators or flutter breathing.

❍   **What is the recommended use of dornase alfa (Pulmozyme)?**

Once daily inhalation in patients with moderately severe cystic fibrosis.

❍   **What are the principal side effects of dornase alfa?**

Hoarseness and occasionally a fall in pulmonary function.

❍   **How is cystic fibrosis sputum abnormal?**

It is hyperadhesive.

○   **What is diffuse panbronchiolitis?**

A chronic hypersecretory, inflammatory and infectious disease seen in Japan and Korea

○   **What is the effect of macrolide antibiotics (erythromycin, clarithromycin) on mucus hypersecretion?**

Some macrolide antibiotics have the ability to down regulate mucus secretion by an unknown mechanism, thought to be do to anti-inflammatory activity.

○   **How is bronchorrhea defined?**

The production of large volumes of watery secretions. This is usually the result of inflammation and has best been described in some patients with asthma.

○   **T/F: Patients with infantile fucosidosis who do not have cellular alpha-L-fucosidase activity produce extremely watery mucus that cannot be cleared by cough or ciliary mechanisms.**

True.

○   **What is plastic bronchitis or fibrinous bronchitis?**

The complete obstruction of the airway by a large mucus cast associated with atopy, asthma and allergic bronchopulmonary aspergillosis.

○   **What are the mucin genes?**

This is a group of genes that control mucin synthesis in the airway, gastrointestinal tract and elsewhere in the body. There are at least nine human mucin genes described thus far. All but two of these have been demonstrated in the human airway and MUC5AC appears to predominate.

○   **A patient presents with well-demarcated swelling of the lips and tongue. She was started on an antihypertensive agent three weeks ago. What is the most likely agent?**

Angiotensin-converting enzyme (ACE) inhibitor. Although angioneurotic edema may occur anytime during therapy, it is most likely to occur within the first month of using an ACE inhibitor.

○   **A foreign body is suspected in the lower airways. What will plain films show?**

Air trapping of the affected side. Inspiration and expiration views demonstrate mediastinal shift away from the affected side.

○   **Grunting is usually more prominent in what type of respiratory pathology?**

Typically in small airway disease such as bronchiolitis, or in diseases with loss of functional residual capacity, such as pneumonia or pulmonary edema, because grunting is an effort to maintain positive airway pressure during expiration.

COLLAGEN VASCULAR DISEASES

"That rheumatic diseases do abound"
A Midsummer Night's Dream, Shakespeare

○ **What drugs can induce a lupus reaction?**

Procainamide, hydralazine, isoniazid and phenytoin.

○ **Patients with the presence of antiphospholipid antibodies in either primary or secondary antiphopholipid syndromes are at increased risk for what diseases?**

1. Risk of thrombotic events
2. Thrombocytopenia
3. Hemolytic anemia
4. Stroke
5. Chorea
6. Transverse myelitis
7. Vascular heart disease

○ **What rheumatologic ailments produce pulmonary hemorrhage?**

Goodpasture's disease, systemic lupus erythematosus, Wegener's granulomatosis and non-specific vasculitides.

○ **What rheumatologic ailments more commonly produce pulmonary fibrosis?**

Ankylosing spondylitis, scleroderma and rheumatoid arthritis.

○ **What rheumatologic ailments more commonly produce respiratory muscle failure?**

Dermatomyositis and polymyositis.

○ **What are the pulmonary manifestations of SLE?**

Acute pneumonitis, diffuse alveolar hemorrhage, pleuritis, interstitial lung disease, pulmonary hypertension, bronchiolitis and weakness of the diaphragm.

○ **What is the underlying histopathology of acute lupus pneumonitis?**

Diffuse alveolar damage, BOOP, cellular interstitial pneumonitis, or a combination of these.

○ **What is the treatment for acute pneumonitis or diffuse alveolar hemorrhage?**

There are no controlled trials. Steroids, azathioprine, cyclophosphamide and plasmapheresis have all been used.

○ **Can one see histopathological changes of both acute pneumonitis and diffuse alveolar hemorrhage (with or without capillaritis) in the same biopsy specimen?**

Yes.

○ **What is the most common pulmonary manifestation of lupus?**

Pleurisy and pleural effusion.

○   **Describe the effusions seen in lupus.**

Exudative, pleural fluid positive for dsDNA and pleural fluid ANA titer greater than 1:160.

○   **What are the histopathological findings of interstitial lung disease in lupus?**

Usual interstitial pneumonitis, lymphocytic interstitial pneumonitis and BOOP.

○   **What is the shrinking lung syndrome in lupus?**

Weakness of the diaphragm that results in reduction of static lung volumes but with a normal DLCO when volumes are taken into account.

○   **What are the pulmonary manifestations of RA?**

Pleurisy, pleural effusions, pulmonary hypertension, rheumatoid nodule, obliterative bronchiolits, interstitial lung disease, BOOP and lymphocytic interstitial pneumonia.

○   **Characterize the pleural fluid seen in RA.**

Exudative, low pH (less than 7.2), low glucose, (often under 50), low complement levels, cytology of necrotic debris, spindle shaped macrophages, multinucleated histiocytes and the presence of rheumatoid factor (RF) in the fluid.

○   **Can a necrobiotic nodule rupture causing a pneumothorax?**

Yes.

○   **Characterize the x-ray findings of a necrobiotic nodule.**

Single or multiple, usually in the upper and mid lung zones, size variable up to 7 cm and spontaneous resolution and recurrence may occur.

○   **What is Caplan's syndrome?**

Sudden appearance of necrobiotic nodules mostly in the upper lung zones in patients who are coal miners and have RA.

○   **Arthritis of what joint may impose difficulty in dealing with airways?**

The cricoarytenoid and atlanto-axial joints.

○   **Describe obliterative bronchiolitis seen in RA.**

Insidious onset, obstructive ventilatory defect, normal or hyperinflated CXR and a minority on patients respond to steroids and cyclophosphamide.

○   **Can the interstitial lung disease of RA present before the articular manifestations occur?**

Yes.

❍ **What are the histopathological findings of interstitial lung disease in RA?**
Mostly usual interstitial pneumonitis with some degrees of cellular interstitial pneumonitis.

❍ **Which drugs, used to treat RA, may cause interstitial lung disease?**

Gold, penicillamine and methotrexate.

❍ **What are the pulmonary manifestations of scleroderma?**

Pleural disease, interstitial lung diseases, pulmonary hypertension and aspiration pneumonitis.

❍ **Is the usual interstitial pneumonitis of scleroderma more likely to occur in the CREST syndrome or the diffuse cutaneous form?**

The diffuse cutaneous form.

❍ **The presence of what autoantibody increases the risk for developing pulmonary fibrosis in a patient with scleroderma?**

Anti-Scl-70.

❍ **What high resolution CT findings are suggestive of responsiveness to steroids in a patient with interstitial lung disease?**

Ground glass attenuation. Honeycomb-type fibrosis is suggestive of nonresponsiveness.

❍ **Which scleroderma syndrome is more associated with pulmonary hypertension?**

CREST.

❍ **Why is aspiration a concern in scleroderma?**

The associated esophageal disorder of decreased peristalsis and dilatation, more commonly seen in the CREST variant, predisposes patients to aspiration.

❍ **What are the pulmonary manifestations of the polymyositis-dermatomyositis syndrome?**

Aspiration pneumonia, diaphragmatic weakness and interstitial lung disease.

❍ **What is the mechanism for aspiration seen in polymyositis-dermatomyositis?**

Inflammatory myositis involving the striated muscle of the hypopharynx and upper esophagus.

❍ **What types of interstitial lung disease can be seen in the polymyositis-dermatomyositis syndrome?**

Usual interstitial pneumonitis, diffuse alveolar damage, BOOP and diffuse alveolar hemorrhage due to capillaritis.

❍ **Can the interstitial lung disease manifest before other manifestations of the polymyositis-dermatomyositis syndrome?**

Yes.

❍ **What autoantibody is associated with the interstitial lung disease of polymyositis-dermatomyositis?**

Anti-Jo-1.

○ **What are the pulmonary manifestations of mixed connective tissue disease (MCTD)?**

Pleural effusion, pleurisy, pulmonary hypertension, aspiration pneumonitis, diaphragmatic weakness, interstitial lung disease.

○ **What autoantibody is associated with MCTD?**

Anti-ribonucleoprotein.

○ **What are the pulmonary manifestations of Sjogren's syndrome?**

Xerostomia, dried airway secretions resulting in atelectasis, lymphocytic interstitial pneumonitis and pseudolymphoma.

○ **What autoantibodies are associated with Sjogren's syndrome?**

RF, ANA (speckled pattern), anti-SSA and anti-SSB.

○ **Describe lymphocytic interstitial pneumonitis.**

Lymphocytes infiltrate the interstitium and alveolar air spaces. The disease responds to steroids and occasionally immunosuppressive therapy and cyclosporine have been used. The development of pleural effusions and hilar or mediastinal adenopathy may indicate the presence of lymphoma.

○ **What is a pseudolymphoma?**

It is not a malignant lymphoma. It is thought to be a type of localized lymphocytic interstitial pneumonitis.

PULMONARY CRITICAL CARE

"For he was great of heart"
Othello, Shakespeare

O   **Weaning from mechanical ventilation is associated with what effect on myocardial oxygen demand?**

Increased MVO_2. Consider weaning to be a cardiac stress test.

O   **In patients with congestive heart failure, cardiovascular insufficiency and respiratory distress, the initiation of positive pressure ventilation is often associated with what hemodynamic response?**

Improvement in overall cardiovascular status due to the combined effects of the associated reduced work of breathing and reduced LV afterload.

O   **In patients with unilateral lung injury, is the effect of positive end-expiratory pressure applied at the trachea the same as in patients with bilateral lung injury?**

No. PEEP may overdistend the healthy lung in subjects with unilateral lung injury causing an increased intrapulmonary shunt and increased pulmonary vascular resistance.

O   **An intubated patient with ischemic heart disease develops mild inspiratory stridor upon extubation associated with severe chest pain and marked ST segment elevations across the precordium.   The immediate treatment of this condition should include what ventilatory therapy?**

Eliminate the markedly negative swings in intrathoracic pressure by re-intubation.

O   **In a patient with impaired right ventricular dysfunction following anterior chest trauma, excessive positive end-expiratory pressure (PEEP) therapy may induce cardiovascular collapse by any of three mechanisms, name one.**

1.   Hyperinflation will increase pulmonary vascular resistance impeding right ventricular ejection.
2.   Hyperinflation will increase intrathoracic pressure reducing venous return and limiting right ventricular filling.
3.   Hyperinflation that compresses the heart is similar to tamponade restricting right ventricular filling.

O   **In a patient with acute lung injury breathing spontaneously, intubation and the application of both an enriched FIO2 and PEEP sufficient to recruit collapse alveolar units should do what to pulmonary vascular resistance?**

Decrease it by reversing hypoxic pulmonary vasoconstriction.

O   **A mechanically ventilated patient with chronic obstructive lung disease is breathing spontaneously on assist-control mode with a measured intrinsic PEEP of 12 cm H_2O. What will the application of 8 cm H_2O extrinsic PEEP (from the ventilatory circuit) do to the patient's work of breathing?**

Decrease it by reducing the amount of airway pressure drop needed to trigger the positive-pressure breath.

O   **A patient returns to the emergency department with fever, nausea, vomiting and hypotension two days after having nasal packing placed for an anterior nosebleed. What potential complication of nasal packing should be considered?**

Toxic shock syndrome.

○ **What are the primary goals of nutritional support in critically ill patients?**

To provide usable substrates to meet energy needs, conserve lean body mass and restore physiologic homeostasis.

○ **What proportion of critically ill and injured patients are catabolic or hypermetabolic?**

Nearly all.

○ **Are immunocompetence and vital organ function dependent upon nutritional support?**

Yes. Both are secondary goals of nutritional support.

○ **What is the predominant energy source used during starvation by a healthy subject?**

Lipids.

○ **How long does the body's reserve of carbohydrates last during starvation?**

Glycogen stores are consumed within 24 hours.

○ **Does the metabolic rate increase or decrease during starvation in a healthy subject?**

Decrease.

○ **Are adaptation mechanisms seen with starvation similar to those seen in critically ill patients?**

No. There is impaired protein conservation and a persistent hypermetabolic response in the critically ill patient.

○ **With the onset of critical illness, what factors are thought to raise resting energy expenditure and protein turnover?**

Catecholamines and cortisol.

○ **How does the insulin resistance associated with critical illness affect substrate use?**

Insulin resistance decreases the peripheral use of glucose and increases proteolysis.

○ **Is there any rationale for overfeeding or underfeeding critically ill patients?**

No. Both have been shown to be detrimental. The goal is to <u>meet</u> the metabolic needs of the patient.

○ What is the utility of anthropometric (e.g., weight change), biochemical (e.g., serum albumin level), or immunologic (e.g., absolute lymphocyte count) indices as measures of nutritional status in the critical care setting?

Low. Too many other factors such as fluid retention, changes in protein synthesis priorities and underlying infections make these indices less reliable than in otherwise healthy patients.

○ **What are the serum half-lives of albumin and prealbumin?**

18 days and 2 to 3 days, respectfully.

O   **What two methods are frequently used to assess nutritional status in critically ill patients?**

Indirect calorimetry and nitrogen balance.

O   **As a patient's FIO2 requirements increase, is indirect calorimetry more or less accurate in measuring energy expenditure?**

Less.

O   **What other factors are sources of errors with indirect calorimetry?**

Air leaks from endotracheal tubes and the need for extrapolation of measurements to 24 hours.

O   **What is the equation for nitrogen balance?**

Nitrogen Balance = Nitrogen intake - Nitrogen loss = (Protein (g) / 6.25) - ((Urine Urea Nitrogen / 0.8) + 3)

O   **How much protein is required for balance in a healthy stable adult?**

Approximately 0.6 g/kg ideal body weight/day.

O   **What is the goal of protein delivery?**

To achieve a positive nitrogen balance.

O   **What is the optimal calorie-to-nitrogen ratio for critically ill patients?**

100 : 1 to 200 : 1.

O   **What is the recommended starting point for non-protein calorie needs for hypermetabolic critically ill patients?**

25 kcal/kg ideal body weight/day.

O   **What is the most common manifestation of excessive carbohydrate administration?**

Hyperglycemia.

O   **Can lipid emulsions be useful in patients needing volume restriction or demonstrating carbohydrate intolerance?**

Yes. Lipids are calorie dense compared to dextrose solutions.

O   **What minimum percentage of total calories should be supplied as lipid to prevent fatty acid deficiency?**

Five percent of total calories at minimum.

O   **How long does it take non-stressed patients receiving lipid-free total parenteral nutrition (TPN) to demonstrate evidence of essential fatty acid deficiency?**

Within four weeks. Hypermetabolic patients within ten days.

O   **Can lipids administered parenterally hurt cellular immunity?**

There is data to suggest lipids cause reticuloendothelial dysfunction and immune suppression.

O   **What clinical symptoms are seen with hypophosphatemia brought on by refeeding a malnourished patient?**

Weakness and congestive heart failure.

O   **Which form of protein, peptides or amino acids, is more uniformly and efficiently absorbed from the gut?**

Peptides.

O   **What is the main energy source of enterocytes?**

Glutamine.

O   **Besides an energy source, what role does glutamine play in the gut?**

It is thought to be important in maintaining intestinal structure and function.

O   **How much glutamine has been included in standard amino acid solutions used with total parenteral nutrition (TPN)?**

None, due to its instability in parenteral solutions.

O   **Is glutamine an essential amino acid?**

No. However, during times of metabolic stress, intracellular glutamine stores are markedly depleted, indicating supplementation may be beneficial.

O   **Arginine, a semi-essential amino acid, is considered to be vital to what body system?**

The immune system.

O   **Can branched-chain amino acids improve the outcome in critically ill patients?**

No. Some suggest it may be helpful in patients with hepatic encephalopathy.

O   **Have immunoenriched diets, containing substrates such as omega-3 fish oils, arginine and RNA nucleotides, been found to improve outcome?**

Yes, a number of recent studies suggest improvement using enteral immunoenriched formulas.

O   **What is the preferred route for the delivery of nutrition, enteral or parenteral?**

The enteral route, although there is still some debate.

O   **When should nutritional support be started?**

As soon as a hypermetabolic state (e.g., trauma or sepsis), underlying malnutrition, or an expected delay in resuming an oral diet of > 5-10 days is recognized.

O   **What complications are associated with enteral nutrition?**

Complications involve routes of access to the GI tract (e.g., feeding tube displacement or obstruction), the GI tract itself (e.g., nausea, vomiting, diarrhea), or the metabolic system (e.g., hyperglycemia, hypophosphatemia).

❍   **T/F: Bowel sounds are a good index of small bowel motility.**

False.

❍   **Has preoperative nutritional support for malnourished patients been shown to be reduce postoperative morbidity?**

Yes, for those with severe malnutrition.

❍   **In which patients is parenteral nutritional support indicated?**

When enteral access is unobtainable, enteral feeding contraindicated, or when level of enteral nutrition fails to meet requirements.

❍   **In which patients is intravenous nutritional support unlikely to be of benefit?**

Those expected to start oral intake in 5 to 7 days or with mild injuries.

❍   **Typically, what feeding route requires a greater length of time to reach full support?**

Enteral.

❍   **Can lipids be given through a peripheral vein?**

Yes. They are iso-osmotic, unlike the concentrated dextrose solutions that should be infused centrally.

❍   **Are omega-3 fatty acids (fish oil) or omega-6 fatty acids thought to be anti-inflammatory?**

Omega-3 fatty acids.

❍   **What are the complications of parenteral nutrition?**

Those associated with catheter insertion (e.g., pneumothorax), the indwelling line (e.g., line sepsis, thrombosis), lipid emulsions (e.g., pancreatitis, reticuloendothelial dysfunction) and GI tract complications (e.g., cholestasis, acalculous cholecystitis).

❍   **Can overfeeding result in difficulty weaning a patient from mechanical ventilation?**

Yes. This is related to increased energy expenditure, oxygen consumption and CO_2 production with a resultant increase in respiratory rate and minute ventilation.

❍   **Can underfeeding result in difficulty weaning a patient from mechanical ventilation?**

Yes. Malnutrition can cause respiratory muscle weakness and ventilator dependence.

❍   **T/F: It is not recommended to place patients simultaneously on enteral and parenteral feedings.**

False. On the contrary, a small amount of nutrition delivered enterally may be all that is required to gain the positive effects of this route while the parenteral route supplies the balance of caloric and protein needs.

❍   **What are the ventilation and perfusion relationships between Zone 1, Zone 2 and Zone 3 of the lung?**

Zone 1 represents dead space (ventilation occurs without perfusion); zone 2 contains high V/Q mismatch (ventilation occurs in excess of perfusion); zone 3 represents areas of optimal V/Q matching.

○   **What is the equation for determining a patient's oxygen extraction ratio?**

Oxygen extraction ratio = $(CaO2 - CvO2)/CaO2$ where CaO2 is arterial blood oxygen content and CvO2 is the mixed venous blood oxygen content.

○   **What is a normal oxygen extraction ratio in a healthy adult?**

25%.

○   **What is the normal whole lung V/Q ratio?**

4 liters of ventilation to 5 liters of blood flow or 0.8.

○   **Blood drawn from the tip of a pulmonary artery catheter wedged in zone III will reflect PO2 from what source?**

Pulmonary capillary.

○   **Which mitral valve abnormalities can lead to large v waves on the pulmonary artery wedge tracing?**

Both mitral stenosis and mitral regurgitation because of overfilling of the left atrium.

○   **How do increases in heart rate alter the systolic and diastolic components of the cardiac cycle?**

As heart rate increases and cardiac cycle time decreases, systolic time remains relatively constant while diastolic time decreases, thereby, increasing the ratio of systole/diastole.

○   **What information regarding flow is obtained from the Reynolds number?**

The Reynolds number is calculated from the equation Re=2rvd/n, where r=radius, v=average velocity, d=density and n=viscosity. When the Reynolds number exceeds 2000, turbulent flow is probable. Less than 2000 indicates probable laminar flow.

○   **What property of helium allows less turbulence in a high flow system?**

Density. The low density of helium yields a lower Reynolds number when compared with a gas of higher density (air or oxygen) in the same system.

○   **What is Boyle's law of gases?**

$P_1V_1=P_2V_2$ where P is pressure, V is volume and temperature is constant.

○   **What is the calculation for mean arterial pressure (MAP) based on systolic (SBP) and diastolic pressure (DBP)?**

MAP=DBP + 1/3(SBP-DBP).

○   **What is the hemodynamic response to an acute complete spinal cord injury at the C7 level?**

Initially there is hypertension and tachycardia secondary to increased circulating catecholamines at the time of the injury followed shortly by hypotension due to vasodilatation and bradycardia secondary to loss of cardiac accelerator input.

○   **During the first minute of apnea, how much would you expect PaCO₂ will rise?**

During apnea, the $PaCO_2$ will increase approximately 6 mmHg during the first minute and then 3-4 mmHg each minute thereafter.

○   **In the resting healthy adult what percentage of total body oxygen consumption is spent on the work of breathing?**

In the resting healthy adult, 2-3% of total oxygen consumption is spent on the work of breathing.

○   **What is the most important factor in control of ventilation under normal conditions?**

Under normal conditions, $PaCO_2$ of the arterial blood is the most important factor in control of ventilation.

○   **What do peripheral chemoreceptors located in the carotid and aortic bodies respond to?**

The peripheral chemoreceptors respond to decreases in arterial PO_2 and pH and increases in arterial PCO_2.

○   **What is functional residual capacity (FRC).**

The volume of gas in the lung after a normal expiration is the FRC and is comprised of residual volume and expiratory reserve volume.

○   **What are the two most important determinants of coronary perfusion pressure?**

The two most important determinants of coronary perfusion pressure are diastolic blood pressure and left ventricular end-diastolic pressure, their relationship being:

CPP = DBP - LVEDP.

○   **What are the determinants of stroke volume?**

Preload, contractility and afterload.

○   **How would you calculate systemic vascular resistance (SVR)?**

$$\frac{MAP - CVP}{CO} \times 80 \; [dyne \times sec/cm^5]$$

○   **How would you calculate pulmonary vascular resistance (PVR)?**

$$\frac{Mean\ PAP - PAOP}{CO} \times 80 \; [dyne \times sec/cm^5]$$

○   **What is the closing capacity of the lungs?**

Closing capacity (closing volume plus residual volume) is the lung volume at which small airways close. Closing capacity is normally well below FRC (functional residual capacity) but rises steadily with age.

○   **What are the four major forms of cellular hypoxia?**

Anemic hypoxia, hypoxemic hypoxia, circulatory hypoxia and histotoxic hypoxia.

○   **What are the major causes of arterial hypoxemia?**

Hypoventilation, ventilation/perfusion inequality, shunt, low FIO_2, and diffusion impairment.

○ **How does one assess oxygenation?**

Skin color, pulse oximetry and blood gas analysis.

○ **How does one assess ventilation?**

End tidal CO_2 monitoring and blood gas analysis.

○ **What is a tension pneumothorax?**

An injury to the lung allowing intrapleural air to collect without escaping via the chest wall or trachea. This accumulation of air compresses the lung and shifts the mediastinum, leading to impaired venous return and hypotension.

○ **What are the physical findings in tension pneumothorax?**

Distended neck veins, hypotension, tracheal deviation and hyperresonant hemithorax.

○ **What is the treatment for tension pneumothorax?**

Immediate needle decompression of the hyperresonant hemithorax, based on clinical suspicion. Radiography should not be used to confirm tension pneumothorax.

○ **What is adequate urinary output to gauge resuscitation in adults?**

0.5 cc/kg or about 50 cc/hr.

○ **How does one assess for disability in ATLS?**

A rapid assessment to establish level of consciousness (alert, arouses to voice, arouses to pain, or unresponsive) and pupillary appearance and reaction constitute the initial assessment. A more detailed examination is performed later.

○ **What is the most common type of intracranial bleeding?**

Subdural hematomas, in about a third of head injuries with positive CT findings.

○ **How does one determine need for transfer?**

Transfer of the patient is needed for definitive care and is dependent on the resources available at the initial treatment area, i.e. availability of surgical care, need for monitoring, need for other specialized care. Such determinations can be made with information obtained during the initial evaluation and resuscitation.

○ **Primary and spontaneous bacterial peritonitis is more frequently seen in patients with what underlying conditions?**

Nephrotic syndrome, chronic liver disease and systemic lupus erythematosus.

○ **What are the MRI findings suggestive of herpes simplex encephalitis?**

Edema or hemorrhage in the temporal lobes.

○ **If herpes simplex encephalitis is suspected, how can the diagnosis be confirmed?**

PCR of CSF, brain culture and biopsy. EEG, CT and MRI show lateralizing findings to temporal lobes.

O **What is the most common cause of fulminant hepatic failure in the U.S.?**

Acute viral hepatitis.

O **What characterizes liver dysfunction in fulminant hepatic failure?**

Uncorrectable coagulopathy, jaundice and encephalopathy. All three occur together in an illness of less than eight-week's duration.

O **What are the risks and complications of pericardiocentesis?**

Cardiac tamponade, myocardial infarction, intra-abdominal injuries and pneumothorax.

O **What are the indications for calcium therapy?**

Documented or suspected hypocalcemia, hyperkalemia, hypermagnesemia and calcium channel blocker overdose.

O **What are the arterial blood gas findings in a patient with salicylate overdose?**

Respiratory alkalosis and an increased anion gap metabolic acidosis.

O **Tumor lysis syndrome is characterized by what lab findings?**

Hyperuricemia, hyperkalemia and hyperphosphatemia.

O **What is the major goal of therapy for tumor lysis syndrome?**

Prevention of acute renal failure. The principles for treatment include alkalization of the urine, vigorous hydration and diuresis and prevention of the formation of toxic metabolites.

O **What are the blood gas findings in a patient with malignant hyperthermia?**

Metabolic and respiratory acidosis.

O **What is the treatment for malignant hyperthermia?**

A change in the anesthetic agent to remove possible triggers, administration of dantrolene and the procedure is terminated.

O **A twenty two year old sickle cell patient presents with pallor, weakness, tachycardia and abdominal fullness. What should you suspect first?**

Acute splenic sequestration.

O **What infectious agents are associated with necrotizing enterocolitis?**

Gram negative enteric bacilli, E. coli, klebsiella and enterococcus.

O **What conditions present with both intracranial calcifications and skin lesions?**

Toxoplasmosis, cytomegalovirus and Sturge-Weber Syndrome.

O **What effect does intrinsic PEEP have on the work of breathing in patients receiving mechanical ventilation?**

Increased elastic work and increased work to trigger assisted breaths.

○   **How can the work of breathing with mechanical ventilation associated with intrinsic PEEP be reduced?**

Add CPAP, reduce tidal volume, reduce inspiratory time and increase expiratory time.

○   **What complications are associated with mask ventilation?**

Skin breakdown, aspiration pneumonia, aerophagia, pneumothorax and barotrauma (volutrauma).

○   **Through what mechanism does PEEP decrease cardiac output?**

Reduced preload.

○   **Through what mechanism does positive pressure ventilation increase cardiac output?**

Decreased left ventricular afterload.

○   **Which lobes of the lung can develop atelectasis from intubation of the right mainstem bronchus?**

Right upper lobe, left upper lobe and left lower lobe.

○   **How can static compliance of the lung/chest wall be approximated from airway pressure measurements during mechanical ventilation?**

Tidal volume/(inspiratory plateau pressure - end expiratory (pause) pressure).

○   **What evidence of barotrauma can be observed on chest x-ray?**

Pneumomediastinum, pneumothorax, pneumopericardium, subcutaneous emphysema and pulmonary interstitial emphysema.

○   **What are the primary determinants of the work of breathing?**

Minute ventilation, lung/chest wall compliance and presence of intrinsic PEEP.

○   **What are the determinants of PaCO2?**

Carbon dioxide production and alveolar ventilation.

○   **What are some conditions under which CO2 production is increased?**

Lipogenesis, fever and hyperthyroidism.

○   **What is the preferred FIO2 for patients with ARDS?**

The lowest that will maintain a hemoglobin oxygen saturation of about 90%.

○   **How is oxygen delivery calculated?**

Cardiac output x arterial blood oxygen content.

○   **What is the primary determinant of the oxygen content of arterial blood?**

The product of hemoglobin concentration and the percent hemoglobin oxygen saturation of arterial blood. The amount of oxygen dissolved in the plasma (a function of the PaO2) is negligible at one atmosphere of pressure.

○ **How can adequate tidal volume be delivered to a patient undergoing volume cycled mechanical ventilation whose endotracheal tube cuff is failing to maintain an adequate seal (without changing the tube)?**

Increase the mandatory tidal volume.

○ **What is the maximal accepted endotracheal tube cuff pressure?**

Approximately 25 cm H2O at the end of expiration.

○ **What is the potential harm of excess endotracheal tube cuff pressure?**

Excess pressure can induce ischemia and necrosis of the underlying tissue resulting in tracheomalacia and tracheal stenosis.

○ **What are indications for stress ulcer prophylaxis in critically ill patients?**

Mechanical ventilation and coagulopathy.

○ **What combination of medications, often used in the treatment of status asthmaticus requiring mechanical ventilation, may result in prolonged weakness?**

Steroids and neuromuscular blocking agents.

○ **What is the principal mechanism of increased PaCO2 with increased FIO2?**

Worsening V/Q mismatch and the Haldane effect.

○ **How does malnutrition contribute to respiratory failure?**

Increase in the oxygen cost of breathing and respiratory muscle weakness.

○ **T/F: Pulse oximetry is a reliable method for estimating oxyhemoglobin saturation in a patient suffering from CO poisoning.**

False. COHb has light absorbance that can lead to a falsely elevated pulse oximeter saturation level. The calculated value from a standard ABG may also be falsely elevated. The oxygen saturation should be determined by using a co-oximeter that measures the amounts of unsaturated O_2Hb, COHb and metHb.

○ **When may end-tidal carbon dioxide detectors prove inaccurate?**

In patients with very low blood flow to the lungs or in those with a large dead space (i.e. following a pulmonary embolism).

○ **What is the most common complication of endotracheal intubation?**

Intubation of a bronchus. Other complications include esophageal intubation, lacerations of the lip, tongue and pharyngeal or tracheal mucosa, resulting in bleeding, hematoma, or abscess. Tracheal rupture, avulsion of an arytenoid cartilage, vocal cord injury, pharyngeal-esophageal perforation, intubation of the pyriform sinus, gastric content aspiration, hypertension, tachycardia, or arrhythmias may also occur.

○ **What oxygen flow rate is recommended for face mask ventilation?**

At least 5 L/min. Recommended flow is 8-10 L/min, which will produce oxygen concentrations as high as 40% to 60%.

O   **What oxygen concentration can be supplied with a face mask and oxygen reservoir?**

6 L/min provides approximately 60% oxygen concentration and each liter increases the concentration by 10%. 10 L/min is almost 100%.

O   **Describe botulism intoxication.**

Acute food poisoning caused by Clostridium botulinum. Neurologic symptoms usually occur within 24 to 48 hours of ingestion of contaminated foods. Muscle paralysis and weakness typically spread rapidly, involving all muscles of the trunk and extremities.

O   **Describe Guillain-Barre syndrome?**

A lower motor neuron disease which commonly affects people in their thirties and forties. Symptoms include ascending weakness in the legs and arms. A sensory component may be present. Bulbar muscles are usually involved late in the course of the disease. Reflexes are affected early. Paralysis can progress rapidly. Recovery is usually slow, but it is almost always complete.

O   **Describe the clinical characteristics of carboxyhemoglobin concentrations, specifically for ranges of 10 to 70%.**

10%: Frontal headache
20%: Headache and dyspnea
30%: Nausea, dizziness, visual disturbance, fatigue and impaired judgment
40%: Syncope and confusion
50%: Coma and seizures
60%: Respiratory failure and hypotension
70%: May be lethal

O   **What causes toxic shock syndrome (TSS)?**

An exotoxin, from certain strains of Staphylococcus aureus. Other organisms that cause toxic shock syndrome are group A streptococci, Pseudomonas aeruginosa and Streptococcus pneumoniae. Tampons, IUD's, septic abortions, sponges, soft tissue abscesses, osteomyelitis, nasal packing and postpartum infections all can house these organisms.

O   **What dermatological changes occur with TSS?**

Initially, the patient will have a blanching erythematous rash that lasts for 3 days. After 10 days from the start of the infection, there will be a full thickness desquamation of the palms and soles.

O   **What criteria are necessary for the diagnosis of TSS?**

All of the following must be present: T > 38.9° C (102° F), rash, systolic BP < 90, orthostasis, involvement of 3 organ systems (GI, renal, musculoskeletal, mucosal, hepatic, hematologic, or CNS) and negative serologic tests for diseases such as rocky mountain spotted fever, hepatitis B, measles, leptospirosis, VDRL, etc.

O   **A 27 year-old male arrives somnolent with vitals of P 130, RR 26, BP 170/80 and T 105° F. You note diffuse muscular rigidity and intermittent focal muscle twitching and/or jerking that lasts for 1 to 2 seconds. As you "work him up," your nurse returns from the waiting area with news from the family that the patient has had a progressive decline of mental status for the last 2 days, after seeing his psychiatrist. The patient has had a history of psychosis for almost a year. What process should be included in your differential diagnosis at this time?**

Neuroleptic malignant syndrome (NMS).

○   **What are the signs indicating a possible basilar skull fracture?**

Bilateral periorbital ecchymosis, mastoid ecchymosis, hemotympanum, cerebral spinal fluid otorrhea and cerebral spinal fluid rhinorrhea.

○   **Describe the oculocephalic maneuver and its interpretation.**

After establishing the absence of a cervical spinal injury, the patient's head is positioned thirty degrees above the horizontal and rotated from side to side. If the neural pathways are intact, the patient's eyes will maintain a forward gaze as if fixed on an object and the eyes will not deviate to the side as the neural pathway adjusts for rotation of the head. Loss of horizontal gaze indicates a significant injury.

○   **Describe ice water caloric testing.**

Caloric testing can be done to confirm the oculocephalic response if there is no evidence of tympanic membrane perforation or dural perforation. In a patient with an intact cervical spine and dural membrane, the head can be positioned thirty degrees above the horizontal plane. Cold water is flushed into the external auditory canal. Within one minute, an intact labyrinthine system, brain stem and cranial nerves will result in a slow deviation of the eyes toward the tested side and a fast return to the midline. If the reticular activating system is injured, there is loss of the fast phase and a tonic deviation of the eyes to the tested side.

○   **What are the advantages and disadvantages of intraventricular catheters for monitoring intracranial pressure?**

An intraventricular catheter not only permits monitoring of the intracranial pressure, but some permit the withdrawal of cerebral spinal fluid to decrease intracranial pressure. The intraventricular catheter is useful in the treatment of hydrocephalus prior to the placement of a permanent shunt. Disadvantages of the intraventricular catheter include infection, bleeding, failure due to occlusion, care required to maintain drainage collection system and difficulty in interpreting waveform.

○   **What signs are associated with increased intracranial pressure?**

Headache, nausea, emesis, papilledema, systemic hypertension, bradycardia, irregular respiratory pattern and paralysis of upward gaze ("setting sun sign").

○   **Name several ways to control intracranial pressure.**

Venous drainage through proper head positioning, hyperventilation, cerebral dehydration with the use of mannitol, cerebral spinal fluid drainage, muscle relaxants and sedation and barbiturate coma.

○   **A trauma victim has sustained injury to her thoracic spine. On examination, there are no reflexes below the level of her injury and she is bradycardic and hypotensive. What is the most likely diagnosis?**

Spinal shock. The reflexes have disappeared as a result of abrupt withdrawal of descending excitatory influences from cerebral centers combined with persistent inhibition from below the injury. A relative hypovolemia has been created by an increased venous capacitance resulting from a traumatic sympathectomy. The patient should be treated with steroids, fluid resuscitation and a vasopressor to maintain pressure and avoid fluid overload.

○   **A multi-trauma patient undergoes extensive surgery and aggressive fluid resuscitation prior to arriving in the ICU. What are the probable metabolic abnormalities?**

Hypokalemia, hyperchloremia, metabolic acidosis, low ionized calcium, hypomagnesemia and hyperglycemia.

○   **Explain the relationship between magnesium and potassium.**

Magnesium depletion promotes the loss of potassium in the urine. Hypomagnesemia also inhibits sodium-potassium transport resulting in decreased intracellular concentrations of potassium.

○ **What are the possibly etiologies of hypernatremia in a multitrauma patient?**

Large volumes or rapid infusion rates of normal saline, use of hypertonic solutions and diabetes insipidus.

○ **What clinical features are associated with hypernatremia?**

Weakness, twitching, lethargy, obtundation, irritability and seizures.

○ **What signs are associated with hypocalcemia?**

Decreased cardiac inotropy, hypotension, ventricular arrhythmias, muscle spasms, laryngospasm, paresthesias and tetany.

○ **Initial assessment of vital signs in the intensive care unit shows the patient to be hypothermic with a temperature of 34.3 degrees Centigrade. What complications are associated with hypothermia?**

Coagulopathy, confusion, disorientation, decreased immune response, platelet dysfunction, reduced cardiac function and output, vasoconstriction and hypertension.

○ **As the patient rewarms, what problems can arise?**

The development of metabolic acidosis with increased serum lactate as perfusion is re-established in areas of intense vasoconstriction and hypoperfusion. Shivering is accompanied by an increase in oxygen consumption as high as 200 to 300%. Hypotension and tachycardia is associated with inadequate fluid resuscitation as the patient vasodilates during rewarming.

○ **The above patient is noted to be oozing from multiple wound sites. What tests and accompanying results would be consistent with disseminated intravascular coagulopathy (DIC)?**

Decreased platelet count, elevated prothrombin time, elevated activated partial thromboplastin time, decreased fibrinogen, elevated fibrin degradation products and presence of D-dimers.

○ **How can DIC be differentiated from bleeding caused primarily by massive transfusion?**

Coagulopathy secondary to massive transfusion is not associated with fibrinogen degradation products or with D-dimers. The coagulopathy is most commonly due to thrombocytopenia. In addition, all factors are reduced. However, DIC can develop in a patient with massive transfusion syndrome and therefore it should be considered if bleeding does not stop after adequate treatment.

○ **What are the four commonly used modes of ventilation?**

Intermittent mandatory ventilation (IMV), pressure support (PS), assist control (AC) and pressure control (PC).

○ **What is the difference between IMV and AC? Can you wean a patient using AC?**

IMV provides a given tidal volume at a set respiratory rate. Any breaths initiated by the patient achieve only the tidal volume the patient is able to generate. In AC, all tidal volumes whether initiated by the patient or by the ventilator, achieve the set tidal volume. Therefore, you cannot wean a patient in the AC mode.

○ **What is the difference between pressure control ventilation and pressure support ventilation?**

In pressure support ventilation, a breath is spontaneously initiated by the patient. The ventilator delivers a flow of gas to reach a target pressure. This flow is maintained until a flow threshold is reached during the decelerating phase of inspiration. At this time expiration begins.

In pressure control ventilation, a patient receives a mechanical breath at a predetermined rate. Once again the ventilator delivers a flow of gas to reach a certain pressure. In this instance, however, flow during inspiration is time-cycled as determined by ventilator settings.

In neither mode is the tidal volume controlled. Instead, the tidal volume is determined by pulmonary compliance, duration of inspiration and synchrony between the ventilator and the patient.

O **Describe the events associated with auto-PEEP.**

Also known as air trapping and intrinsic PEEP (positive end-expiratory pressure), auto-PEEP occurs mostly in patients with asthma, chronic obstructive pulmonary disease and acute respiratory distress syndrome. Auto-PEEP occurs when a patient suffering from severe airway obstruction is unable to completely exhale each tidal volume. The gradual accumulation of air and pressure results in a persistent difference between alveolar pressure and external airway pressure at end expiration. The persistent pressure difference results in continuing airflow at end exhalation.

O **What are the consequences of auto-PEEP?**

Auto-PEEP results in tidal volumes that occur at the upper limit of total lung capacity where compliance is low. Thus higher pressures are required to achieve a given tidal volume and the patient is at increased risk for barotrauma. In a patient who is initiating breaths on the ventilator (e.g. spontaneous breaths supported by pressure support), auto-PEEP increases the work of breathing. Like extrinsic PEEP, auto-PEEP can compromise cardiac function by decreasing venous return and cardiac output.

O **An intubated patient is left on 100% oxygen for 20 hours. Describe changes that can be attributed to oxygen toxicity.**

Tracheobronchial irritation (coughing, substernal discomfort), decreased vital capacity, decreased lung compliance, decreased diffusing capacity, decreased tracheal mucus velocity, increased arteriovenous shunting, absorption atelectasis and increased dead space to tidal volume ratio.

O **What is the pathophysiology of oxygen toxicity?**

At high partial pressure of inspired oxygen, the rate of highly reactive oxygen metabolite production is increased. Production of free radicals exceeds the detoxification capacity of the superoxide dismutase system. The cytotoxic metabolites impair enzyme function and protein synthesis leading to decreased surfactant production, increased alveolar-capillary leakage, pulmonary edema and destruction of the capillary endothelium.

O **A patient has been ventilator dependent for almost four weeks. She appears to be making slow progress in weaning from the ventilator. What are the advantages and disadvantages of undergoing a tracheotomy?**

A tracheotomy may help by decreasing dead space, improving clearance of secretions and improving patient comfort. It also partially restores glottic function. Assuming the patient progresses well, a tracheotomy also offers the potential to be able to verbally communicate and to tolerate oral feedings.
However, a tracheotomy requires the patient to undergo another surgical procedure. It is also associated with the risks of stoma granulation, tracheal erosion, tracheal stenosis and tracheo-innominate fistula.

O **What are the traditional criteria for extubation?**

Tidal volume of at least 5ml/kg, vital capacity at least 10-15 ml/kg, negative inspiratory force less than –25 cm of water, respiratory rate greater than 10 and less than 30, adequate oxygenation on an inspired oxygen concentration of 40% or less and ability to protect the airway.

O   If a patient aspirates, what treatment steps should be taken?

Secure the airway, administer oxygen, suction any aspirate, consider bronchoscopy and lavage if large particulates are present in aspirate, ventilatory support and bronchodilators as needed for bronchospasm. Corticosteroids should be avoided. Antibiotics should be deferred until clinical evidence of infection occurs and culture results are available. Prophylactic antibiotics may, however, be useful if the aspirate is grossly infected or feculent.

O   A patient is admitted to the ICU after surgical debridement for necrotizing pancreatitis. Over the next several hours, the patient's oxygenation deteriorates, with oxygen saturation of 90% on 75% inspired oxygen and 10 of PEEP. What is your diagnosis? What clinical findings are consistent with this diagnosis?

Acute respiratory distress syndrome. Common findings include hypoxia (PaO_2/FIO_2 ratio ≤ 200), diffuse bilateral infiltrates on chest roentgenogram, pulmonary artery occlusion pressure < 18 mmHg and decreased lung compliance.

O   What are possible causes of ARDS?

Sepsis, pneumonia, trauma, pulmonary contusion, multiple transfusions, aspiration of gastric contents and near drowning.

O   What ventilatory steps can be taken to optimize an ARDS patient's respiratory function?

Using pressure control to minimize barotrauma, decreasing tidal volume to minimize volutrauma, using inverse ratio ventilation and permissive hypercapnia to maximize inspiration time. None of these strategies have been proven by clinical trials.

O   What is nitric oxide?

Nitric oxide (NO) is a specific pulmonary vasodilator which helps to improve ventilation-perfusion matching and oxygenation. It is useful in treating pulmonary hypertension in pediatric patients and in patients with persistent pulmonary hypertension after cardiac surgery. Its use in the treatment of ARDS continues to be investigated. NO is inactivated by rapid binding to hemoglobin.

O   What is partial liquid ventilation?

Partial liquid ventilation is a technique that involves filling the functional residual capacity (FRC) of the lungs with a perfluorocarbon liquid and ventilating the lungs using conventional mechanical ventilation. The perfluorocarbon liquid acts as a liquid PEEP, stenting the lung open. The perfluorocarbon liquid also has a high oxygen carrying capacity facilitating gas exchange, a good spreading coefficient and evaporates fairly quickly thus acting like surfactant.

O   What is the equation for calculating arterial oxygen content (CaO_2)?

$CaO_2 = (1.39 \times Hgb \times$ arterial O_2 Sat$) + (.003 \times PaO_2)$ where Hgb is hemoglobin, O_2 sat is oxygen saturation and PaO_2 is arterial partial pressure of oxygen.

O   What is the equation for calculating oxygen consumption (VO_2)?

$VO_2 = CO \times (CaO_2-CvO_2)$ where CO is cardiac output, CaO_2 is arterial oxygen content and CvO_2 is venous oxygen content.

O   What factors shift the oxygen-hemoglobin dissociation curve to the right?

Acidemia, increased 2,3 DPG and increased temperature

○   **What hemodynamic changes are associated with sepsis?**

Increased cardiac index, decreased systemic vascular resistance (early stage), increased systemic vascular resistance (late stage), normal to decreased cardiac filling pressures and normal or elevated mixed venous oxygen saturation (early stage).

○   **What metabolic changes occur with acute illness?**

Catabolism, negative protein balance, hypermetabolic states and hyperglycemia.

○   **Hypermetabolic states commonly occur in what patients?**

Patients with burns, neurological injury, sepsis and multiple trauma.

○   **What are the nutritional parameters that can be followed in a critically ill patient?**

Indirect calorimetry, protein measurements (albumin, prealbumin, transferrin, retinol binding protein), 24-hour nitrogen balance study and daily weights.

○   **When is indirect calorimetry inaccurate?**

If the patient is hyperactive, hyperventilating, when the inspired oxygen concentration is above 60% and in the presence of an air leak.

○   **Using indirect calorimetry, how is resting energy expenditure calculated?**

Resting Energy Expenditure (kcal/day) = 3.94 x VO2 (L/day) + 1.11 x VCO2 (L/day)

○   **What is basal energy expenditure predicted by the Harris-Benedict equation?**

Men: 66.473 + (13.7516 x weight in kg) + (5.0 x height in cm) – (6.8 x age in years)
Women: 655.0955 + (9.563 x weight in kg) + (1.8496 x height in cm) – (4.6756 x age in years)

○   **In a 70 kg man in acute renal failure and unable to tolerate enteral feedings, what considerations should be accounted for in ordering total parenteral nutrition?**

Minimize fluids, avoid excess protein content (1.0-1.5 g/kg/day), unless the patient is on hemodialysis, and closely monitor and adjust daily potassium, calcium and magnesium.

○   **What is in a nutritional formula designed for patients with hepatic failure?**

Higher levels of branched chain amino acids and lower concentrations of aromatic amino acids. This is to minimize the development of encephalopathy.

○   **How much glucose per day is needed to reduce protein losses?**

The infusion of 100 to 150 g of glucose per day can decrease urine urea nitrogen losses to less than 5 g per day.

○   **What are the goals of nutritional therapy?**

Maintain lean body mass, minimize catabolism, preserve organ function and promote immune function.

○   **When should enteral nutrition be started?**

Most proponents believe enteral nutrition should be started as soon as possible, preferably in the first 24 hours after injury or surgery.

○   **What is acalculous cholecystitis?**

It occurs in patients with bile stasis from narcotics or fasting, patients on total parenteral nutrition, those who have suffered hypotension and patients with increased pigment load after multiple blood transfusions. Patients often have localized tenderness in the right upper quadrant and may develop jaundice. In some patients, sepsis is the only symptom. Diagnosis is made by ultrasound evidence of a thickened gallbladder wall and pericholecystic fluid. The treatment is either cholecystostomy or cholecystectomy. The former is often done percutaneously at the patient's bedside.

○   **What factors are associated with the development of stress ulcers?**

Sepsis, shock, major trauma, burns greater than 35% of body surface area, head trauma, history of ulcers, use of steroids, respiratory failure, renal failure and hepatic insufficiency.

○   **Prophylaxis for stress ulcers include what agents?**

Sucralfate, antacids and H-2 receptor antagonists. The first should be used cautiously, if at all, in patients with renal failure given their aluminum content. When using the latter two agents, one should check the pH to ensure that it is greater than 5.0. Enteral feedings have not been shown to definitively decrease the risk for gastric stress ulcers.

○   **What are the most common causes of rhabdomyolyis?**

Crush injury, muscular ischemia, trauma, compression (compartment syndrome), alcohol, seizures, cocaine, heroin, amphetamines, burns, gas gangrene and malignant hyperthermia.

○   **What laboratory tests show significant changes in rhabdomyolyis?**

Hyperkalemia and hypocalcemia. Other abnormalities include hyperphosphatemia, hyperuricemia, widened anion gap and elevated serum CK levels. In the urine, myoglobin is detected once serum levels exceed 1500 to 3000 ng/ml.

○   **How do you calculate the fractional excretion of sodium (FENa)?**

FENa = [(Urine sodium/Plasma sodium)/(Urine creatinine/Plasma creatinine)] x 100. When the value is less than 1%, it is suggestive of prerenal azotemia. When the value is greater than 2%, it is suggestive of renal parenchymal disease.

○   **A patient in the ICU develops acute renal failure, what are the indications for emergency hemodialysis?**

Elevated potassium, decreased pH, pericarditis, mental status changes and severe volume overload.

○   **What other methods are available to replace renal function? What are the advantages and disadvantages of each?**

Continuous arteriovenous hemofiltration (CAVH), continuous arteriovenous hemodiafiltration (CAVHD), continuous venovenous hemofiltration (CVVH), continuous venovenous hemodiafiltration (CVVHD) and peritoneal dialysis (PD).

CAVH is driven by arterial blood pressure, eliminates fluid and solutes and avoids hemodynamic instability, but requires arterial access and heparinization. CAVHD is similar to CAVH except that it removes fluids and solutes to a greater degree.

CVVH is driven by a pump, eliminates fluids and solutes, avoids hemodynamic instability, requires less heparin than CAVH (D) and does not require arterial access. CVVHD is similar to CVVH except that it eliminates more fluids and solutes than CVVH.

PD uses the peritoneum and oncotic pressure to remove fluids and to a lesser degree solutes. Unlike the other modalities, PD does not require venous or arterial access or heparin. However, PD is less effective and has potential for infection. More often, PD is used in an outpatient setting rather than in the ICU.

○   **A patient has the following pulmonary artery catheter readings: cardiac index (CI) 2.0 L/min, central venous pressure (CVP) 2 mmHg, pulmonary artery occlusion pressure (PAOP) 7 mmHg and systemic vascular resistance (SVR) 1600 dyne sec cm^{-5}. What is the most consistent diagnosis and appropriate therapy?**

The patient is hypovolemic and would benefit from fluid resuscitation.

○   **A patient's pulmonary artery catheter readings are CVP 12 mmHg, PAOP 18 mmHg, CI 1.7 L/min, SVR 1650 dyne sec cm^{-5}. What is the most likely diagnosis? What therapy should be considered?**

The patient is probably suffering from cardiogenic shock. Using echocardiography to further evaluate the patient's cardiac function can be very useful. The patient will benefit from inotropic support to improve the cardiac output. However, this must be judiciously balanced against increasing myocardial oxygen demand. Intra-aortic balloon pumping may be useful.

○   **Compare and contrast epinephrine and norepinephrine.**

Epinephrine has both alpha and beta effects as does norepinephrine. However, alpha effects are greater than beta effects with norepinephrine. Both drugs will increase SVR and BP. Epinephrine is also associated with an increase in HR whereas norepinephrine often has an associated reflex bradycardia.

○   **How does phenylephrine differ from norepinephrine?**

Phenylephrine is a pure alpha agonist. It can be used to increase SVR and BP. Like norepinephrine it is associated with a reflex bradycardia.

○   **Compare nitroglycerin and sodium nitroprusside.**

Both are vasodilators. Nitroglycerin is a greater venous vasodilator than an arterial vasodilator. In contrast, nitroprusside is primarily an arterial vasodilator. Unlike nitroprusside which is used primarily to manage hypertension and hypertensive crisis, nitroglycerin is also used to treat angina and congestive heart failure. Prolonged nitroprusside administration is limited by the risk of thiocyanate toxicity.

○   **Discuss amrinone and milrinone.**

Both are phosphodiesterase inhibitors which have a relative selectivity for phosphodiesterase III, the predominant cAMP-specific form in cardiac tissue. They have an inotropic as well as a vasodilatory effect. A major drawback is the development of thrombocytopenia. Milrinone is at least as effective if not more potent than amrinone. Another benefit of milrinone is that its incidence of thrombocytopenia is much lower than amrinone.

○   **Name three limitations of pulmonary artery catheter (PAC) readings.**

PAC readings can fluctuate during respiratory variations and should therefore be read at end expiration. High PEEP can falsely elevate PAC readings, particularly PAOP. Heart rates exceeding 120 beats/minute can also falsely elevate pulmonary artery diastolic pressure readings. A pressure change should be greater than 4 mmHg to be considered clinically significant.

○   **What catheter tip culture results are suggestive of catheter sepsis?**

More than 15 colonies of the same organism grown from the catheter tip suggest that septicemia is related to an infected catheter.

O   **What risks are associated with using aminoglycosides?**

The development of prolonged neuromuscular blockade, ototoxicity and nephrotoxicity.

O   **For what bacteria is vancomycin effective?**

Gram-positive cocci, including methicillin-resistant Staphylococcus aureus (MRSA), staphylococcus epidermidis, enterococcus, diphteroids and Clostridium difficile.

O   **If the patient is being treated for Clostridium difficile, can vancomycin be given orally?**

Yes, vancomycin must be given orally. Metronidazole can be given effectively orally or intravenously.

O   **What is Red Man's Syndrome?**

Red Man's Syndrome is produced by rapid infusion of vancomycin, which is associated with histamine release. The clinical features include flushing of the face and neck, pruritis and hypotension. The incidence can be reduced by slow infusion of vancomycin.

O   **What more recent problem has arisen with the use of vancomycin?**

There has been the widespread development of vancomycin resistant enterococci (VRE). A VRE infection is associated with a high mortality rate because there are few antimicrobial agents that have activity against VRE.

O   **What is the equation that relates total pulmonary compliance to lung compliance and chest wall compliance?**

1/total pulmonary compliance = 1/lung compliance + 1/chest wall compliance

O   **During sleep what is the normal, expected change in PaCO2 and PaO2 from the baseline, awake state?**

Normally, PaCO2 increases 4-8mmHg and PaO2 decreases 3-10mmHg.

O   **What is a normal oxygen extraction ratio in a healthy adult?**

20 vol%-15 vol%/20 vol% = 5/20 or 25%

O   **What is the interrelationship described by the Bowditch effect?**

As heart rate increases myocardial contractility increases.

O   **How does a cardiac output thermistor resting on a vessel wall alter the cardiac output calculation based on the Stewart-Hamilton equation for thermodilution cardiac output?**

It isolates the thermistor from temperature change causing less of a temperature change, causing less of a temperature change in the thermodilution solution thereby overestimating the patient's cardiac output.

O   **What is Beck's triad for the diagnosis of cardiac tamponade?**

Hypotension, elevated CVP and a quiet precordium on auscultation

O   **What is Graham's law of gases?**

The rate of diffusion of a gas is inversely proportional to its molecular weight.

○   What is the Hering-Breuer inflation reflex?

Inhibition of inspiratory muscle activity by inflation of the lungs. In newborns overinflation of the lungs during controlled or mechanical ventilation may lead to apnea. This reflex does not appear to be as active in adults.

○   What is the Bohr effect?

Enhanced release of oxygen from hemoglobin in the presence of carbon dioxide.

○   What is the Haldane effect?

Enhanced release of carbon dioxide from hemoglobin in the presence of oxygen

○   What is transpulmonary pressure?

Transpulmonary pressure is the pressure gradient across the lung measured as the pressure difference between the airway opening and the pleural surface.

○   What factors shift the hemoglobin dissociation curve for oxygen to the right?

An increase in hydrogen ion concentration, $PaCO_2$, temperature and the concentration of 2,3-diphosphoglycerate in the red cells.

○   Define compliance.

The change in volume divided by the change in distending pressure. Elastic recoil is usually measured in terms of compliance. Compliance measurements can be obtained for the chest, the lung or both together.

○   What is afterload?

Afterload is either ventricular wall tension during systole or arterial impedance to ejection. Wall tension is usually described as the pressure the ventricle must overcome to reduce cavity size.

○   What is the baroreceptor reflex?

Increase in blood pressure stimulates peripheral baroreceptors located at the bifurcation of the common carotid arteries and the aortic arch. These baroreceptors then send afferent signals to the brainstem circulatory centers via the glossopharyngeal and vagus nerves, allowing an increase in vagal tone and, consequently, vasodilatation and a decrease in heart rate.

○   What is the predominant stimulus for activation of hypoxic pulmonary vasoconstriction?

Decreased alveolar oxygen tension.

○   What components contribute to physiologic shunting (venous admixture)?

The bronchial, pleural and thebesian veins and abnormal arterial to venous communications in the lungs.

○   What is the primary form of carbon dioxide transport?

Carbon dioxide hydrolyzed by carbonic anhydrase to carbonic acid.

○   What is the respiratory quotient?

The rate of carbon dioxide production divided by the rate of oxygen consumption.

❍   **What is the primary mechanism responsible for postoperative atelectasis?**

Decreased expiratory reserve volume relative to closing volume.

❍   **What is the distribution of alveoli in relation to their size at end-exhalation in dependent vs. nondependent lung regions?**

Alveoli in dependent lung regions are smaller than nondependent alveoli at end-exhalation.

❍   **Write a recognized form of the shunt equation.**

$$\frac{CcO_2 - CaO_2}{CcO_2 - CvO_2}$$

CaO_2 = arterial oxygen content
CvO_2 = mixed venous oxygen content
CcO_2 = oxygen content of ideal pulmonary end-capillary blood

Pulmonary end-capillary blood is considered to the have the same concentration of oxygen as alveolar gas.

❍   **Write a recognized form of the Bohr equation.**

$$Vd/Vt = \frac{PaCO_2 - PeCO_2}{PaCO_2}$$

Vd/Vt = Dead space ventilation
$PaCO_2$ = Arterial partial pressure of CO_2
$PeCO_2$ = End-tidal CO_2

❍   **What factors can potentially contribute to the difficulty in weaning critically ill patients from mechanical ventilation?**

Lack of central ventilatory drive due to encephalopathy, primary myopathy, muscle fatigue or weakness and neuropathy of critical illness.

❍   **What is the neuropathy of critical illness?**

Primary axonal degeneration of motor and sensory fibers.

❍   **Respiratory failure is worsened in spinal injuries at or above which nerve root?**

C2.

❍   **What is the mechanism of diaphragm dysfunction following open heart surgery?**

Thermal or mechanical injury to the phrenic nerve.

❍   **What infectious syndromes can lead to ventilatory insufficiency?**

Botulism, tetanus, campylobacter, polio, diphtheria and Guillain-Barré syndrome.

○ **Which neuromuscular and spinal diseases can lead to ventilatory insufficiency?**

Muscular dystrophy, polymyositis, myotonic dystrophy, polyneuritis, Eaton Lambert syndrome, myasthenia gravis, amyotrophic lateral sclerosis, trauma, Guillain-Barré syndrome, multiple sclerosis, Parkinson's Disease and stroke.

○ **Inherited abnormalities in which enzyme contribute to respiratory insufficiency after succinylcholine administration?**

Serum cholinesterase.

○ **Adequacy of alveolar ventilation is reflected by which component of arterial blood gas analysis?**

P_aCO_2.

○ **PaCO₂ is mathematically related to alveolar ventilation in what manner?**

Inverse proportion.

○ **Patients on mechanical ventilation can develop hypoventilation based on what factors?**

Increased deadspace (including length of ventilator circuit proximal to the "Y" piece separating the inspiratory and expiratory limbs), decreased tidal volume, overdistention of lung, air leaks and massive pulmonary embolism.

○ **What factors can interfere with the bellows function of the chest?**

Abdominal binding, massive obesity, trauma with flail chest, massive effusion, massive ascites, pneumothorax, thoracic burn with eschar, neuromuscular blockade and strapping of ribs.

○ **What constitutes post polio syndrome?**

Thirty to forty years afterwards, polio survivors experience reduced endurance, reduced ambulation and increased weakness of previously affected limbs.

○ **Patients with failure of which organs are at increased risk of developing prolonged paralysis following neuromuscular blocker administration?**

Liver and kidney.

○ **How is the neuropathy of critical illness diagnosed?**

EMG.

○ **What methods rapidly confirm that an endotracheal tube was not placed in the esophagus.**

Auscultation, capnography and fiberoptic bronchoscopy.

○ **What are the principal complications of nasal endotracheal intubation (as opposed to oral)?**

Maxillary sinusitis, amputation of turbinates, septal perforation and increased airway resistance associated with a more narrow tube.

○ **How is the work of breathing affected by patient triggered positive pressure ventilation?**

It can increase, decrease, or remain the same.

○   **What should be done first when tension pneumothorax is suspected?**

Needle thoracostomy followed by tube thoracostomy.

○   **How can the presence of intrinsic PEEP be confirmed in patients undergoing mechanical ventilation?**

Observing that expiratory flow has not ceased prior to the onset of inspiration, measurement of persistent positive pressure just prior to inspiration by an esophageal balloon, or airway occlusion pressure measurements at end expiration.

○   **What are the determinants of P_aCO_2?**

Carbon dioxide production and alveolar ventilation.

○   **Under what circumstances should deadspace be added to the ventilator circuit?**

None.

○   **What is the FIO2 at the top of Mount Everest?**

21%.

○   **What are the two components of tidal volume?**

Alveolar volume (V_a) and dead space volume (V_d).

○   **What is the potential harm of excess endotracheal tube cuff pressure?**

Excess pressure can induce ischemia and necrosis of the underlying tissue.

○   **What position is preferred for patients suspected of having an air embolism?**

Left lateral decubitus/Trendelenberg position.

○   **What are the signs and symptoms of rabies?**

Incubation period of 12 to 700 days with an average of 20 to 90 days. Initial signs and systems include fever, headache, malaise, anorexia, sore throat, nausea, cough and pain or paresthesias at the bite site.

In the CNS stage, agitation, restlessness, altered mental status, painful bulbar and peripheral muscular spasms, bulbar or focal motor paresis and opisthotonos are exhibited. As in the Landry-Guillain-Barre syndrome, 20% develop ascending, symmetric flaccid and areflexic paralysis. In addition, hypersensitivity to water and sensory stimuli to light, touch and noise may occur.

The progressive stage includes lucid and confused intervals with hyperpyrexia, lacrimation, salivation and mydriasis, along with brainstem dysfunction, hyperreflexia and extensor planter response. Final stages include coma, convulsions and apnea, followed by death between the fourth and seventh day for the untreated patient.

○   **What is a paradoxical embolus?**

A venous thrombus that goes through a right-to-left intra-cardiac shunt to the arterial side.

○   **Why is a paradoxical embolus able to cause septic end-organ disease?**

An infected venous thrombus can enter the arterial circulation via the right-to-left intra-cardiac shunt and be sent distal to affect end organs.

○   **Splinter hemorrhages, Osler's nodes, Janeway lesions, petechiae and Roth spots can be indications of what process?**

Infective endocarditis.

○   **T/F: Osler nodes are usually nodular and painful.**

True. In contrast, the macular Janeway lesions are painless.

○   **What is the sensitivity rate of two-dimensional transesophageal echocardiograms for detecting vegetations?**

95%.

○   **Who is at high risk for developing endocarditis?**

People with prosthetic heart valves, previous incidents of endocarditis, complex congenital heart disease and surgically constructed systemic pulmonic shunts.

○   **Who is at moderate risk for developing endocarditis?**

Moderate risk factors include acquired valvular dysfunction, hypertrophic cardiomyopathy and uncorrected congenital conditions. These latter conditions include patent ductus arteriosus, ventricular septal defect, primum atrial septal defect, coarctation of the aorta and bicuspid aortic valve.

○   **What are the bacteremia inducing procedures that increase the risk for developing bacterial endocarditis?**

Procedures of the dental, oral, respiratory, gastrointestinal, and genitourinary tracts and vaginal delivery.

○   **What is the appropriate prophylaxis for these procedures?**

Depending upon the nature of the procedure, amoxicillin, ampicillin, gentamicin, clindamycin, or a combination of these antibiotics.

○   **What is the clinical picture of a myocardial abscess?**

Low-grade fevers, chills, leukocytosis, conduction system abnormalities and nonspecific ECG changes.

○   **What is Streptococcal Toxic Shock Syndrome?**

The recent emergence of highly virulent strains of Group A Streptococcus pyogenes has been associated with severe invasive disease and a mortality rate of approximately 30%. This fulminant process may be precipitated by seemingly minor trauma to skin or mucosal surfaces and is rarely associated with streptococcal pharyngitis. Exotoxin production by these strains, especially exotoxin A, has been implicated as the cause of tissue injury, which often includes organ failure, ARDS and necrotizing fasciitis. Patients with prior exposure to streptococcal M proteins are relatively protected from this syndrome.

The definite case definition is: Isolation of group A streptococci from a normally sterile site (eg, blood, CSF, pleural or peritoneal fluid) and the presence of hypotension or shock plus at least two of the following signs: renal impairment, disseminated intravascular coagulation, abnormal liver function, ARDS, erythematous rash with or without desquamation and soft tissue necrosis (eg, necrotizing fasciitis, myositis and gangrene).

A probable case has group A streptococcus isolated from a normally nonsterile site (eg, pharynx, skin and sputum), in addition to hypotension, shock and at least two of the above listed signs.

O   **What are risk factors for developing sinusitis in the intensive care unit?**

Nasally intubated patients develop sinusitis with an incidence that has been quoted as anywhere from 2-25%. This complication is related to trauma, edema and obstruction of drainage from the ostia in the lateral nasal wall. Trauma patients with facial fractures, patients with limited head mobility and those who require nasal packing and nasogastric tubes are also especially prone.

O   **What is the clinical scenario in which sinusitis occurs in the ICU?**

Though sinusitis develops relatively early after nasal intubation, the diagnosis may not be readily apparent as it is often not accompanied by purulent nasal drainage. Most typically patients present with fever and leukocytosis and may progress to sepsis.

O   **How is sinusitis that occurs in the ICU diagnosed and treated?**

Sinus CT scans will confirm the diagnosis, but antral taps for gram stain and culture are recommended to guide treatment. Unlike community acquired sinusitis, Staphylococcus aureus and gram negatives are the most common organisms. Polymicrobial infections are frequently seen. Removal of the foreign body is key for recovery. Phenylephrine nasal drops may help decrease edema and promote drainage. Some patients may require repeated antral lavage. Patients who are nasotracheally intubated should be reintubated orally as soon as possible if it appears that they will require intubation for more than a few days (five days is often used as a guideline).

O   **What are the characteristics of drug fever?**

Patients with a drug-related fever often will appear relatively well, despite a high temperature. Those with a known history of atopy are more susceptible. Usual temperatures are in the range of 102-104 degrees Fahrenheit, though low-grade and extreme elevations may also be seen. Sustained fevers are more typical, with variations of less than 1 degree Fahrenheit per day. A "relative bradycardia" is characteristic. Besides antibiotics, other common causes of drug fever include amphotericin, procainamide, salicylates, barbiturates, phenytoin, quinidine and interferon. Drug fever is not always accompanied by rash.

O   **Who is especially at risk for developing meningococcal disease?**

Neisseria meningitidis, a gram-negative diplococcus, classically strikes children and young adults, especially military recruits and those in crowded living conditions. The reservoir of the meningococcus is in the nasopharynx of asymptomatic carriers, who are felt to be the major source of transmission of the disease. Congenital deficiencies of complement, especially terminal complement components C5 to C9 or properdin, impact a significantly increased risk of developing invasive disease. Acquired complement deficiencies related to nephrotic syndrome, liver disease, systemic lupus erythematosus, as well as asplenia and immunoglobulin deficiencies also result in increased risk.

O   **Who should receive meningococcal vaccination?**

Vaccination is recommended for patients 2 years of age or older with functional or anatomic asplenia, complement deficiencies and military recruits. The currently available vaccine is tetravalent and contains the polysaccharides groups A, C, Y and W135. Unfortunately, there is no effective vaccine available for serogroup type B, which accounts for almost half of the infections in the United States.

O   **What are the risk factors for developing primary peritonitis?**

Primary peritonitis, also known as spontaneous bacterial peritonitis, is an acute or subacute bacterial infection of the peritoneum unrelated to the usual causes of peritonitis, such as a perforated viscus or intrQ:bdominal abscess. The vast majority of cases occur in patients with alcoholic cirrhosis, but patients with cirrhosis and ascites from other causes are also predisposed.

O   **What are the clinical findings and treatment for primary peritonitis?**

Fever and abdominal pain are present in most patients, but peritoneal signs may not be appreciable. Most cirrhotic patients with primary peritonitis will have advanced liver disease and present with coexisting encephalopathy. The most useful findings on analysis of peritoneal fluid include an elevated polymorphonuclear count > 250/mm3. Gram staining of peritoneal fluid may be negative up to 80% of cases, so empiric treatment should be begun while awaiting culture results if there is sufficient suspicion. The infections tend to be due to a single organism in most cases, commonly Escherichia coli and Streptococcus pneumoniae, unlike secondary peritonitis which is usually polymicrobial.

O   **What are the clinical findings of herpes simplex encephalitis?**

Herpes Simplex encephalitis is the most common cause of nonepidemic encephalitis in the United States. Patients will generally present with headache, fever, anosmia, memory or personality changes and a decreased level of consciousness. Focal signs are common, including hemiparesis, seizures, or an ataxic gait. Herpes Simplex Type 1 is ordinarily responsible in the adult population.

O   **What is the pathophysiology of HSV encephalitis?**

Unlike the arthropod-borne viruses, which spread to the CNS hematogenously, HSV 1's mode of entry is neuronal, often due to reactivation of latent virus present in the trigeminal ganglia, which sends fibers to the frontal and temporal lobes. This may explain why these sites seem to be preferentially involved. This disease has an extremely high morbidity and mortality.

O   **How is HSV encephalitis diagnosed and treated?**

Focal findings on electroencephalography may show characteristic periodic spike waves and slow waves in the temporal zones. MRI and CT may also show abnormalities in these areas. Routine CSF findings are nonspecific. The diagnosis may be made by CSF polymerase chain reaction for HSV. Brain biopsy is useful to help distinguish HSV encephalitis from other potentially treatable syndromes, including bacterial brain abscesses, cryptococcal disease, tuberculosis, toxoplasmosis and malignancies. Brain biopsy is most typically performed in those patients who are not responding to empiric therapy.

Early treatment is critical and will salvage some patients. IV acyclovir is generally nontoxic and should be instituted empirically and promptly in patients in whom there is a clinical suspicion for Herpes Simplex encephalitis. Unfortunately, it has not been shown to be useful as a treatment for other viral encephalitides.

O   **What is necrotizing fasciitis?**

Necrotizing fasciitis is a severe infection distinguished by necrosis of the fascia and subcutaneous tissues, resulting in undermining of the skin. Onset is abrupt and is more common in diabetics, alcoholics and IV drug abusers, usually precipitated by a traumatized area of skin. Initial physical findings may mimic cellulitis with swollen, tender and erythematous skin. Unlike cellulitis however, the margins are usually not well demarcated. Prior to emergence of grossly necrotic skin or bulla formation, the involved area typically becomes anesthetic due to the destruction of cutaneous nerves by the inflammatory process. This is a feature not typical of cellulitis. A certain percentage of cases have subcutaneous gas formation. Very high fever and signs of toxicity disproportionate to the physical findings should raise suspicion. The superficial skin findings are the tip of the iceberg with this infection which is often fulminant in nature.

Early diagnosis, which can be definitively made by biopsy of the subcutaneous tissue, fascia and muscle, may help decrease the mortality rate (from up to 50% in the untreated patient) by enabling appropriate treatment with surgical debridement. Common antibiotic regimens include ampicillin/clindamycin/gentamicin to cover anaerobes, facultative anaerobes and Enterobacteriaceae.

O   **What ultrasound findings suggest the diagnosis of acalculous cholecystitis?**

These include thickening of the gallbladder wall > 4 mm, intramural gas, subserosal edema without ascites, or a sloughed gallbladder mucosal membrane. The diagnosis can be difficult to make. Gallbladder sludging, wall thickening and hydrops have been found to be common findings in asymptomatic medical intensive care unit patients. The presence of sepsis, new-onset jaundice and ultrasound-induced Murphy's sign help to confirm the significance of suggestive ultrasound findings.

O   **What are the risk factors for acalculous cholecystitis?**

Patients in the intensive care unit are at increased risk for gallbladder stasis or acute acalculous cholecystitis, related to fasting, hyperalimentation, opioid use and infectious processes. Polytrauma patients and those with recent major surgery are especially at risk to develop acute acalculous cholecystitis.

O   **How is acalculous cholecystitis treated?**

Percutaneous cholecystostomy, laparoscopic cholecystectomy, or traditional cholecystectomy for the more stable patient.

O   **What is Chariot's triad?**

Fever, right upper quadrant pain and jaundice are the three classic signs in patients with acute cholangitis. Chills are also typical. Biliary decompression, either surgically, via stent placement, or percutaneous drainage techniques, is essential in addition to appropriate antibiotic coverage.

O   **Which antibiotics are most frequently implicated as precipitants for Stevens-Johnson syndrome?**

Stevens-Johnson syndrome, or erythema multiforme major, is a serious hypersensitivity reaction which presents with a generalized vesiculobullous eruption of the skin, mouth, eyes and genitals. Many drugs have been identified as triggering this reaction, but the most common antibiotics named are the sulfa drugs and the penicillins. Stevens-Johnson syndrome has also been seen in patients with recent mycoplasma infections.

O   **Barotrauma in a mechanically ventilated patient may result in what syndromes?**

Alveolar rupture may lead to pulmonary interstitial emphysema, systemic air embolism, pneumothorax, subcutaneous emphysema, pneumomediastinum, pneumopericardium, pneumoretroperitoneum and pneumoperitoneum.

O   **What are the chest x-ray findings of pneumothorax in a mechanically ventilated patient?**

Deep sulcus sign, relative lucency of one or part of one lung and increase in volume of one hemithorax.

DRUG INDUCED LUNG DISEASE

"Here's to my love! O true apothecary!
Thy drugs are quick. Thus with a kiss I die.
Romeo & Juliet, Shakespeare

○   **What is the typical time period during which acute radiation pneumonitis develops?**

Within the first eight weeks after radiation.

○   **What is the earliest radiographic abnormality in bleomycin lung toxicity?**

Bibasilar reticular infiltrates.

○   **What is the mortality of patients with bleomycin lung toxicity?**

25%.

○   **What are the proven risk factors for the development of bleomycin lung toxicity?**

Total accumulative dose, older age (rare<70), radiation therapy, multidrug regimens and high FIO2.

○   **What is the most characteristic presentation of bleomycin lung toxicity?**

Pulmonary fibrosis.

○   **T/F: The return of pulmonary function abnormalities to normal after withdrawal of bleomycin is the rule.**

False.

○   **What are four distinct presentations of bleomycin lung toxicity?**

Chronic pulmonary fibrosis, hypersensitivity lung reaction, acute pneumonitis and acute chest pain syndrome.

○   **What dose of radiation is generally required to cause the synergistic effect of bleomycin and radiotherapy on the incidence of bleomycin lung toxicity?**

5000 to 6000 rads.

○   **An acute chest pain syndrome can occur with which chemotherapeutic agents?**

Methotrexate and bleomycin.

○   **What drug will produce hilar and mediastinal adenopathy as a toxic reaction?**

Methotrexate.

○   **Hemolytic-uremic syndrome has been associated with what chemotherapeutic agent?**

Mitomycin. This complication has a high mortality and can cause a microangiopathic hemolytic anemia, renal failure, cerebrovascular events and other manifestations of a vasculopathy. Blood transfusions are often associated with this disorder.

○   **What is the most common presentation for lung toxicity caused by cytosine arabinoside?**

Non-cardiogenic pulmonary edema. Fever, dyspnea and cough typically appear within 4 weeks of completing drug therapy. Acute pulmonary disease with diffuse alveolar infiltrates and pleural effusions occur, mechanical ventilation is often required and mortality approaches 50%.

○   **Chronic interstitial pneumonitis can be caused by cyclophosphamide. What physical finding is more common with cyclophosphamide-induced lung injury than other chemotherapy-related lung injuries?**

Fever.

○   **Radiation therapy is a potent risk factor for the development of pulmonary toxicity due to which chemotherapy agents?**

Cyclophosphamide, busulfan and bleomycin.

○   **What is the nature of the lung toxicity associated with the cytokine, interleukin-2?**

Fluid retention and pulmonary edema.

○   **What toxicity has been observed with the use of all-transretinoic acid for the treatment of acute leukemia?**

Acute lung disease associated with massive fluid retention.

○   **Which is more common, cough induced by enalapril or captopril?**

Enalapril.

○   **T/F: Generally, the cough related to ACE inhibitors resolves within a few days of withdrawal of the drug.**

False. The resolution of cough may be slow, taking several weeks.

○   **Is ACE inhibitor cough more common in men or women?**

Male : female = 1:2.

○   **What is the usual time course for lung toxicity with gold salts?**

Several days of fever, cough and dyspnea.

○   **What are the bronchoalveolar lavage findings in patients with gold salt induced hypersensitivity pulmonary disease?**

Increased numbers of lymphocytes.

○   **What are four syndromes of penicillamine induced lung toxicity?**

Chronic pneumonitis, hypersensitivity lung disease, bronchiolitis obliterans and pulmonary-renal syndrome.

○   **A syndrome similar to Goodpasture's disease has been reported with what drug?**

Penicillamine.

○   **What drugs are known to have caused bronchiolitis obliterans organizing pneumonia?**

Bleomycin, penicillamine, amiodarone, cocaine, cyclophosphamide, mitomycin C, methotrexate, sulfasalazine and gold.

○   **What acute pulmonary reaction might one encounter at the time of a persantine-thallium study for cardiac ischemia?**

Bronchospasm due to dipyridamole.

○   **After removal from cardiopulmonary bypass during coronary revascularization surgery, a patient develops severe wheezing. What drug might be responsible?**

Protamine.

○   **Alveolar proteinosis has been described in association with the use of what drug?**

Busulfan.

○   **A sarcoidosis-like lesion has been described with use of which chemotherapeutic agent?**

Nitrosoureas.

○   **A mid-inspiratory squeak while non-specific may be auscultated with what pathologic lesion occasionally seen as an adverse effect of certain drugs?**

Bronchiolitis obliterans, e.g. penicillamine.

○   **T/F: Clubbing is very unusual with drug-induced interstitial lung disease.**

True.

○   **Which of the following drugs have dose dependent lung toxicity: cyclophosphamide, bleomycin, or BCNU?**

Bleomycin and BCNU.

○   **What are the historical findings in patients with an acute pleuripulmonary reaction to nitrofurantoin?**

Fever, dyspnea, cough and pleuritic pain, typically within hours or several days of starting the drug.

○   **T/F: Untreated acute nitrofurantoin lung toxicity will progress to the chronic form within several months.**

False. There seems to be no overlap between the acute and the chronic forms.

○   **Acute respiratory failure occurring in patients taking amiodarone is associated with what two procedures?**

Cardiovascular surgery and angiography.

○   **What risk factors predispose to a higher incidence of pulmonary injury with amiodarone?**

A maintenance dose of amiodarone in excess of 400 mg/day, use of angiography, cardiac or lung surgery and concomitant lung disease.

○   **The presence of foamy appearing macrophages and infiltration of inflammatory cells including lymphocytes, plasma cells, histiocytes and neutrophils suggests lung injury from what drug?**

Amiodarone.

○   **What laboratory and radiological findings help distinguish amiodarone lung toxicity from CHF?**

Elevated ESR, reduced DLCO, abnormal gallium-67 uptake and high attenuation of infiltrates on CT scan of lungs.

○   **Pulmonary reactions often occur when drugs or agents combine synergistically with each other. Fill in the associated agent causing the pulmonary lesion listed to the right.**

Bleomycin	**+**	**a**	**=**	**NCPE (non-cardiogenic pulmonary edema)**
Mitomycin	**+**	**b**	**=**	**NCPE**
Mitomycin	**+**	**c**	**=**	**NCPE**
Amphotericin B	**+**	**d**	**=**	**NCPE**
Vinblastine	**+**	**e**	**=**	**Asthma**
Nitrofurantoin	**+**	**f**	**=**	**Pulmonary granulomas**
Amiodarone	**+**	**g**	**=**	**NCPE**

a-oxygen, b-5-fluorouracil, c-leukocyte transfusion, d-leukocyte transfusion, e-mitomycin, f-low dose methotrexate, g-oxygen.

○   **What chemotherapeutic agents are associated with pulmonary veno-occlusive disease?**

Bleomycin, mitomycin, BCNU, etoposide and cyclophosphamide.

○   **What is the incidence of aspirin-induced bronchospasm in patients with nasal polyps?**

Up to 75%.

○   **T/F: In aspirin-induced bronchospasm there can be cross-reactivity with non-steroidal anti-inflammatory drugs.**

True.

○   **What are the risk factors for the development of tocolytic-induced pulmonary edema?**

Use of corticosteroids, fluid overload, twin gestation, multiparous state, anemia and silent cardiac disease.

○   **A lymphocytic interstitial pneumonitis has been associated with which antiarrhythmic?**

Flecainide.

○   **Mediastinal lipomatosis is associated with what drug class?**

Corticosteroids.

○   **What laboratory finding distinguishes patients with primary SLE and drug-induced lupus?**

Drug- induced lupus has a positive ANA but a <u>negative</u> ds-DNA.

○ **T/F: Beta-adrenergic antagonists in massive overdose may cause severe bronchospasm in normal individuals.**

False.

○ **T/F: Cardioselective beta-blockers avoid precipitation of bronchospasm in asthmatic individuals.**

False.

○ **What is the therapeutic drug of choice for beta-blocker-induced bronchospasm?**

Inhaled ipratropium bromide.

○ **What is the pulmonary lesion associated with overdosage of phenothiazine?**

Non-cardiogenic pulmonary edema.

○ **What drugs are associated with bronchospasm?**

Salicylates, NSAIDs, beta-blockers, protamine, contrast media, neuromuscular blocking agents and interleukin-2.

EXERCISE TESTING AND PRE-OP TESTING

"I have of late - but wherefore I know not -
lost all my mirth, foregone all custom of exercises"
Hamlet, Shakespeare

○ **What is the physiologic limiting factor in a normal adult, exercising at his maximal capacity?**

The cardiac output. At that point, the lungs, if normal, should not be functioning at more than 60% of their maximal capacity (expressed as minute O_2 consumption).

○ **What preoperative arterial blood gas value implies an increased risk of respiratory insufficiency following pulmonary resection?**

PCO2 > 45 torr.

○ **T/F: A preoperative maximal voluntary ventilation (MVV) of < 50% predicted has no impact on the decision to proceed with a pulmonary resection.**

False. It implies an increased risk of postoperative respiratory insufficiency.

○ **T/F: A 60 year old patient with a preoperative FEV_1 of 1.6 l and a pulmonary ventilation-perfusion scan showing 60% function from the left lung is at increased risk of postoperative respiratory insufficiency following left pneumonectomy.**

True. The calculated postoperative FEV_1 is < 0.8 l implying an increased risk of respiratory insufficiency.

○ **T/F: A patient with a preoperative maximal voluntary ventilation of 75% predicted, a normal arterial blood gas and an FEV_1 of 1.7 l requires no further evaluation prior to pulmonary resection.**

False. Patients with a preoperative FEV_1 < 2.0 l should undergo a preoperative ventilation - perfusion lung scan to ensure that the intended pulmonary resection will not result in a postoperative FEV_1 < 0.8 l.

○ **Does incentive spirometry prevent post-operative pulmonary function abnormalities?**

No. However, complications are reduced.

○ **What are the common pulmonary complications after upper abdominal surgery?**

Atelectasis, bronchitis, cough, pneumonia, pleural effusion and respiratory failure.

○ **Are pulmonary complications reduced after laparoscopic cholecystectomy compared to standard cholecystectomy?**

Yes, pulmonary function abnormalities are also reduced.

○ **What studies best predict the risk of post-operative pulmonary complications?**

Arterial blood gases and spirometry. CO2 retention, FEV1 less than 70% of predicted, FVC less than 70% of predicted and MVV less than 50% of predicted indicate high risk.

○   **Is regional anesthesia preferred in patients with COPD?**

No.

○   **Is cessation of smoking 24 hours pre-operatively beneficial?**

Yes, by reduction in pulse, blood pressure and carboxyhemoglobin level.

○   **What is the pre-operative therapy for patients with COPD?**

Bronchodilators, hydration, chest physiotherapy/incentive spirometry and antibiotics if sputum is purulent. For maximum benefit, smoking cessation 4 to 8 weeks prior to surgery (if possible).

○   **Which produces more hypoxemia - intravenous or inhalation anesthesia?**

Inhalation.

○   **What is the purpose of the pre-operative assessment of lung function prior to pulmonary resection?**

Prediction of long term respiratory status.

○   **How is lung function assessed prior to lung resection?**

Spirometry and blood gas. If FEV1 is greater than 2L or 80% predicted of normal and pCO_2 less than 45 mmHg, then no further testing is required.

○   **What is the further assessment of patients with operable lung cancer who fail to meet the blood gas and spirometric criteria for resection?**

Quantitative lung scanning, to assess the relative contribution of each lung to overall function.

○   **What is the minimum postoperative FEV1 following resection?**

800 cc or 40% of predicted normal FEV1.

○   **What are the criteria for pulmonary resection by exercise testing?**

Maximal oxygen consumption more than 20 ml/kg/min.

○   **What is the ratio of CO_2 produced to O_2 consumed called?**

The respiratory quotient.

○   **What is the point where exercising muscle begins anaerobic metabolism?**

Anaerobic threshold (AT).

○   **What happens to $PaCO_2$ in exercise?**

Below AT it is normal. It is reduced above the AT due to the ventilatory response to lactic acidosis. In COPD, $PaCO_2$ may rise with exercise.

○   **What happens to PaO_2 in exercise?**

It is usually normal but may decrease in patients with lung disease.

○ **What is the maximal O2 consumption?**

The O2 consumption at which O2 consumption plateaus despite increased power. This is the most important measure of fitness, but may be difficult to achieve. The peak O2 consumption at maximal exercise is often used instead.

○ **What are the criteria for peak O2 consumption?**

The patient should appear tired, be near predicted maximal heart rate, or near predicted maximal minute volume. A lactate level over 8 mEq/L or a RQ over 1.15 are other criteria.

○ **How does interstitial lung disease (ILD) affect maximal work rate and O2 consumption?**

Both are reduced.

○ **What happens to minute ventilation at submaximal work rates in ILD?**

Increased due to increased dead space ventilation. Respiratory rate increases and tidal volume decreases.

○ **What happens to maximal voluntary ventilation and breathing reserve in ILD?**

Both are reduced.

○ **Do patients with ILD desaturate during exercise?**

Yes.

○ **T/F: Anaerobic threshold less than 40% in patients with COPD suggests concomitant cardiovascular disease.**

True.

○ **What is the best test of impairment in disability testing?**

Peak or maximal O2 consumption. Anaerobic threshold may also be used. If maximal consumption is less than 15 ml/kg/min, the patient is unable to do most jobs. 15 to 25 correlates with moderate work. Over 25, the patient can do most jobs.

○ **What improvements can be expected from pulmonary rehabilitation?**

Increased peak oxygen consumption and maximum work capacity, improved efficiency (decreased O2 consumption for a given task) and improved motivation.

○ **What is the most common postoperative respiratory complication?**

Atelectasis. Respiratory failure and aspiration pneumonia are other postoperative complications.

○ **What percentage of patients who have had abdominal surgery develop atelectasis?**

> 25%.

○ **Atelectasis accounts for what percentage of postoperative fevers?**

90%.

○   **Why do we care about postoperative atelectasis?**

If it persists for more than 72 hours, pneumonia may develop. Perioperative mortality rates are then 20%. Incentive spirometry is an important therapy for the prevention of atelectasis.

○   **What supplies the energy for muscle contraction?**

ATP.

○   **When oxygen transport is insufficient, 1 unit of glycogen is metabolized to 2 pyruvates, producing 3 ATPs. This is called _____ metabolism, as oxygen is not used.**

Anaerobic. The pyruvate is metabolized to lactic acid, which is buffered by bicarbonate, producing CO_2.

○   **At the anaerobic threshold, pulmonary CO_2 output increases with respect to O_2 consumption, what is another name for this threshold?**

This is also called the lactate threshold as lactate rises or the bicarbonate threshold as bicarbonate decreases.

○   **In exercise, oxygen consumption and cardiac output (CO) increase. Oxygen consumption increases more, so the (a-v) O_2 difference _____.**

Increases, due to decreased mixed venous O_2. Fit subjects achieve greater increases in both oxygen consumption and CO and have a more reduced mixed venous O_2 at maximal exercise.

○   **Increased cardiac output in exercise is due to increased _____ _____ and _____ _____.**

Stroke volume (SV) and heart rate. Stroke volume increases over the lower one third of the work range, further increases in cardiac output is by rate only. Cardiac output is the cardiovascular limit to exercise.

○   **What is the O_2 pulse?**

The O_2 pulse may be thought of as the oxygen consumption per heart beat. It can be described as oxygen consumption divided by heart rate or as stroke volume x (a-v) O_2 difference. The oxygen pulse is a reflection of stroke volume.

○   **The _____ _____ is the cardiovascular limit to exercise.**

Cardiac output.

○   **The highest sustainable work rate above the anaerobic threshold is the _____ _____.**

Critical power, usually about halfway between anaerobic threshold and maximum O_2 consumption.

○   **Alveolar ventilation in exercise rises to maintain gas exchange in proportion to ____ _____ and ____ _____.**

CO_2 production and O_2 consumption. The coupling is closer to CO_2 production.

○   **What is the initial ventilatory response to increased work – an increase in respiratory rate or tidal volume?**

Tidal volume.

○   **What apparatus is used for exercise tests?**

Treadmill or cycle ergometer. The cycle is easier for most patients with lung disease.

○   **What is power?**

Work done per unit time, in watts.

○   **What is the duration of an exercise test?**

Testing is incremental, increasing power by 5 to 25 watts per minute, for about 10 minutes. The test is stopped if there is chest pain, severe dyspnea, or desaturation.

○   **At anaerobic threshold, minute ventilation and CO_2 output increase with respect to O_2 consumption. The ratio of minute ventilation to O_2 consumption rises, while the ratio of minute ventilation to CO_2 output is stable. This method of determining anaerobic threshold is the _____ _____.**

Ventilatory equivalent or ventilatory threshold.

○   **T/F: Another method of estimating the anaerobic threshold is to calculate the respiratory quotient. The anaerobic threshold is met when the respiratory quotient exceeds 1.0.**

True.

○   **The difference between the maximal voluntary ventilation (measured or calculated) and the minute volume at maximal exercise is the _____ _____.**

Breathing reserve (BR). Patients with lung disease have a low BR. At maximal exercise, they are near their maximal ventilatory volume.

○   **What is the heart rate reserve?**

The heart rate reserve (HRR) is the difference between the predicted maximum heart rate and the rate at maximal exercise.

○   **O_2 delivery is reduced in heart disease, so anaerobic threshold is _____.**

Reduced. Anaerobic metabolism begins at lower work loads. Either AT or maximal O_2 consumption can be used to classify severity of heart disease.

○   **What is the normal AT (anaerobic threshold)?**

50-60% of predicted maximum O_2 consumption. Less than 40% implies circulatory impairment or deconditioning.

○   **How are heart rate and O_2 consumption related?**

Linearly. Cardiac patients may have a high rate for a given load, resulting in a left shifted heart rate - O_2 consumption relation.

○   **What does the O_2 pulse reflect?**

Stroke volume. O_2 pulse is reduced in cardiac disease.

○   **Why is a peak O_2 consumption less than 10 ml/kg/min an indication for heart transplant?**

When due to cardiac disease, this level shows severe impairment and predicts poor survival without intervention. Levels more than 20 indicate minimal functional impairment.

○   **What is the usual reason for an ILD patient to discontinue an exercise test?**

Dyspnea.

○   **ILD patients may have an increased heart rate and reduced stroke volume for a task. What happens to the O_2 pulse in such circumstances?**

It decreases.

○   **What are the clinical uses of cardio-pulmonary exercise testing in lung disease?**

Evaluation of dyspnea and exercise limitation, assess severity, response to therapy, disability evaluation and oxygen titration.

○   **What happens to maximal work rate and oxygen consumption in COPD?**

It decreases. This pattern is common to COPD, ILD, cardiac disease and the unfit.

○   **What happens to maximum heart rate in COPD?**

It is normal or reduced. The heart rate for submaximal work is increased but maximum rate achieved is often lower than predicted.

○   **What happens to the oxygen saturation during exercise in patients with COPD?**

It increases, decreases, or remains unchanged.

○   **T/F: In patients with COPD, breathing reserve is reduced and heart rate reserve is usually increased.**

True. This is generally true in chronic lung disease. Cardiac patients have a normal breathing reserve and reduced heart rate reserve.

○   **Why does the ratio of dead space to tidal volume (VD/VT) decrease in exercise in normal individuals?**

Because of increased tidal volume and recruitment of pulmonary capillaries. Anatomic dead space does not change, so increasing tidal volume decreases the proportion of dead space ventilation. Recruitment of pulmonary capillaries decreases physiologic dead space.

○   **What happens to VD/VT during exercise in patients with lung disease?**

It increases. Unlike normals and patients with cardiac disease in whom it decreases.

○   **Does pulmonary rehabilitation improve spirometry and blood gases?**

No.

○   **What are the components of a training program (the exercise prescription)?**

An exercise, which the patient can perform comfortably, 3 to 4 times weekly, lasting 20 to 30, minutes at a time and achieving a target heart rate.

○   **What is the target heart rate?**

Normally about 60% of the maximal heart rate.

○ **What is the effect of general anesthesia on lung function?**

A 20% decrease in functional residual capacity.

○ **What is the average reduction in vital capacity after upper abdominal surgery?**

50%.

○ **What is the postoperative FEV_1 (predicted) from quantitative lung scanning?**

Post-op FEV_1 (predicted) = Pre-op FEV_1 x % of function in lung (or segments) remaining after resection.

EXTRAPULMONARY CAUSES OF LUNG CONDITIONS

"I come not, friends, to steal away your hearts"
Julius Caesar, Shakespeare

○ **What is the differential diagnosis of pulmonary edema with a normal size heart?**

Constrictive pericarditis, massive MI, non-cardiogenic pulmonary edema and mitral stenosis (not mitral regurgitation).

○ **T/F: Most episodes of transfusion associated acute lung injury (TRALI) are caused by donor antibodies reacting with recipient neutrophil or HLA antigens.**

True.

○ **What are the pulmonary manifestations of polycythemia?**

Pulmonary vascular sludging related to hyperviscosity and pulmonary hemorrhage related to an increased bleeding tendency.

○ **What is the differential diagnosis of pulmonary infiltrates in patients with hematological malignancies?**

Infections, treatment related (radiation, chemotherapy), hemorrhage, malignant infiltration and hyperleukocytosis.

○ **What is pseudohypoxemia?**

Hypoxemia from consumption of oxygen by cells in blood during transport, as can occur with hyperleukocytosis.

○ **What is acute chest syndrome in sickle cell lung disease?**

Fever, chest pain, leukocytosis and pulmonary infiltrates. The major dilemma is in distinguishing infarction from pneumonia. Fat embolism is a less common cause.

○ **What is sickle cell chronic lung disease?**

It is thought to be the result of years of uncontrolled and often asymptomatic sickling and is characterized by pulmonary hypertension, cor pulmonale and ventilatory defects.

○ **What is the most common cause of pneumonia in sickle cell disease?**

Streptococcus pneumoniae.

○ **What are the preventive measures commonly employed in sickle cell disease?**

Pneumococcal vaccine, Hemophilus influenza b vaccine and yearly influenza vaccine.

○ **What are the pulmonary manifestations of pancreatitis?**

Hypoxemia with normal CXR, ARDS and pleural effusions.

125

○   **Contrast acute versus chronic effusions associated with pancreatitis.**

Acute: occur when abdominal symptoms are present and dominate, the effusion is small to moderate.
Chronic: may occur when abdominal symptoms have resolved, chest symptoms predominate and the effusion is large. It may be due to a fistula from the pancreas to the pleural space.

○   **What are the pulmonary manifestations of primary biliary cirrhosis?**

Interstitial pulmonary fibrosis (rare), chest wall deformity due to osteopenia and Sjogren's syndrome.

○   **What are the pulmonary manifestations of cirrhosis?**

Hypoxemia (due to V/Q mismatching and microvascular shunting), pleural effusions (transudative, usually right sided, usually associated with ascites), reduction in static lung volumes due to ascites and pulmonary hypertension.

○   **Approximately how many patients with chronic cough have gastroesophageal reflux?**

20%.

○   **What are the pulmonary manifestations of chronic renal disease?**

Pulmonary edema, pleural effusions, uremic pleuritis, metastatic calcifications, urinothorax, pO_2 reduction during hemodialysis and atelectasis associated with peritoneal dialysis.

○   **What is the mechanism for pO_2 reduction during hemodialysis?**

The primary mechanism is hypoventilation resulting from less CO_2 production associated with the oxidation of acetate. Secondarily, complement is activated resulting in leukocyte and platelet aggregation, which alters V/Q.

○   **What are the pulmonary manifestations of sickle cell disease?**

Acute chest syndrome, bacterial pneumonia, cor pulmonale, upper airway obstruction, reduction in DLCO, reduced static lung volumes and a right shifted oxygen dissociation curve.

○   **What is the mechanism for the acute chest syndrome?**

Microvascular occlusion by sickle cells resulting in alveolar wall destruction and subsequent fibrosis.

○   **What is the treatment for a severe case of acute chest syndrome?**

Exchange transfusion.

○   **What are the common pathogens causing pneumonia in sickle cell patients?**

S. Pneumoniae, H. Influenzae, alpha-hemolytic streptococcus and salmonella.

○   **What is the hyperleukocytic syndrome?**

Vascular occlusion due to high numbers of circulating leukemic cells. Pulmonary manifestations include hypoxemia, dyspnea, infiltrates and fever in the absence of infection. The treatment is emergent leukapheresis.

○   **What are the pulmonary manifestations of Hodgkin's disease?**

Parenchymal infiltration by tumor cells, infection (due to immunocompromised state), radiation pneumonitis, lung cancer after radiation therapy and drug toxicity from agents as bleomycin.

○ **What is the cutoff for platelets before lung biopsy can be performed?**

50,000 or more platelets for biopsy.

○ **What are the pulmonary manifestations of multiple myeloma?**

Pleural effusion (malignant from direct involvement and benign from amyloid heart disease), weak respiratory muscles, extrapleural mass from rib lesion, pneumonia with encapsulated organisms, infiltrative parenchymal disease, extramedullary plasmacytoma involving the lung parenchyma, diffuse amyloidosis, airway mass (usually supralaryngeal) and amyloidosis of the tongue.

○ **What are the pulmonary manifestations of amyloidosis?**

Tracheobronchial submucosal amyloidosis (discrete or diffuse), nodular or diffuse parenchymal involvement and pleural effusion.

○ **What are the pulmonary function changes seen with cardiac disease?**

Reduction in static lung volumes and DLCO. A decrease in FEV1/FVC is seen in acute heart failure.

○ **What is the normal PCO2 in pregnancy?**

30-34 mmHg from chronic mild hyperventilation, presumably as a result of progesterone.

○ **What is the predominant change in the lung volumes in pregnancy?**

Decrease in functional residual capacity by as much as 15-25%.

○ **T/F: In pregnacy, the elevated diaphragm depresses tidal breathing.**

False. The tidal volume actually increases and accounts for much of the increased minute ventilation and mild respiratory alkalosis.

○ **T/F: The decreased functional residual capacity results in early airway closure in pregnancy.**

False.

○ **Why is the incidence of thromboembolism increased in pregnancy?**

Venous stasis from uterine pressure on the inferior vena cava, increase in clotting factors, increased fibrinogen and decreased fibrinolysis.

○ **What are some of the risk factors for thromboembolism in pregnancy?**

Ceasarian section, multiparity, bed rest, obesity, increased maternal age and surgical procedures.

○ **What are the predisposing factors for amniotic fluid embolism?**

Older maternal age, multiparity, Ceasarian section, amniotomy and insertion of intrauterine fetal monitoring devices.

○ **How does amniotic fluid enter the maternal circulation?**

Through uterine tears, injury, or endocervical veins.

○   **What are the major consequences of amniotic fluid embolism?**

Cardiorespiratory collapse and DIC.

○   **What are the potential mechanisms of cardiorespiratory collapse?**

Mechanical obstruction of pulmonary vasculature, alveolar capillary leak, pulmonary edema from LV failure and anaphylaxis.

○   **How is amniotic fluid embolism diagnosed?**

By demonstrating fetal squames in the sputum or buffy coat preparations of blood and by pulmonary microvascular cytology of blood drawn from the distal lumen of a PA catheter.

○   **What is the treatment for amniotic fluid embolism?**

Supportive.

○   **What is the mortality rate in amniotic fluid embolism?**

About 80%.

○   **What is the classic presentation of a venous air embolism?**

Sudden hypotension with a mill wheel murmur audible over the precordium.

○   **What factors in pregnancy increase the risk of aspiration of gastric contents?**

Increased intragastric pressure from the gravid uterus, progesterone induced relaxation of the lower esophageal sphincter, delayed gastric emptying in labor and depressed mental status from analgesia.

○   **What is the role of prophylactic antibiotics for aspiration in pregnancy?**

None.

○   **What is the general outcome of asthma in pregnancy?**

Generally good, similar to non-pregnant patients. The course of asthma in pregnancy may be the same, worse or better.

○   **What are some of the common misconceptions about the management of asthma during pregnancy?**

That dyspnea is common in pregnancy and that medications should be sparsely used.

○   **Should immunotherapy be used in pregnant asthmatics?**

Immunotherapy may be continued if felt to be useful but should not be initiated during pregnancy.

○   **T/F: An arterial PCO2 of 35 mmHg does not represent severe asthma.**

False. This may represent pseudonormalization since there is chronic mild hyperventilation in pregnancy.

○   **What is the pulmonary complication of tocolytic therapy?**

Tocolytic induced pulmonary edema.

O   **Which agents are associated with this syndrome?**

Terbutaline, ritadrine and magnesium sulfate.

O   **What are some of the proposed mechanisms for tocolytic induced pulmonary edema?**

Fluid overload, myocardial toxicity, reduced oncotic pressure and increased capillary permeability.

O   **What is the therapy for this syndrome?**

Stop the tocolytics and supportive care.

O   **What factors should be taken into account during intubation in pregnancy?**

Upper airway hyperemia may require a smaller endotracheal tube and the decreased FRC may lower oxygen reserve. Therefore, patients should be adequately preoxygenated with 100% followed by a quick apnea time during intubation.

O   **What anticoagulant is safe in pregnancy?**

Heparin. Warfarin is contraindicated.

O   **Can influenza vaccine be used in pregnancy?**

Yes.

O   **What antituberculous drugs should be avoided in pregnancy?**

Streptomycin and ethionamide.

O   **T/F: Therapy of active tuberculosis in pregnancy should be postponed until after** delivery.

False.

O   **What adjunctive therapy for chronic cough could precipitate thyroid storm?**

SSKI.

O   **What is the most common location of ectopic parathyroids?**

The mediastinum.

O   **What is the mechanism of alveolar hypoventilation (manifested by high PCO2) in myxedema?**

Depression of the hypoxic and hypercapnic respiratory drive. Respiratory muscle myopathy and phrenic neuropathy are uncommon.

O   **Compare and contrast primary and secondary myxedema.**

	Primary	Secondary
Source	Thyroid	Pituitary
Frequency	Common (95%)	Uncommon (5%)
Heart	Big	Small
TSH	High	Low
Iodine	< 2µg/dL	> 2µg/dL
Coarse voice	Yes	No
Goiter	Yes	No
Pubic hair	Yes	No

○   **T/F: All individuals with chronic unexplained alveolar hypoventilation should be tested for hypothyroidism.**

True.

○   **Is obstructive sleep apnea common in hypothyroidism?**

Yes. Contributing factors include enlarged tongue and myopathy. Hypothyroidism should be excluded in most patients with sleep apnea.

○   **What other endocrine disorder is associated with an increased frequency of sleep apnea?**

Acromegaly. Sleep apnea may be central or obstructive in origin.

○   **Can beta-adrenergic agonists result in tolerance?**

Yes. Repeated administration of beta agonist bronchodilators can result in hyposensitization of the receptors but this should not preclude their use. Glucocorticoids have been shown to restore the depressed receptor responsiveness.

○   **Prior steroid administration can precipitate adrenal insufficiency under conditions of stress. How long can this effect last?**

Up to one year.

○   **What pulmonary infection is a common cause of adrenal insufficiency, especially in third world countries?**

Tuberculosis.

○   **What is the common mechanism of hyponatremia in pulmonary tumors and infections?**

Syndrome of inappropriate anti-diuretic hormone production (SIADH).

○   **What type of lung cancer is commonly associated with hypercalcemia?**

Squamous cell carcinoma. The production of parathormone related peptide can produce hypercalcemia even without bony metastases.

○   **What non-neoplastic pulmonary disease is often associated with hypercalcemia and hypercalciuria?**

Sarcoidosis.

○ **What type of lung tumors can cause excessive ACTH production and Cushing's syndrome?**

Small cell carcinoma and carcinoid tumors.

○ **What are the neuroendocrine tumors of the lung?**

Typical carcinoid, atypical carcinoid and small cell carcinoma.

○ **T/F: Carcinoid syndrome is common with pulmonary carcinoid.**

False. It is rare, with incidence ranging from 2 to 7%.

○ **Does diabetes predispose to the development of pulmonary tuberculosis?**

Yes, especially when poorly controlled.

○ **In thyroid carcinoma, what factors favor metastasis to the lung?**

Follicular subtype, inadequate treatment of the primary and cervical lymph node involvement.

○ **What are the pulmonary manifestations in Paget's Disease?**

High output cardiac failure with pulmonary edema, impaired respiratory control from bony involvement at the base of the skull, vertebral fractures leading to kyphosis and restrictive lung disease.

○ **What type of pneumonia is often associated with cold agglutinins?**

Mycoplasma pneumoniae.

○ **What hypercoagulable states predispose to thrombosis and pulmonary embolism.**

Deficiencies of protein C, protein S and antithrombin III; factor V mutation; antiphospholipid syndrome; malignancy particularly adenocarcinoma; nephrotic syndrome; protein losing enteropathy; extensive burns; paroxysmal nocturnal hemoglobinuria; and oral contraceptives.

○ **What interstitial lung diseases are associated with diabetes insipidus?**

Eosinophilic granuloma or histiocytosis X.

○ **What factors increase the bleeding complications after transbronchial lung biopsy?**

Renal failure, hemorrhagic diathesis, amyloidosis, bronchiectasis and pulmonary hypertension.

○ **What are the most common causes of acute pancreatitis?**

Alcohol and gallstones.

○ **Mention some other causes of pancreatitis.**

Surgery, trauma, ERCP, viral and mycoplasma infections, hypertriglyceridemia, vasculitis, drugs, penetrating peptic ulcer, anatomic abnormalities near the ampulla of Vater, hyperparathyroidism, end stage renal disease, organ transplantation and idiopathic.

○ **What drugs are known to cause pancreatitis.**

Sulfonamides, estrogens, tetracyclines, pentamidine, azathioprine, thiazides, furosemide and valproic acid.

O   **What is the pathological spectrum in acute pancreatitis?**

Edematous pancreatitis (mild cases) and necrotizing pancreatitis (severe cases). Hemorrhagic pancreatitis may evolve from either of them.

O   **What are the septic complications of pancreatitis?**

Pancreatic abscess, infected pseudocyst and infected fluid collections.

O   **What pleuropulmonary abnormalities may be seen in pancreatitis?**

Elevated hemidiaphragm, atelectasis, pleural reaction or effusion, hypoxemia and acute lung injury including ARDS.

O   **What is the nature of pleural fluid in pancreatitis?**

It is an exudate with high amylase levels.

O   **T/F: Pleuropulmonary complications in pancreatitis indicate severe disease.**

True.

O   **What is the mortality rate for patients with pancreatitis who require mechanical ventilation?**

About 75%

O   **Deep tendon reflexes are usually maintained in which of the following diseases: myasthenia gravis, Guillain-Barr, or Eaton-Lambert syndrome?**

Myasthenia gravis. Reflexes are usually depressed in Eaton-Lambert syndrome and absent in Guillain-Barr.

O   **A patient presents with ocular, bulbar and limb weakness that worsens during the day and decreases with rest. What is the most likely diagnosis?**

Myasthenia gravis.

O   **What is the most common cause of thoracic outlet syndrome?**

A cervical rib.

O   **Which cervical nerves innervate the diaphragm?**

C3 to C5.

O   **What are the causes of phrenic nerve injury?**

Cardiac surgery, trauma, cervical osteoarthritis, tumors, herpes zoster, vasculitis and diabetes.

O   **What is the most common presentation of unilateral diaphragmatic paralysis?**

It is often asymptomatic or with mild dyspnea. In patients with lung disease, the symptoms are more severe.

○ **How does bilateral diaphragmatic paralysis present?**

With significant dyspnea that is worse in the supine position.

○ **How is unilateral diaphragmatic paralysis diagnosed?**

Usually with a sniff test under ultrasonic or fluoroscopic observation.

○ **How is bilateral diaphragmatic paralysis diagnosed?**

The sniff test is difficult, as there is no good side to compare to. PFTs in sitting and supine position show a large difference in the two positions.

○ **How is diaphragmatic paralysis treated?**

Usually unilateral involvement requires no treatment. Bilateral paralysis can be treated with mechanical ventilatory support (e.g., BiPAP, rocking bed, or negative pressure ventilation).

○ **In low cervical and upper thoracic spinal injuries, the diaphragm is intact. What occurs to the cough mechanism?**

It is decreased because the expiratory muscles are innervated below C8.

○ **What diffuse neuromuscular diseases can cause respiratory muscle weakness and are acute in onset?**

Myasthenia gravis, Eaton-Lambert syndrome, organophosphate poisoning, botulism and aminoglycosides toxicity.

○ **What diffuse neuromuscular diseases can cause respiratory muscle weakness and are gradual in onset?**

ALS, muscular dystrophies and myopathies (e.g., alcohol and diabetes).

○ **What measurements should be assessed in these patients?**

Vital capacity and inspiratory and expiratory maximal pressures.

○ **When is electrophrenic nerve stimulation useful?**

When the lesion does not involve either the phrenic nerve or the diaphragm.

○ **Which conditions can cause respiratory distress because of repeated ineffective contractions of all the respiratory muscles?**

Status epilepticus, tetanus and strychnine poisoning.

○ **What is kyphosis and scoliosis?**

Kyphosis refers to anteroposterior angulation of the spine. Scoliosis describes the lateral displacement of the spine.

○ **How many Cobb angle degrees define severe kyphoscoliosis?**

Greater than 100 degrees.

○ **What are the complications of severe kyphoscoliosis?**

Respiratory failure, hypoxemia and cor pulmonale.

○   **T/F: Severe kyphoscoliosis can be treated with BiPAP.**

True.

○   **T/F: Respiratory muscle weakness is a contributor to the development of respiratory failure in kyphoscoliosis.**

True.

○   **What are the pulmonary manifestations of ankylosing spondylitis?**

Chronic inflammation which causes fibrosis and ossification of the ligaments of the spine, sacroiliac joint and ribs. This limits rib cage expansion. A minority of patients will develop fibrobullous disease of the upper lobes. These bullae may become infected with aspergillus or atypical mycobacteria.

○   **What is a flail chest?**

When a segment of the thoracic cage becomes anatomically and functionally separated from the rest of the cage. It is caused by double fractures of 3 or more contiguous ribs, most often due to blunt trauma. The flail segment moves outward when the rest of the chest moves inward.

○   **What is the major cause of hypoxemia in patients with flail chest?**

Pulmonary contusion.

○   **How is flail chest treated?**

Analgesics and ventilatory support when respiratory failure occurs. The use of stabilizing devices is controversial.

○   **What is pectus excavatum?**

The sternum is depressed, resulting in exercise intolerance and mild reductions in static lung volumes.

○   **What is the physiology of chest wall disorders.**

These are extraparenchymal restrictive ventilatory defects.

○   **What is the primary pulmonary function abnormality associated with severe scoliosis?**

Curvatures above 60 degrees are usually associated with significant restrictive lung disease. The decreased flow rates are mostly proportional to the limited lung volumes and not due to obstruction. Patients with curvatures above 90 degrees are at risk of cardiorespiratory failure.

HYPERSENSITIVITY PNEUMONITIS

"Go thrust him out at gates and let him smell
His way to Dover"
King Lear, Shakespeare

○ **How many hours after an acute exposure to an antigen may a patient develop the signs and symptoms of hypersensitivity pneumonitis?**

Four to six hours.

○ **What is the most common misdiagnosis given to patients with hypersensitivity pneumonitis?**

Bacterial or viral pneumonia.

○ **The chronic form of hypersensitivity pneumonitis usually presents with gradual onset of symptoms including?**

Cough, dyspnea, malaise, weakness and weight loss.

○ **Most of the etiological agents associated with hypersensitivity pneumonitis are secondary to occupational exposure. Farmer's lung disease is secondary to what organism?**

Thermophilic actinomyces such as Micropolyspora faeni or Thermoactinomyces vulgaris.

○ **Bagassosis is secondary to what organisms?**

Thermophilic actinomyces sacchari or vulgaris.

○ **What occupation is bagassosis seen in?**

Sugarcane workers.

○ **Moldy composts contaminated with thermophilic actinomyces can cause what syndrome?**

Mushroom worker's disease.

○ **Moldy cork contaminated with Penicillium species can cause what syndrome?**

Suberosis.

○ **Malt worker's lung is secondary to what organism?**

Aspergillus clavatus contaminated barley.

○ **Which organism is responsible for Maple bark disease?**

Maple logs contaminated with Cryptostroma corticale.

○ **Which organism causes Wood pulp worker's disease?**

Wood pulp contaminated with Alternaria species.

O   **Contaminated humidifiers, dehumidifiers and air conditioning cooling systems can result in humidifier lung when contaminated by which organisms?**

Thermophilic actinomyces, Penicillium species, Cephalosporium species and Amebae.

O   **Bacillus subtilis can contaminate detergents.   What disease can it cause?**

Detergent worker's disease.

O   **By what mechanism do the reactive simple chemicals such as TDI (Toluene diisocyanate) and TMA (Trimellitic anhydride) cause hypersensitivity pneumonitis?**

Binding to proteins and altering the protein that induces the reaction.

O   **What is the size of the spores released from actinomyces?**

Smaller than six microns.

O   **What organism is the most important source of antigen from moldy hay?**

Micropolyspora faeni.

O   **What is the most common tissue reaction seen in hypersensitivity pneumonitis?**

An alveolar and interstitial inflammation with marked predominance of lymphocytes.

O   **What is a common pathologic feature of most cases of hypersensitivity pneumonitis?**

Macrophages with foamy cytoplasm.

O   **Airway obstruction that can be seen on pulmonary function testing is thought to be secondary to what condition?**

Obstructive bronchiolitis.

O   **The non-caseating granuloma seen in hypersensitivity pneumonitis may mimic those seen in what disease?**

Sarcoidosis.

O   **Which portion of the lung is affected with advanced disease interstitial fibrosis?**

The upper zones of the lung field.

O   **Less than 10% of the exposed workers to a particular antigen will develop disease. This suggests there is an HLA susceptibility to developing the disease. Which HLA antigens are associated with hypersensitivity pneumonitis?**

None have been demonstrated.

O   **What are the usual levels of IgE and eosinophils in patients with hypersensitivity pneumonitis?**

Within normal limits.

○ **What do precipitating antibodies seen in patients with hypersensitivity pneumonitis suggest?**

Exposure to an antigen.

○ **What happens to most patients with precipitating antibodies and continued exposure?**

They do not develop the disease.

○ **What are the complement levels in patients who have hypersensitivity pneumonitis?**

Normal.

○ **What type of immune reaction does hypersensitivity pneumonitis probably represent?**

Type four Gel and Coombs hypersensitivity reaction.

○ **Asymptomatic patients that are exposed to antigens responsible for hypersensitivity pneumonitis may be found to have what on their lavage specimens?**

An increase in lymphocytes.

○ **What are the three clinical forms of hypersensitivity pneumonitis?**

Acute, subacute and chronic.

○ **The manifestations of hypersensitivity pneumonitis and which form it presents as is dependent on what features?**

The intensity and frequency of exposure to the antigen.

○ **Large amounts of antigen over a short period of time with intermittent exposure usually results in which form of the disease?**

Acute disease.

○ **Continuous exposure to very low levels of antigen over prolonged periods of time probably results in which type of disease?**

Subacute disease.

○ **What form of disease results from exposure over long periods of time?**

Chronic irreversible disease.

○ **What are the symptoms seen in acute hypersensitivity pneumonitis which occur four to six hours after antigen exposure?**

Fever, chills, dyspnea and malaise.

○ **What physical findings are seen in acute hypersensitivity pneumonitis?**

Fever, pulmonary crackles and possibly cyanosis.

○ **What is the most common physical abnormality in subacute disease?**

Diffuse rales or crackles.

○   **In which fashion do the symptoms in the subacute form develop?**

With an insidious onset.

○   **What are the chest x-ray findings in hypersensitivity pneumonitis?**

Non-specific and variable.

○   **Where are the infiltrates in hypersensitivity pneumonitis?**

Usually bilaterally and equally distributed (involving the upper lobes).

○   **What is the chest x-ray finding in the early stages of the disease?**

It is often within normal limits.

○   **What is the chest x-ray finding in chronic disease?**

Diffuse interstitial fibrosis.

○   **Pulmonary function tests during an acute attack usually show what changes in lung volumes and vital capacity?**

Usually lung volumes and vital capacity are decreased.

○   **What is the usual pulmonary function pattern seen in chronic disease?**

Restrictive.

○   **When should you suspect the diagnosis of hypersensitivity pneumonitis?**

In those patients with respiratory symptoms and restrictive lung disease.

○   **What is the key to the diagnosis of hypersensitivity pneumonitis?**

The establishment of a relationship between exposure to an antigen and the development of symptoms.

○   **90% of the patients with Farmer's lung have precipitating antibodies against what organism?**

Thermophilic actinomyces.

○   **What percentage of pigeon breeders are expected to have precipitant antibodies with or without hypersensitivity pneumonitis?**

40% of pigeon breeders will develop precipitants against birds without evidence of lung disease.

○   **Although there is no correlation between having precipitating antibodies and symptoms there is a certain relationship noted in patients who have active disease.   What is this relationship?**

Patients with active disease have significantly higher antibody titers against the antigens.

○   **What is the drawback to using Ouchterlony double diffusion analysis to determine immuno-precipitants?**

It is relatively insensitive.

○   **T/F: Skin tests are helpful in diagnosing hypersensitivity pneumonitis.**

False. Positive skin tests are seen even in asymptomatic individuals.

○   **If you suspect a patient is having hypersensitivity pneumonitis and decide to naturally challenge the patient by re-exposing them to the area that their symptoms occurred in, you should follow their clinical parameters, laboratory parameters and pulmonary function tests closely for what period of time?**

24 hours.

○   **Under which circumstances should intentional laboratory inhalation challenge be performed?**

Only by those who have a specialized laboratory and resuscitation equipment available.

○   **What is the only method to prove a direct relationship between a suspected offending agent and disease process?**

Controlled laboratory challenge.

○   **T/F: Challenge materials can cause false positives in controlled laboratory challenges.**

True, if they contain endotoxins or other irritants.

○   **What may occur after controlled laboratory challenge?**

Severe acute pneumonic process that might permanently damage the patient or even lead to fatality.

○   **What is the predominate cell type found in bronchoalveolar lavage (BAL) sampling during a challenge test?**

The CD8 positive suppressor cell.

○   **Very early after challenge a patient with hypersensitivity pneumonitis may present with a predominance of what cell type?**

Neutrophils.

○   **After prolonged avoidance from the antigen that caused hypersensitivity pneumonitis, the bronchoalveolar lavage may return to what ratio of CD4:CD8 cells?**

The ratio may return to a CD4 predominant cell type.

○   **What is the IgG:albumin ratio in patients with hypersensitivity pneumonitis?**

Significantly elevated.

○   **People exposed to bacteria or animal protein that cause hypersensitivity pneumonitis and are asymptomatic may have what predominance of cell type on their lavage?**

Lymphocytes of the CD8 type.

○   **Unlike in hypersensitivity pneumonitis, what is the predominant cell type in sarcoidosis?**

CD4 positive lymphocytes.

O   **The manifestations of hypersensitivity pneumonitis are modulated by what factors?**

The extent and degree of exposure to the inhaled organic dust antigen.

O   **What levels may asymptomatic healthy farmers regularly exposed to organic dust antigen be elevated?**

The bronchoalveolar lavage may have elevated levels of albumin, fibronectin, angiotensin converting enzyme and lymphocytes.

O   **What may healthy farmers exposed to organic dust antigens exhibit?**

Subclinical lymphocytic alveolitis.

O   **What is the key therapeutic goal in patients with hypersensitivity pneumonitis?**

To recognize the offending agent and eliminate it.

O   **In industries in which actinomyces spores may be present, what activities can reduce exposure to workers?**

Wetting the composts or other agents prior to working may decrease the aerosol of the actinomyces spore.

O   **What inhibits the growth of the actinomyces organisms?**

A non-toxic 1% solution of propionic acid.

O   **To reduce the occurrence of humidifier lung, what techniques can be used to decrease the growth of thermophilic organisms?**

Frequent cleaning and changing of the water in humidifiers.

O   **What would be a proper approach for a patient with hypersensitivity pneumonitis if the antigen cannot be identified or avoided?**

Remove the patient from the work environment.

O   **What is a treatment for a mild and acute episode of hypersensitivity pneumonitis?**

Removal from the environment.

O   **What is the treatment for severe acute attacks?**

Corticosteroid therapy at 60 mg per day.

O   **How long should prednisone be administered in patients with acute hypersensitivity pneumonitis?**

The dose of predisone should be continued until there is significant clinical improvement, clearing of the x-ray and return of the pulmonary function tests to normal.

O   **How long is the usual course of steroids?**

Four to eight weeks.

○   **What is the main cause of respiratory disability in patients with hypersensitivity pneumonitis?**

Pulmonary fibrosis.

○   **Do all patients who have hypersensitivity pneumonitis and are exposed to antigen progress to chronic lung disease?**

No, a sub-population may have continued exposure without decompensation or progression of their lung disease.

○   **What organisms cause Sequoiosis?**

Graphium and Pullularia species.

○   **What is the cause of epoxy resin lung?**

Phthalic anhydride.

○   **What causes MDI hypersensitivity pneumonitis?**

Diphenylmethane diisocyanate.

○   **Wheat weevils (Sitophilus granarius) can cause which hypersensitivity pneumonitis?**

Miller's lung.

○   **What is the etiology of pituitary snuff takers lung?**

Bovine and porcine proteins in pituitary powder.

○   **What causes laboratory worker's hypersensitivity pneumonitis?**

Male rat urine.

○   **What organism causes paprika splitters lung?**

Mucor stolonifer.

○   **What causes familial hypersensitivity pneumonitis?**

Bacillus subtilis growing on wood in walls.

○   **What is the source of Japanese summer-type hypersensitivity pneumonitis (Trichosporon cutaneum)?**

Contaminated home environments.

○   **Basements contaminated with sewage can cause what type of hypersensitivity pneumonitis?**

Cephalosporium hypersensitivity pneumonitis.

○   **Sauna taker's disease is caused by what organism?**

Pullularia species.

○   **Which organism in contaminated fertilizer may cause hypersensitivity pneumonitis?**

Streptomyces albus.

O   **What disease is caused by dried grasses and leaves contaminated with Saccharomonospora viridis?**

Thatched roof disease.

O   **Rhizopus and Mucor growing on wood can cause what disease?**

Wood trimmer's disease.

O   **Cheesemakers can develop hypersensitivity pneumonitis because of what organism?**

Penicillium species (that grew on cheese casings).

O   **What is the etiology of Soybean Worker's lung disease?**

Soybean hulls.

O   **Bacteria and fungi growing in aerosolized metal working fluid can cause what disease?**

Machine operator's lung.

O   **What is the best way to diagnose hypersensitivity pneumonitis?**

A good environmental and occupational history.

O   **What cell type is most commonly isolated in hypersensitivity pneumonitis?**

CD8 positive lymphocytes.

O   **What is the classic x-ray finding in hypersensitivity pneumonitis?**

Reticular nodular pattern.

O   **The differential on a blood sample during an acute episode of hypersensitivity pneumonitis will demonstrate an increase in which cells?**

Neutrophils.

O   **What is the classic PFT abnormality in hypersensitivity pneumonitis?**

A restrictive pattern.

O   **What will the DLCO be in hypersensitivity pneumonitis?**

Reduced.

O   **What is the most sensitive test for hypersensitivity pneumonitis?**

Exercise stress test for oxygen desaturation.

O   **Which medications cause drug induced hypersensitivity pneumonitis?**

Amiodarone, gold and procarbazine

○   **Describe the histological picture of advanced chronic hypersensitivity pneumonitis?**

Extensive fibrosis involving alveolar walls and peribronchial tissues. Many alveolar spaces are completely obliterated.

○   **Can the number of lymphocytes on BAL distinguish between asymptomatic, exposed patients and patients with hypersensitivity pneumonitis?**

No, both may have increased lymphocytes with CD8>CD4 cells.

○   **When should hypersensitivity pneumonitis be considered?**

In patients with unexplained pulmonary symptoms or interstitial lung disease.

○   **Evidence supports which type of immune mediated reaction as key in hypersensitivity pneumonitis?**

Cell mediated hypersensitivity.

○   **T/F: High resolution CT scan is diagnostic of hypersensitivity pneumonitis.**

False. No pathognomic CT features have been described.

○   **Symptoms of acute hypersensitivity pneumonitis are expected to resolve how long after an isolated acute exposure?**

A few days.

○   **What is another name for hypersensitivity pneumonitis?**

Extrinsic allergic alveolitis.

INFECTIOUS DISEASES

"Poor worm, thou art infected"
The Tempest, Shakespeare

❍   **What pulmonary fungal infection grows in soil, is endemic to the Mississippi River basin and rarely results in symptoms?**

Histoplasmosis.

❍   **What fungus is endemic to the deserts of the southwestern United States, produces a granulomatous tissue reaction and can cause the triad of pneumonitis, erythema nodosum and arthralgias known as "valley fever"?**

Coccidioidomycosis.

❍   **What ubiquitous protozoan is responsible for a diffuse interstitial pneumonitis in immunocompromised patients?**

Pneumocystis carinii.

❍   **What is the standard therapy for a lung abscess?**

Systemic antibiotics. Bronchoscopy may be necessary to remove any foreign body and to exclude endobronchial tumor or obstruction.

❍   **Which microaerophillic bacterium can produce lung abscesses and sinus tracts that drain yellow-brown material resembling sulfur granules?**

Actinomycosis.

❍   **What fungus has a propensity to colonize a pre-existing pulmonary cavity?**

Aspergillus.

❍   **What are the current indications for surgical resection of pulmonary tuberculosis?**

Persistent or recurrent infection despite adequate multi-drug therapy, massive or recurrent, severe hemoptysis, inability to exclude carcinoma and bronchopleural fistula unresponsive to tube thoracostomy.

❍   **Among patients with cystic fibrosis, what bacteria are seen with increased frequency as causes of pneumonia?**

Pseudomonas aeruginosa and Staphylococcus aureus.

❍   **What is the most common cause of community-acquired pneumonia among alcoholic patients?**

Streptococcus pneumoniae.

❍   **Which other bacteria are seen with increased frequency as causes of pneumonia among alcoholic patients?**

Klebsiella pneumoniae and Hemophilus influenzae.

O   **What pathophysiologic process is suggested by infiltrates in the right upper lobe or the apical segment of the lower lobe?**

Aspiration.

O   **The number of epithelial cells seen on microscopic examination of sputum smears is indicative of the presence or absence of significant contamination of the specimen with oral secretions. How many epithelial cells per high power field are considered indicative of such contamination?**

Ten or more.

O   **What degree of leukocytosis is considered a risk factor for poor outcome among patients with bacterial pneumonia?**

Greater than 30,000 cells/cubic mm.

O   **What lower limit of leukocyte count portends an unfavorable prognosis in bacterial pneumonia?**

Less than 4,000 cells/cubic mm.

O   **What bacteria are associated with pneumonia following influenza?**

Streptococcus pneumoniae, Staphylococcus pneumoniae and Hemophilus influenzae.

O   **What is the leading identifiable cause of acute community-acquired pneumonia in adults?**

Streptococcus pneumoniae.

O   **In addition to Streptococcus pneumoniae, what other bacteria are associated with acute lobar pneumonia in adults?**

Hemophilus influenzae, Staphylococcus aureus, Klebsiella pneumoniae and Streptococcus pyogenes.

O   **How long before elective splenectomy should pneumococcal vaccine be administered in order to achieve an adequate antibody response?**

Two weeks or more.

O   **What two underlying medical conditions are associated with Hemophilus influenzae pneumonia?**

Chronic obstructive lung disease and HIV infection.

O   **What is the treatment of choice (antibiotic and dose) for Legionella pneumonia?**

Erythromycin, one gram intravenously every six hours.

O   **What three stains may be used to identify Legionella organisms on sputum smear?**

Modified acid fast stain, Dieterle silver stain and direct fluorescent antibody stain.

O   **T/F: The pneumococcal vaccine may be given simultaneously with influenza vaccine.**

True.

❍ **How many of the more than 80 antigenic capsular types of Streptococcus pneumoniae are included in the current pneumococcal vaccine?**

23.

❍ **At what age should pneumococcal vaccine be administered among healthy adults with no comorbid condition?**

65 or greater.

❍ **T/F: Patients who received the prior 14-valent vaccine should be given the 23-valent vaccine now available.**

True.

❍ **Are any extrapulmonary manifestations specific for the diagnosis of Legionnaire's disease?**

No.

❍ **What category of bacteria is most important in community-acquired aspiration pneumonia?**

Anaerobes.

❍ **What category of bacteria is most important in hospital-acquired aspiration pneumonia?**

Gram negative bacilli and Staphylococcus aureus.

❍ **What is the antibiotic of choice for patients with community-acquired aspiration pneumonia?**

Clindamycin.

❍ **What antibiotic has been consistently effective against highly penicillin-resistant Streptococcus pneumoniae?**

Vancomycin.

❍ **T/F: Infection with penicillin-resistant Streptococcus pneumoniae can be recognized on clinical grounds.**

False.

❍ **T/F: The pneumococcal vaccine is equally effective against penicillin-resistant and penicillin-sensitive strains of Streptococcus pneumoniae.**

True.

❍ **What is the most important risk factor for Moraxella catarrhalis pneumonia?**

Chronic obstructive lung disease.

❍ **T/F: Penicillin is effective in this treatment of pneumonia due to Moraxella catarrhalis.**

False.

○   **What two new macrolide antibiotics offer broad coverage of the following common causes of community-acquired pneumonia: Streptococcus pneumoniae, Hemophilus influenzae, Legionella pneumophila, Moraxella catarrhalis and Mycoplasma pneumoniae?**

Azithromycin and clarithromycin.

○   **What common type of community-acquired pneumonia is typically spread by aspiration of microdroplets from common water supplies?**

Legionnaire's disease.

○   **What is the most common etiologic agent of atypical pneumonia?**

Mycoplasma pneumoniae.

○   **What is considered to be the second most common cause of atypical pneumonia?**

Chlamydia pneumoniae.

○   **T/F: Mycoplasma pneumoniae is commonly spread by person-to-person contact.**

True.

○   **T/F: Single antibiotic therapy is typically effective in the treatment of Klebsiella pneumoniae pneumonia.**

True.

○   **What is the common cause of community-acquired bacterial pneumonia among patients with HIV?**

Streptococcus pneumoniae.

○   **What other forms of bacterial pneumonia appear to occur with increased frequency among patients infected with HIV?**

Hemophilus influenzae and Pseudomonas aeruginosa.

○   **What three roentgenographic findings are associated with a poor outcome in patients with pneumonia?**

Multiple lobe involvement, pleural effusion and cavitation.

○   **What is the single most important risk factor for hospital-acquired bacterial pneumonia?**

Endotracheal intubation.

○   **What are the two most important risk factors for the development of anaerobic lung abscess?**

Poor oral hygiene and a predisposition toward aspiration.

○   **Which lung is most often the site of anaerobic lung abscess formation?**

The right lung.

○   **Which lung segments are most often the sites of lung abscess formation?**

The posterior segments of the upper lobes and superior segments of the lower lobes.

○ **What are the characteristic findings on sputum gram stain in cases of anaerobic lung abscess?**

Numerous polymorphonuclear cells and both gram-positive and gram-negative bacteria of various morphologies.

○ **What is the antibiotic of choice for the treatment of anaerobic lung abscess.**

Clindamycin.

○ **What anaerobic respiratory infection is associated with slowly enlarging pulmonary infiltrates, pleural effusions, rib destruction and fistula formation?**

Actinomycosis.

○ **What are the most important anatomical defenses of the lower respiratory tract?**

The vocal cords and epiglottis.

○ **What are the indications for drainage of a pleural effusion associated with pneumonia?**

Positive gram stain or culture, presence of gross pus, pleural fluid glucose less than 40 mg/dl or fluid pH of less than 7.0.

○ **What pathological process is suggested by an air-fluid level in the pleural space?**

A bronchopleural fistula.

○ **What is the definition of nosocomial pneumonia?**

Pneumonia occurring in patients who have been hospitalized for at least 72 hours.

○ **What are the two most important routes of transmission of nosocomial bacterial pneumonia?**

Person-to-person transmission via healthcare workers and contaminated ventilator tubing.

○ **How may stress ulcer prophylaxis in ICU patients contribute to the development of nosocomial pneumonia?**

By raising the gastric pH and increasing bacterial colonization rates.

○ **What agent used for the prevention of stress ulcers in ICU patients is associated**

with the lowest risk of nosocomial pneumonia?

Sucralfate.

○ **T/F: Anaerobic lung infections do not occur in edentulous patients.**

False.

○ **Hematogenous embolization from a septic jugular thrombophlebitis is a rare cause of anaerobic lung infection. What is the organism?**

Fusobacterium necrophorum (Lemiere's syndrome).

○ **What are the most common bacterial genera known to cause anaerobic lung infections?**

Peptostreptococcus, fusobacterium and bacteroides.

○ **When should bronchoscopy be used in the setting of a lung abcess?**

In atypical presentations, failure to respond to therapy or in situations where there is no apparent risk factor for aspiration.

○ **Which gram-negative aerobes are known to cause lung abscess?**

Pseudomonas and klebsiella.

○ **T/F: The presence of a cuffed endotracheal tube makes aspiration pneumonia an unlikely cause of new pulmonary infiltrates.**

False.

○ **With aspiration pneumonias manifesting as lobar infiltrates, which are the most common sites?**

The superior segments of the lower lobes and posterior segments of the upper lobes.

○ **What is the drug of choice for pneumonias acquired in the outpatient setting due to anaerobic bacteria?**

Clindamycin.

○ **What are the predominant organisms that complicate aspiration in a hospital setting?**

S. aureus, E. coli, Ps. aeruginosa, Klebsiella, or Proteus.

○ **Why is clindamycin superior to penicillin in the treatment of anaerobic lung abcess?**

The presence of penicillin-resistant Bacteroides melaninogenicus.

○ **What factor determines the magnitude of injury in gastric acid aspiration?**

The gastric pH. A pH of less than 2.5 produces the most severe injury.

○ **Empyema in the absence of a parenchymal lung infiltrate suggests what underlying process?**

Subphrenic or other intra-abdominal abscess.

○ **What is the incidence of Bacteroides fragilis in anaerobic lung infections?**

5 to 7%.

○ **What is the recommended duration of antibiotic therapy for necrotizing anaerobic pneumonia, lung abcess, or empyema?**

4 to 8 weeks.

○ **T/F: Nasogastric and gastric tubes increase the risk of aspiration.**

True.

○   **T/F: Healthy individuals may aspirate small amounts of oral contents without developing clinical complications.**

True.

○   **What determines the likelihood of pulmonary complications from aspiration?**

Frequency of aspiration, volume of aspirate and character of aspirate.

○   **Currant jelly sputum is indicative of what kind of pneumonia?**

Klebsiella. Currant jelly stools are associated with intussusception.

○   **What are the most common causes of Staphylococcal pneumonias?**

Drug use and endocarditis. This pneumonia produces high fever, chills and a purulent productive cough.

○   **A 23 year-old male presents with a dry cough, malaise, fever and a sore throat that developed in the past two weeks. What is the most likely diagnosis?**

Mycoplasma pneumonia. This condition usually has a slow onset and occurs in the young. Treat the patient with erythromycin or tetracycline.

○   **What are the extrapulmonary manifestations of mycoplasma?**

Erythema multiforme, pericarditis, GI and CNS disease.

○   **A 67 year-old alcoholic was found in an alley, covered in his own vomit and beer.   Upon examination, he is shaking, has a fever of 103.5° F and is coughing up currant jelly sputum. What is the most likely diagnosis?**

Pneumonia induced by Klebsiella pneumoniae. This is a likely etiology in alcoholics, the elderly, the very young and immunocompromised patients. Other gram-negative bacteria, such as E. coli and other Enterobacteriaceae, may cause pneumonia in alcoholics who have aspirated.

○   **A 46-year-old smoker comes to your office bragging about a three day business convention he attended last week in Las Vegas. He is nauseated and coughing, has chills, and a fever of 103. 5° F and his pulse is 68. Should you be concerned about your own health, as he has just given a mighty cough in your direction?**

No. This patient probably has Legionnaires' disease. Unless you attended the same convention in Las Vegas, you are unlikely to catch pneumonia from him. Legionella pneumophila contaminates the water in air conditioning towers and moist soil. It is not easily transmitted from person to person.

○   **Match the pneumonia with the treatment.**

1) Klebsiella pneumoniae   a) Erythromycin, azithromycin, or doxycycline
2) Streptococcal pneumoniae   b) Penicillin G
3) Legionella pneumophila   c) Cefuroxime
4) Haemophilus influenza   d) Erythromycin and rifampin
5) Mycoplasma species

Answers: (1) c, (2) b, (3) d, (4) c and (5) a.

○   **What are the classic chest x-ray findings in a patient with mycoplasma pneumonia.**

Patchy diffuse densities involving the entire lung. Pneumatoceles, cavities, abscesses and pleural effusions can occur but are uncommon.

○   **What is the classic chest x-ray finding associated with Legionella pneumonia.**

Dense consolidation and bulging fissures. Expect elevated liver enzymes and hypophosphatemia. Patients with Legionella pneumonia classically present with a relative bradycardia.

○   **A 43 year-old male presents with pleurisy, sudden onset of fever and chills and rust colored sputum. What is the most likely diagnosis?**

Pneumococcal pneumonia caused by Streptococcus pneumoniae, the most common community-acquired pneumonia. It is a consolidating lobar pneumonia and can be treated with penicillin G (if not resistant) or erythromycin.

○   **A 20 year old college student is home for winter break and presents complaining of a 10-day history of a non-productive dry hacking cough, malaise, a mild fever and no chills. What is the most likely diagnosis?**

Mycoplasma pneumoniae, also known as walking pneumonia. Although this is one of the most common pneumonias that develops in teenagers and young adults, it is an atypical pneumonia and most frequently occurs in close contact populations, i.e., schools and military barracks.

○   **A 56 year-old smoker with COPD presents with chills, fever, green sputum and extreme shortness of breath. An x-ray shows a right lower lobe pneumonia. What is expected from the sputum culture?**

Haemophilus influenza. This organism is generally found in pneumonia and bronchitis patients with COPD. The two other common organisms in COPD patients are Streptococcus pneumoniae and Moraxella catarrhalis. Ampicillin/clavulanate (Augmentin) is the drug of choice.

○   **Describe the different presentations of bacterial and viral pneumonia.**

Bacterial pneumonia is typified by a sudden onset of symptoms, including pleurisy, fever, chills, productive cough, tachypnea and tachycardia. The most common bacterial pneumonia is Streptococcus pneumoniae.
Viral pneumonia is characterized by gradual onset of symptoms, general malaise and a non-productive cough.

○   **What two antimicrobial agents are broadly effective against organisms that cause both typical and atypical pneumonias?**

Azithromycin and clarithromycin.

○   **What percentage of upper-respiratory infectious agents are non-bacterial?**

Over 90% of pharyngitis, laryngitis, tracheobronchitis and bronchitis.

○   **What two anti-viral medications are useful for viral pneumonia.**

Amantadine, for influenza A and aerosolized ribavirin, for RSV.

○   **If a patient has a patchy infiltrate on chest x-ray and bullous myringitis, what antibiotic should be prescribed?**

Erythromycin for mycoplasma.

O **What secondary bacterial infection often occurs following a viral pneumonia?**

Staphylococcal pneumonia.

O **What three findings should be present to consider a sputum sample adequate?**

1. 25 PMN's
2. < 10 squamous epithelial cells per low-powered field
3. A predominant bacterial organism

O **In what season does Legionella pneumonia most commonly occur?**

Summer. Legionella pneumophila thrive in environments such as the water cooling towers that are used in large buildings and hotels. Staphylococcal pneumonias also occur more frequently in summer.

O **An older patient with GI symptoms, hyponatremia and a relative bradycardia probably has which type of pneumonia?**

Legionella.

O **T/F: Steroids should be used in aspiration pneumonia.**

False.

O **The initial therapy for PCP includes which antibiotics?**

Trimethoprim-sulfamethoxazole (Bactrim) or pentamidine.

O **What other medication should be prescribed to a patient with PCP?**

Corticosteroids, when the pO_2 is < 70 mmHg or an A-a gradient > 35 mmHg.

O **T/F: The flora of lung abscesses are usually polymicrobial.**
True.

O **What percentage of people in the Ohio and the Mississippi valleys are infected with histoplasmosis?**

100% in endemic areas. However, only 1% of these individuals develop the active disease. The spores of H. capsulatum can remain active for 10 years. For unknown reasons, bird and bat feces promote the growth of the actual fungus. The disease is transmitted when the spores are released and inhaled.

O **Hantavirus occurs most commonly in what geographic location?**

Southwestern US, especially in areas with deer mice.

O **Which organisms are most commonly associated with acute exacerbations of bronchitis in smokers?**

S. pneumoniae, H. influenzae and M. catarrhalis.

O **Where in the US is coccidioidomycosis most prevalent?**

The Southwest.

○　**Which populations are predisposed to progressive infection with coccidioidomycosis?**

African Americans and diabetics.

○　**What common nosocomial respiratory pathogens would not be adequately covered by second generation cephalosporins?**

Methicillin-resistant Staphylococcus aureus, enterococcus and highly resistant gram negative bacilli.

○　**History of contact with mammals and /or birds may suggest infection by what organisms?**

Coxiella burnetii (Q fever), Brucella species, or Chlamydia psittaci.

○　**A nosocomial cluster of cases postoperatively may be caused by what organisms?**

Legionella species or mycobacterium species.

○　**What causes Q fever?**

Coxiella burnetii, also known as Rickettsia burnetii. It is found in the Dermacentor tick.

○　**What signs indicate an HIV positive patient is at increased risk for opportunistic infections like PCP?**

An absolute CD-4 count of less than 200 and a CD-4 lymphocytic percentage of less than 20.

○　**What types of pneumonia are often contracted during the summer months?**

Staphylococcal and legionella pneumonia.

○　**What are the classic symptoms of TB?**

Night sweats, fever, weight loss, malaise, cough and greenish yellow sputum most commonly seen in the mornings.

○　**Describe the skin lesions associated with a Pseudomonas aeruginosa infection.**

Pale, erythematous lesions, 1 cm in size, with an ulcerated necrotic center.

○　**A patient with AIDS presents with a grayish-white plaque on the lateral borders of her tongue that does not scrape off. What is the most likely diagnosis?**

Hairy leukoplakia.

○　**Where are Kaposi's sarcoma lesions found?**

Everywhere—inside and out. They typically occur on the face, neck, arms, back, thighs and in the lungs, lymphatic system and GI system.

○　**Staphylococcal pneumonia frequently develops pleural effusion or empyema. Which lung is most frequently involved?**

The right lung is involved in 65% of the cases. 80% of these pneumonias are unilateral. 25% of the patients will go on to develop pyopneumothorax.

○　**What is the most important risk factor for Moraxella catarrhalis pneumonia?**

Chronic obstructive lung disease.

O   **Contrast pneumonia due to Mycoplasma sp. with pneumonia due to Streptococcal pneumoniae.**

	S. pneumoniae	M. pneumoniae
Prodrome	Little	Mild fever, malaise, cough, HA
Onset	Rapid	Gradual
Severe respiratory symptoms	Tachypnea, cough, occasional pleuritic pain	Little
Associated findings	High fever	Exanthem, arthritis, GI complaints, neurologic complications
Pleural effusion	Occasional	Rare
Lab	Leukocytosis	WBC normal or slight elevation
Treatment	Penicillin	Erythromycin

O   **What organisms are most commonly responsible for overwhelming postsplenectomy sepsis?**

Encapsulated organisms: pneumococcal (50%), meningococcal (12%), E. coli (11%), H. influenza (8%), staphylococcal (8%), and streptococcal (7%).

O   **A patient presents with fever and shoulder pain 4 days following a splenectomy. What is the most probable postoperative complication?**

Subphrenic abscess. This condition can cause fever as well as irritation to the diaphragm and to the branch of the phrenic nerve that innervates it.

O   **What is the most common infectious disease complication of measles and influenza?**

Pneumococcal pneumonia.

O   **What is the most common complication of AIDS?**

Pneumocystis carinii pneumonia (PCP). Kaposi's sarcoma is the second most common.

O   **Patients with HIV infections, who go on to develop AIDS, are most commonly infected with what organisms?**

Pneumocystis carinii, cytomegalovirus, candida, aspergillus, nocardia, cryptococcus and mycobacteria.

O   **Adults with sickle cell disease are most commonly affected with what organisms?**

Streptococcus pneumoniae, Haemophilus influenzae B and Mycoplasma pneumoniae.

O   **How is the diagnosis of histoplasmosis made?**

By culture or staining from sputum, bronchoalveolar lavage or tissue and by a positive serology.

O   **How is the diagnosis of coccidiomycosis made?**

By culture or staining of sputum, bronchoalveolar lavage or tissue and by a positive serology.

O   **How does one diagnose invasive aspergillosis?**

By biopsy.

O **What is the evaluation of foreign body in the lung?**

Chest x-ray and bronchoscopy.

O **What is the evaluation for candida of the lung?**

Fresh sputum or transtracheal aspirate should reveal yeast and pseudohyphae. Mycelia and blastospores will be seen in established colonization, so a tissue exam is needed for definitive proof.

O **What are some of the most convenient ways to make the diagnosis of Mycoplasma pneumonia?**

The gold standard for diagnosis is a 4 fold rise in the complement fixation titer between the acute and convalescent sera. A single titer of 1:128 or greater for either cold agglutinins or the complement fixation antibody in the right clinical setting is highly suggestive of active disease.

O **What are the most common causes of non-infectious stomatitis?**

Behcet's syndrome, Stevens-Johnson syndrome, cancer chemotherapy and Kawasaki syndrome.

O **What infectious agents are associated with erythema nodosum?**

Group A streptococcus, meningococcus, syphilis, Mycobacterium tuberculosis and Mycobacterium leprae, as well as histoplasmosis, coccidiomycosis, blastomycosis and herpes simplex virus.

O **In a patient with a chest x-ray typical of tuberculosis, the PPD is negative. A repeat PPD after two weeks is still negative. A panel of skin tests is placed and all of them prove to be positive. Does this rule out tuberculosis as a cause of the chest x-ray abnormality?**

No. Patients with tuberculosis can be selectively anergic. If TB is suspected, one must continue to maintain a high index of suspicion for that disease. Other more aggressive approaches will need to be taken to prove the diagnosis such as gastric washings, or if the patient's condition warrants, bronchoscopy or lung biopsy.

O **A patient from the Philippines has a hypo-pigmented patch that is lacking in sensation. What is the most likely cause of his problem?**

Leprosy (Mycobacterium leprae).

O **What is the most feared complication of infection in the retropharyngeal space?**

Mediastinitis.

O **What fascial space is involved in Ludwig's angina?**

The submandibular space.

O **What is the most common origin of infection in patients with Ludwig's angina?**

Dental abscesses.

O **What are the most common local findings in patients with Ludwig's angina.**

Swelling of the floor of the mouth and tongue.

O   **What is the most common cause of death in Ludwig's angina?**

Asphyxiation.

O   **What is the most common indication for surgical drainage in patients with Ludwig's angina?**

Failure of antibiotic therapy.

O   **What are the most important organisms in Ludwig's angina?**

Oral anaerobes.

O   **What are the antibiotics of choice for Ludwig's angina?**

Penicillin and metronidazole.

O   **What are the most common presenting signs of anterior lateral pharyngeal space infections?**

Trismus, swelling at the angle of the mandible and medial bulging of the pharyngeal wall.

O   **What is the most feared complication of lateral pharyngeal space infections?**

Septic thrombophlebitis of the jugular vein.

O   **What are the most common findings on lateral neck x-ray in patients with a retropharyngeal abscess?**

Prevertebral soft tissue widening, air-fluid levels and loss of cervical lordosis.

O   **What is the imaging modality of choice for the diagnosis of septic thrombophlebitis of the jugular vein?**

Computed tomography with contrast.

O   **What is Lemierre's syndrome?**

Septic thrombophlebitis of the internal jugular vein with septic pulmonary emboli associated with anaerobic oropharyngeal infection.

O   **What are the most common bacterial causes of acute sinusitis?**

Pneumococcus and Hemophilus influenzae.

O   **What is the most important risk factor for malignant external otitis?**

Diabetes mellitus.

O   **What is the most common bacterial cause of malignant external otitis?**

Pseudomonas aeruginosa.

O   **What is the most characteristic physical finding associated with malignant external otitis?**

Granulation tissue in the external auditory canal.

❍   **What is the most frequent neurological complication of malignant external otitis?**

Facial nerve palsy.

❍   **What antibiotic regimen is most appropriate in the treatment of malignant external otitis?**

Broad spectrum combination therapy with activity against Pseudomonas aeruginosa continued for 4-6 weeks.

❍   **What is the most important risk factor for the development of acute bacterial parotitis?**

Dehydration.

❍   **What local physical findings are associated with acute bacterial parotitis?**

Tender swelling of the parotid and pus expressible from Stenson's duct.

❍   **What are the two most important risk factors for rhinocerebral mucormycosis?**

Neutropenia and diabetic ketoacidosis.

❍   **What local findings are most characteristic of rhinocerebral mucormycosis?**

Black nasal discharge and cranial nerve palsies.

❍   **Which antifungal agent is considered the drug of choice for rhinocerebral mucormycosis?**

Amphotericin B.

❍   **T/F: Surgical debridement is required for effective management of rhinocerebral mucormycosis.**

True.

❍   **What two other organisms may produce a clinical picture similar to that of rhinocerebral mucormycosis?**

Aspergillus and Pseudomonas aeruginosa.

❍   **What infection precedes acute orbital cellulitis in the majority of cases?**

Acute sinusitis.

❍   **What class of bacteria is most commonly isolated from brain abscesses secondary to chronic sinusitis or otitis?**

Anaerobes.

❍   **What is the most common local complaint in adults with acute epiglottitis?**

Dysphagia.

❍   **What organism is most often associated with a bacterial infection of the thyroid?**

Staphylococcus aureus.

❍   **What condition typically precedes the development of a peritonsillar abscess?**

Tonsillitis.

○ **What local sign is most commonly associated with a peritonsillar abscess?**

Unilateral swelling of the soft palate.

○ **What is the preferred method of treatment for a peritonsillar abscess?**

Incision and drainage.

○ **Through what anatomical space must a peritonsillar abscess extend to involve the carotid sheath?**

The lateral pharyngeal space.

○ **What infection is associated with the "lumpy jaw" syndrome?**

Actinomycosis.

○ **What organism is most often associated with Lemierre's syndrome?**

Fusobacterium necrophorum.

○ **Which views on routine x-ray are most sensitive in the diagnosis of acute infection in the paranasal sinuses?**

The Caldwell and Waters view.

○ **What time after insertion are pulmonary artery catheters considered at high risk to be infected?**

After approximately 72 hours.

○ **What are the most common organisms involved with line infections?**

Staphylococcus epidermidis and Staphylococcus aureus.

○ **What is the etiologic agent of Pittsburgh pneumonia?**

Legionella micdadei.

○ **Of the 14 serogroups of Legionella pneumoniae, how many are detected by the urinary antigen test (EIA)?**

One (serogroup 1).

○ **What factors affect the outcome in cases of invasive aspergillosis?**

Patient characteristics associated with a poor response to treatment included persistent neutropenia, no reduction in immunosuppression, diffuse pulmonary disease, recurrent leukemia, major hemoptysis and angioinvasion seen on histological examination.

Treatment factors affecting outcome include a delay in initiating treatment, low dosages of amphotericin, very low serum levels of itraconazole and lack of secondary antifungal prophylaxis during subsequent neutropenic episodes.

Of transplant recipients, heart, lung and renal transplant patients tend to have better outcomes than bone marrow transplant and liver transplant patients. Site of infection affects outcome with cerebral aspergillosis having 99% mortality and pulmonary aspergillosis claiming an 86% mortality. Invasive rhinosinusitis, which occurred mostly in bone marrow transplant recipients and leukemics, has better outcome with crude mortality rates of 66%.

O   **Which antibiotics are recommended as adjunctive therapies in combination with macrolides (erythromycin, azithromycin, or clarithromycin) in the treatment of Legionellosis?**

Rifampin or ciprofloxacin.

O   **Which of the above antibiotics is the treatment of choice in transplant patients with Legionellosis?**

Ciprofloxacin, since both macrolides and rifampin interact pharmacologically with immunosuppressives, such as tacrolimus.

O   **Rifampin has bactericidal activity against which microorganisms?**

Besides mycobacterium tuberculosis, it is a very effective agent against both coagulase-positive and negative staphylococci. It is often used in antibiotic regimens for complications of endocarditis such as myocardial and peripheral abscesses, in conjunction with surgical drainage. Rifampin is also effective treatment for many other gram-positive organisms and some gram-negatives, most notoriously as prophylactic therapy after exposure to Neisseria meningitidis. It is even more active against Legionella than erythromycin and is commonly used as an adjunctive treatment. Unfortunately, bacteria rapidly develop resistance to rifampin. Thus, with the exception of short-term prophylactic treatment protocols, rifampin's use is limited to adjunctive treatment.

O   **Which drugs have shown promise in the treatment of Mycobacterium avium complex (MAC) infections?**

MAC has traditionally been a frustrating disease to treat, due to its resistance to the standard, first-line antimycobacterial agents, such as isoniazid and rifampin. Newer regimens, including various combinations of clarithromycin or azithromycin, rifabutin, streptomycin and ethambutol have higher response rates than before.

O   **What adverse reactions should you be alert for when using dapsone as salvage therapy for pneumocystis carinii pneumonia?**

Dapsone produces dose-dependent hemolysis which is ordinarily of an insignificant degree except in patients with glucose 6-phosphate dehydrogenase deficiency. Patients should be screened for this disorder prior to initiating treatment. Rash is fairly common and usually well tolerated. Bone marrow suppression and mild hyperkalemia is occasionally seen. Methemoglobinemia is very common during treatment with dapsone. Guidelines for discontinuing treatment, other than lack of response after four days of treatment, include rash intolerable to the patient or involving mucous membranes and a methemoglobin level of greater than 20%.

O   **What is the differential diagnosis of extreme hyperthermia?**

Fevers greater than 106 degrees Fahrenheit (extreme pyrexia) are usually not infectious in nature. Causes include heat stroke, malignant hyperthermia, hyperpyretic rigidity syndrome (neuroleptic malignant disease), HIV disease, central fevers and drug fever.

O   **What are the manifestations of chickenpox in the adult?**

Extracutaneous involvement is more common and associated with a significant increase in morbidity and mortality. Varicella pneumonia occurs in up to 1 out of 400 adult cases of chickenpox. Some cases will be manifest only by chest x-ray, typically findings being diffuse interstitial or nodular infiltrates. Cough, dyspnea, hemoptysis and respiratory failure may develop. Thrombocytopenia is common. Sputum Tzanck smear may be positive. Mortality may be as high as 30%, even in the normal host. Encephalitis, myocarditis and hepatitis may also complicate the infection. Treatment is IV acyclovir.

O   **What is reliable treatment for pneumococcal infections?**

Streptococcus pneumoniae had maintained exquisite sensitivity to penicillin for decades. In the past few years, there has been an increasing incidence of intermediate penicillin resistance as well as the emergence of strains with multiple drug resistance. In a recent series, 57% of isolates in Spain were found to be drug-resistant. Resistance is less of a problem in the United States, but has been shown to be increasing. The mechanism for intermediate penicillin resistance is related to a mutation that results in a higher concentration of penicillin being necessary to saturate the penicillin-binding proteins of the bacteria.

Multiple-drug resistance appears to occur via transfer of genetic material from other species of bacteria. Many strains are resistant to penicillin, erythromycin, sulfa drugs, cephalosporins and tetracycline. This can be quite problematic, especially in the treatment of meningitis, where antibiotic selection is also limited by a drug's ability to obtain sufficient concentrations in the CSF. At the present time, the drug-resistant strains are still susceptible to vancomycin and at least in vitro to chloramphenicol.

O   **What are the classic chest x-ray findings of Klebsiella pneumonia?**

Lobar pneumonia with the "bulging fissure" sign. Patients are often alcoholics or have other underlying chronic disease and may produce "currant-jelly" sputum.

O   **What is the significance of a retropharyngeal infection and how is it diagnosed?**

The retropharynx is bounded by the pharynx anteriorly and the spine posteriorly. Between the retropharyngeal space and the prevertebral space in the "danger space" which extends to the base of the skull and to the diaphragm via the posterior mediastinum. The retropharyngeal space may become infected via penetrating injuries or contiguous spread of infection from the lateral pharyngeal space, which can result from tonsillitis, parotitis, mastoiditis and odontogenic infections.

Retropharyngeal space infection may result in acute mediastinitis and result in a fulminant infection with a high mortality rate. Meningitis and pericarditis are other potential complications. Respiratory distress may occur due to compression of the supraglottic structures.

O   **What patients are at increased risk for developing sternal wound infections and mediastinitis after cardiac surgery?**

Patients at increased risk include diabetics, those with bilateral inferior mammary takedowns, reoperations and patients with a low cardiac output state.

O   **What are the clinical findings and treatment for sternal wound infections?**

Symptoms usually are manifest a week or more postoperatively and include fever, drainage, inability to wean from mechanical ventilation and an unstable sternum. Responsible microorganisms are predominately Staphylococcus aureus, Staphylococcus epidermidis, Pseudomonas species and Enterobacteriaceae. Sternal wound infections are commonly managed with operative debridement and muscle flaps.

O   **How does a subphrenic abscess present?**

They usually follow surgery for a ruptured viscus, cholecystitis, or penetrating abdominal wound. Patients may complain of right upper quadrant or shoulder pain in addition to fever and chills. Subphrenic abscesses occur far more commonly on the right. The chest x-ray typically reveals an elevated hemidiaphragm and may show a pleural effusion, or an air/fluid level below the diaphragm in more advanced cases. CT or ultrasound is diagnostic. US or CT-guided drainage is successful in many patients.

O   **What is the clinical presentation of influenza?**

Influenza is responsible for taking approximately 10,000 lives per year, with 80 – 90% of the deaths in patients greater than 65 years of age. Patients present with the abrupt onset of fever and chills, myalgia, fatigue, headache and cough. Elderly patients may present with fever and confusion.

O   **What is the treatment for influenza?**

Amantadine or rimantidine should ideally be initiated within 48 to 72 hours from the onset of symptoms. Complicating bacterial pneumonias are common, especially Streptococcal pneumoniae and Staphylococcus aureus and need to be specifically treated as well.

O   **What laboratory findings are typical in patients with hantavirus pulmonary syndrome?**

Elevated hematocrits are commonly seen in these patients due to pronounced endothelial dysfunction and capillary leak that results in the patients literally drowning in the extravasated fluid. Thrombocytopenia is seen in over 75% of patients. Dramatically elevated serum LDH is often present. Diagnosis is confirmed by Western Blot or polymerase chain reaction.

O   **What mechanism is felt to be responsible for the association of aminoglycoside and muscle weakness?**

Aminoglycosides can prevent calcium uptake into the presynaptic membrane at the neuromuscular junction which can inhibit acetylcholine release. They also can blunt the effects of acetylcholine at the postsynaptic membrane.

The likelihood of muscle weakness is increased in patients who have received neuromuscular blockers, in patients who have muscle disorders, or are hypocalcemic or hypomagnesemic. Calcium channel blockers may also potentiate this effect.

O   **How is "ventilator associated pneumonia" diagnosed?**

Clinical signs that are ordinarily suggestive of pneumonia, including the presence of fever, elevated white blood cell count, worsening oxygenation, progression of pulmonary infiltrates and presence of organisms on sputum culture, are unreliable markers for the diagnosis of ventilator associated pneumonia.

The First International Consensus Conference on Clinical Investigation of ventilator-associated Pneumonia recommended bacterial counts of 10 to the fourth cfu per ml as a criteria to distinguish colonization from infection with bronchoalveolar lavage (BAL) samples. The specificity of BAL samples, however have been somewhat inferior to protected specimen brushing (PSB) in most studies. Bacterial growth of greater than 10 to the third cfu per ml on quantitative culture has been recommended as the criteria of significance for PSB.

Recovery of greater than 1% squamous epithelial cells in a centrifuged BAL sample was an accurate prediction of contamination with oropharyngeal secretions. Neutrophil predominance in BAL samples is present with pneumonia but is not a specific finding. The Consensus Conference recommended the combination of PSB and BAL as the most accurate diagnostic technique. These tests, however, are often confounded when the patient is already on antibiotic treatment.

O   **What adverse reactions may be seen with amphotericin infusion?**

Release of tumor necrosis factor has been postulated to cause the fever, rigors and a drop in blood pressure commonly seen with administration of Amphotericin B. Hypotension occurs more frequently and is often more pronounced in the debilitated patients, especially in the early stages of treatment. This is the reason why a 1mg test dose is given by some practitioners prior to proceeding with a full daily treatment dose. True allergic reactions to Amphotericin B are felt to be uncommon.

O   **What is an effective method to clean one's stethoscope?**

Isopropyl alcohol swabs significantly reduces bacterial loads on the stethoscope. Soap and water are ineffective.

○ **What is the likelihood of a positive bronchoalveolar lavage sample for cytomegalovirus in the presence of HIV disease?**

Lavage samples frequently are culture positive for cytomegalovirus (CMV) in AIDS patients, regardless of the presence or absence of pulmonary symptomatology. CMV is uncommonly a pulmonary pathogen in this population. Those patients with significant CMV pulmonary disease almost always have extremely low CD4 counts.

○ **Why is Kaposi's sarcoma difficult to diagnose histologically?**

Large pieces of tissue are required to demonstrate the spindle-shaped cells.

○ **How is Kaposi's sarcoma diagnosed?**

Usually bronchoscopically in the correct clinical setting. Endobronchial Kaposi's appears as violaceous or bright red irregularly shaped lesions that are flat or mildly raised.

○ **What are the chest x-ray findings of cryptococcus in a patient who is HIV positive?**

Diffuse interstitial infiltrates, focal air space disease, single or multiple nodules and small pleural effusions.

○ **What are the chest x-ray findings of histoplasmosis in a patient who is HIV positve?**

Focal infiltrate with or without adenopathy, small coin lesion, diffuse micronodular infiltrate and cavitation.

○ **What is the yield of sputum induction for PCP in a patient with AIDS?**

70 to 90%.

INTERSTITIAL LUNG DISEASE

"He jests at scars that never felt a wound."
Romeo and Juliet, Shakespeare

○ **Which non-neoplastic pulmonary disease is often associated with hypercalcemia and hypercalciuria?**

Sarcoidosis.

○ **Sarcoidosis is most common in what race and age group?**

African Americans between 20 and 40 years of age.

○ **What are the classic chest x-ray findings in a patient with sarcoidosis?**

Bilateral hilar and paratracheal adenopathy with diffuse nodular appearing infiltrates. Sarcoidosis can be staged by the chest x-ray:

Stage 0:   Normal
Stage 1:   Hilar adenopathy
Stage 2:   Hilar adenopathy and parenchymal infiltrates
Stage 3:   Parenchymal infiltrates only
Stage 4:   Pulmonary fibrosis

○ **What other systems can be affected by sarcoidosis?**

The cardiovascular, gastrointestinal, immunological, integumental, lymphatics and ocular systems.

○ **What are the most common symptoms of idiopathic pulmonary fibrosis (IPF)?**

Cough and dyspnea.

○ **Which patient is least likely to have IPF: a 30 year old man, a 50 year old woman, or a 70 year old man?**

The 30 year old man. IPF is most commonly diagnosed in individuals between the ages of 40-70 years.

○ **How many patients with IPF experience symptoms for less than one year prior to diagnosis?**

Fifty percent.

○ **Approximately 60% of patients with IPF have what extremity finding?**

Clubbing.

○ **Which of the following supports the diagnosis of IPF: Age 70, woman, adenopathy, reduced total lung capacity, slowly progressive radiologic changes, or a brother with IPF.**

All of the above supports the diagnosis of IPF except adenopathy. You should think of an alternative or concurrent diagnosis.

○ **Where are opacities usually observed on chest radiographs of patients with IPF?**

In the lower lung zones and are peripheral.

O   **How often are pleural effusions noted in IPF?**

They're not. You should think of another diagnosis.

O   **What other interstitial lung diseases cause peripheral lung opacities?**

Cryptogenic organizing pneumonitis (i.e., bronchiolitis obliterans with organizing pneumonia) and eosinophilic pneumonia.

O   **What is the most common finding on pulmonary function testing in patients with IPF?**

Decreased total lung capacity.

O   **With what common conditions is obstructive airflow observed in IPF?**

Emphysema and chronic bronchitis.

O   **Which histopathology is specific for IPF: usual interstitial pneumonia or desquamative interstitial pneumonia?**

Neither. Both may be observed in patients with IPF and in many other interstitial lung diseases.

O   **What percentage of patients with IPF improve with oral corticosteroids?**

Only about 30%.

O   **What is the most important benefit a patient can be offered through lung biopsy for suspected IPF?**

Other more easily treatable interstitial lung diseases may be excluded.

O   **What type of lung biopsy is preferred for diagnosis of IPF, transbronchial biopsy or open lung biopsy?**

Open lung biopsy is preferred, as there are no specific histopathologic findings for IPF. IPF is a diagnosis of exclusion. The possibility of sampling error dictates that a larger biopsy specimen is more likely to exclude other more treatable diagnoses.

O   **T/F: A positive antinuclear antibody titer supports the diagnosis of IPF.**

False. A low ANA titer is often observed in patients with IPF, but it is nonspecific. Besides antinuclear antibodies, rheumatoid factors, circulating immune complexes and elevation of serum LDH may be observed but are nonspecific.

O   **Which is more helpful in the management of IPF: gallium scan or high resolution CT scan?**

Gallium scans have not proven useful in either diagnosis or management of IPF. High resolution CT scans are helpful in staging activity and extent of disease.

O   **An 80 year old presents with a 6 month history of progressive dyspnea and peripheral interstitial pulmonary radiographic abnormalities. She has no other collagen-vascular diseases, pleural involvement, or extrapulmonary physical exam signs. PFTs demonstrate severe restriction (decreased lung capacity). What is the next step in management?**

Some would argue this patient does not require biopsy given age, lack of collagen-vascular disease and typical physiologic abnormalities. A trial of prednisone could be given.

○ **What is the mean survival of patients diagnosed with IPF?**

Four to six years.

○ **What histopathological finding in IPF correlates with better treatment response?**

Active inflammation with a cellular infiltrate suggests a better prognosis than acellular fibrosis.

○ **What factor is associated with decreased survival in patients with IPF?**

Smoking.

○ **A 54 year old patient with IPF has been on oral prednisone (1 mg per kg) for 12 weeks and PFTs continue to deteriorate. What is the appropriate treatment?**

Azathioprine or cyclophosphamide can be added to prednisone, or can be used alone.

○ **Another 12 weeks pass and the rate of TLC deterioration has not slowed. Besides changing from azathioprine to cyclophosphamide (or vice–versa), what else should be done?**

This patient should be referred immediately for lung transplant evaluation, if receptive.

○ **A patient with IPF on steroids, previously stabilized on prednisone, begins to deteriorate over a two week period. What is the next step in management?**

Evaluate for infection and augment immunosuppression, if necessary.

○ **T/F: Bronchogenic carcinoma is more common in patients with IPF.**

True. It is fourteen times more common. Bronchogenic carcinoma accounts for approximately 10% of total mortality from IPF.

○ **What do sarcoidosis and tuberculosis have in common?**

Both are multisystem granulomatous diseases.

○ **Which of the following patients is least likely to have sarcoidosis: a 20 year old African–American woman with a cough and mediastinal adenopathy, a 35 year old Finnish woman with sore red shins and joint aches, or a 70 year old man with cough, fever and hemoptysis?**

The older gentleman is least likely to have sarcoidosis. Presentation of sarcoidosis with hemoptysis is unusual but can occur.

○ **What percentage of patients diagnosed with sarcoidosis are over 40 years old?**

Only about 25%.

○ **What percentage of patients with sarcoidosis have intrathoracic pathology at the time of diagnosis?**

90%.

○ **Other than the lymphatic system, what is the most common extrathoracic site of disease involvement in sarcoidosis?**

The liver.

○   **What percentage of patients with sarcoidosis are asymptomatic at the time of diagnosis?**

Approximately 50%.

○   **A patient of Scandinavian ancestry presents with erythema nodosum, bilateral pulmonary hilar adenopathy and polyarthritis. What is the most likely diagnosis?**

Lofgren's syndrome.

○   **In western countries, what percentage of patients die from complications of the sarcoidosis?**

Five to 10 percent.

○   **T/F: Sarcoidosis can run in families.**

True. Familial aggregation may occur but no genetic factors have been consistently confirmed.

○   **How may sarcoidosis affect the heart?**

Sarcoidosis can cause a cardiomyopathy, pericarditis, tachyarrythmias, (including sudden death) and bradyarrythmias (including complete heart block).

○   **Exposure to what periodic table element can lead to a disease process that clinically resembles sarcoidosis?**

Beryllium.

○   **Which is more common in patients with sarcoidosis, hypercalciuria or hypercalcemia?**

Hypercalciuria, which can lead to nephrocalcinosis.

○   **A 30 year old woman with a persistent cough was found to have unilateral pulmonary hilar adenopathy on chest radiograph. She is referred to you for treatment of her sarcoidosis. What is the appropriate management plan?**

Biopsy to confirm the diagnosis, as unilateral pulmonary hilar adenopathy only occurs in 5-10% of patients with sarcoidosis. Lymphoma or bronchogenic carcinoma are more likely diagnoses in this case.

○   **T/F: Angiotensin converting enzyme (ACE) levels are commonly elevated in patients with sarcoidosis and is specific for the disease.**

False. While ACE levels are elevated in 60% or more of patients with sarcoidosis, they are elevated in other unrelated disorders, including HIV infection, atypical mycobacterial disease and silicosis.

○   **What is the most common lesion of neurologic sarcoidosis?**

Cranial neuropathy.

○   **The finding of air bronchograms within lung masses strongly suggests which two diagnoses?**

Lymphoma or sarcoidosis.

○   **Which organs are spared involvement by sarcoidosis?**

None.

O **What characteristic change is noted in serum T–cell lymphocyte subsets of patients with sarcoidosis?**

The CD4/CD8 ratio is increased, as much as 10:1.

O **Transbronchial lung biopsy is the diagnostic procedure of choice in sarcoidosis patients with abnormal chest radiographs. What is the yield of transbronchial biopsies?**

60 to 90%. Better yield if biopsies are performed in regions of abnormal lung parenchyma and lower yield if only hilar adenopathy is present.

O **What percentage of patients with sarcoidosis will experience spontaneous remission of the disease?**

About 50%. This depends on the stage of disease for a given patient.

O **What is the treatment of choice for an asymptomatic patient with sarcoidosis and bilateral hilar adenopathy on chest radiograph?**

Observation.

O **What is the treatment of choice for an asymptomatic sarcoidosis patient with radiographic pulmonary opacities and normal pulmonary function tests?**

Most would say close observation, with initiation of prednisone therapy for the onset of symptoms or progressive objective deterioration of pulmonary function.

O **What is the appropriate dosing regimen for prednisone in patients with sarcoidosis?**

40 mg per day is sufficient for the average patient as induction therapy. It should be slowly tapered to 10-15 mg per day over the first two months and continued at that dose for 4-6 months before gradual withdrawal.

O **Which patients require more intensive corticosteroid therapy?**

Sarcoidosis patients with neurologic, opthalmologic, cardiac, renal and hematologic involvement require higher dose prednisone induction and longer courses, with appropriate clinical monitoring to gauge response and guide the decision to reduce dose.

O **Where are abnormalities commonly noted on chest CT of patients with sarcoidosis?**

Lung abnormalities are generally noted along the distribution of the lymphatics, mostly peribronchovascular and subpleural in location. The abnormalities can vary from small nodules to coarse reticular markings.

O **Name the anti–infective agent that may be helpful in management of dermal sarcoidosis.**

Chloroquine.

O **What percentage of patients with sarcoidosis have disease progression despite corticosteroid treatment?**

Up to 20% of patients.

O **What percentage of patients require retreatment for a relapse soon after corticosteroids are discontinued?**

Up to 75%.

O   **What is the earliest PFT abnormality in patients with IPF?**

A decreased DLCO.

O   **What is the most common symptom of hepatic sarcoid?**

Prolonged fever.

O   **Which serum electrolyte abnormality in patients with sarcoid would prompt treatment with corticosteroids?**

Hypercalcemia.

O   **In patients with sarcoidosis, what are the 3 components of uveoparotid fever or Heerfordt's Syndrome?**

Facial nerve palsy, uveitis and parotitis.

O   **Which population of T lymphocytes is increased in the BAL fluid of patients with sarcoidosis?**

CD 4 + or T helper cells.

O   **What is the typical pathologic finding on a biopsy specimen in a patient with sarcoid?**

Noncaseating granulomas.

O   **Diffuse Alveolar Hemorrhage (DAH) may be seen with which type of cardiac valvular lesion?**

Mitral stenosis.

O   **What is the renal lesion typically seen with DAH?**

Focal segmental necrotizing glomerularnephritis.

O   **What is the pattern of immunoglobulin deposition in the basement membranes of the kidneys and lungs in Goodpasture's disease?**

Linear.

O   **DAH occurs most commonly in which connective tissue disorder?**

SLE (may also complicate scleroderma, rheumatoid arthritis and mixed connective tissue disorders).

O   **Which interstitial lung disease occurs in premenopausal women and has an associated airflow obstruction and hyperinflation?**

Lymphangiomyomatosis (LAM).

O   **What chest complications of LAM may occur at the time of presentation or during the patient's course?**

Chylous pleural effusion, pneumothorax and hemoptysis.

O   **What drug that may be given orally or as an IM injection may result in prolonged periods of disease stability in patients with LAM?**

Medroxyprogesterone.

O   **An autosomal recessive disease, which in its adult form presents with hepatosplenomegaly, thrombocytopenia, anemia, long bone erosions and an elevated serum acid phosphatase, may also rarely be associated with interstitial lung disease. This disorder is caused by a deficiency in which enzyme?**

Glucocerebrosidase (Gaucher's disease). The pathologic hallmark is the Gaucher's cell which is a reticuloendothelial cell with a foamy cytoplasm.

O   **An interstitial lung disease which is pathologically identical to LAM may occur in patients who survive to adulthood and is characterized by mental retardation, adenoma sebaceum and epilepsy. What is this condition?**

Tuberous sclerosis.

O   **Bronchiolitis obliterans may occur as a complication in which type of transplants?**

Bone marrow, heart-lung and lung transplantation.

O   **Which connective tissue disorder is most associated with bronchiolitis obliterans?**

Rheumatoid arthritis.

O   **What percentage of patients with graft versus host disease (GVHD) following allogenic bone marrow transplant (BMT) develop bronchiolitis obliterans?**

10%.

O   **In patients with allogenic BMT, what are the risk factors for the development of bronchiolitis obliterans?**

Chronic GVHD and prior treatment with methotrexate (viral infection may also play a role).

O   **What are the typical pulmonary function study abnormalities in patients with BOOP?**

A restrictive pattern with a decreased DLCO.

O   **Infection with what organism is associated with pulmonary alveolar proteinosis (PAP)?**

Nocardia asteroides.

O   **The amorphous material found in the alveolar space in PAP resembles what normally occurring substance?**

Surfactant.

O   **This amorphous material stains positive (pink) with what type of stain?**
Periodic-Acid Schiff (PAS) stain.

O   **What type of cells may be seen on the BAL fluid of patients with PAP?**

Macrophages.

○   **Which two inorganic dusts have been associated with PAP?**

Silica and aluminum.

○   **What serum chemistry abnormality may be expected in PAP?**

An elevated LDH.

○   **What is the only definitively beneficial treatment for PAP?**

Whole lung lavage.

○   **Uptake on Gallium scan of the lung in a patient with PAP should suggest what?**

Superimposed infection.

○   **What interstitial lung disease is characterized by relatively preserved lung volumes radiographically, is complicated by pneumothorax and occurs more commonly in cigarette smokers?**

Eosinophilic granuloma.

○   **What percentage of patients with eosinophilic granuloma are current or former cigarette smokers?**

90%.

○   **What cell is the histopathologic hallmark of eosinophilic granuloma?**

Langerhan's histiocyte.

○   **What interstitial lung diseases may be inherited as an autosomal dominant trait?**

Familial IPF, tuberous sclerosis and neurofibromatosis.

○   **What interstitial lung diseases may be inherited as an autosomal recessive trait?**

Neimann-Pick disease, Gaucher's disease and Hermansky-Pudlack syndrome.

○   **T/F: Patients with Goodpasture's Syndrome who smoke are more likely than non-smokers to have pulmonary involvement.**

True.

○   **Spontaneous pneumothorax frequently complicates which ILDs?**

LAM and eosinophilic granuloma.

○   **Which ILDs may have increased lung volumes?**

LAM, eosinophilic granuloma, neurofibromatosis, tuberous sclerosis, chronic hypersensitivity pneumonitis and chronic sarcoidosis.

○   **What is the only CXR finding in IPF which is predictive of lung histopathology and prognosis?**

Honeycombing.

❍ **What is the major mechanism for resting hypoxemia in IPF?**

Ventilation-perfusion mismatch.

❍ **An increased percentage of what cell type on BAL in patients with IPF correlates with a better prognosis and better response to corticosteroids?**

Lymphocytes.

❍ **What is the term for the form of idiopathic pulmonary fibrosis which is characterized by a more cellular alveolar infiltrate and a better response to corticosteroids?**

Desquamative interstitial pneumonitis (DIP).

❍ **Digital clubbing may be present in patients with IPF. However, the presence of new clubbing in a patient with long standing IPF should prompt the consideration of what complication?**

Bronchogenic carcinoma.

❍ **10% of patients with IPF develop primary bronchogenic carcinoma. What cell type is most common?**

Adenocarcinoma.

❍ **An increase in which two cell populations in BAL fluid in patients with IPF is predictive of a poor response to corticosteroids?**

Polymorphonuclear leukocytes and eosinophils.

❍ **Infectious bronchiolitis in adults has been associated with what two bacterial pathogens?**

Legionella pneumophila and mycoplasma pneumoniae.

❍ **T/F: The BAL fluid from patients with PAP is usually sterile.**

True.

❍ **Which interstitial lung disease may be associated with diabetes insipidus?**

Eosinophilic granuloma or histiocytosis X.

❍ **A patient presents with cough, lethargy, dyspnea, conjunctivitis, glomerulonephritis, fever and purulent sinusitis. What is the probable diagnosis?**

Wegener's granulomatosis. This is a necrotizing vasculitis and pulmonary granulomatosis that attacks the small arteries and veins.

❍ **What serological test is diagnostic for Wegener's granulomatosis?**

c-ANCA in association with appropriate clinical evidence. A renal, lung, or sinus biopsy may also be helpful in making the diagnosis.

❍ **What are the most common causes of interstitial lung disease?**

In order: interstitial pulmonary fibrosis, collagen-vascular disease related, hypersensitivity pneumonitis, sarcoidosis, BOOP, eosinophilic granuloma and asbestosis.

○   **What interstitial lung diseases have a predilection for the upper lobes?**

Sarcoidosis, chronic hypersensitivity pneumonitis, eosinophilic granuloma, silicosis, berylliosis, ankylosing spondylitis and chronic eosinophilic pneumonia.

○   **What interstitial lung diseases cause subcutaneous calcinosis?**

Scleroderma and polymyositis-dermatomyositis.

○   **What interstitial lung diseases cause a miliary pattern on chest x-ray?**

Sarcoidosis, silicosis, eosinophilic granuloma, acute hypersensitivity pneumonitis, bronchiolitis obliterans, amyloidosis, lymphoma, breast carcinoma and hypernephroma.

○   **What interstitial lung diseases cause a neurologic abnormality?**

Sarcoidosis, lymphangitic carcinomatosis, neurofibromatosis, tuberous sclerosis, collagen-vascular disease related and Wegener's granulomatosis.

○   **What interstitial lung disease cause a granulomatous reaction?**

Sarcoidosis, hypersensitivity pneumonitis, drug reactions, talc, berylliosis and lymphomas.

○   **What is the predominate cell type in a bronchoalveolar lavage in a normal person?**

Alveolar macrophages comprise 85% or more of the cells in such a person, with the remainder being lymphocytes.

○   **What is the treatment for amiodarone-induced drug toxicity?**

The preferred treatment is discontinuation of the drug and corticosteroids. Cases have been reported in which the patient was maintained on a lower dose of amiodarone with corticosteroids.

○   **What is lymphocytic interstitial pneumonia?**

It is a diffuse infiltrate in the interstitium with lymphocytes, plasma cells and histiocytes. It usually presents with a reticulonodular appearance on CXR. Adenopathy is usually absent. It is associated with a variety of autoimmune conditions, including connective tissue diseases, primary biliary cirrhosis, Hashimoto's thyroiditis and HIV (especially in children). Occasionally it is associated with lymphoma. The treatment is steroids.

MEDIASTINUM AND SURGICAL CONSIDERATIONS

"This was the most unkindest cut of all"
Julius Caesar, Shakespeare

○   **T/F: At the level of the carina, the pulmonary arteries lie anterior to the mainstem bronchi and posterior to the aortic arch.**

True.

○   **What is the best initial method for localizing hemoptysis in a patient who is actively bleeding?**

Bronchoscopy.

○   **Which type of bronchopulmonary sequestration has a distinct pleural investment, no communication with the tracheobronchial tree, an arterial supply derived from small systemic arteries and systemic venous drainage?**

Extralobar sequestration.

○   **Which form of bronchopulmonary sequestration shares a common pleural investment with normal pulmonary tissue, derives its blood supply from a large systemic artery and may communicate with the tracheobronchial tree?**

Intralobar sequestration.

○   **Following blunt trauma to the chest, pneumomediastinum, subcutaneous emphysema and a large air leak following tube thoracostomy all imply what type of injury?**

Tracheobronchial tear or disruption.

○   **What is the definitive method for diagnosing a tracheobronchial injury?**

Bronchoscopy.

○   **The sudden onset of a continuous cough with copious serosanguinous or purulent sputum while a patient is recovering from a pneumonectomy is pathognomic for what condition?**

Postoperative bronchopleural fistula.

○   **What are the risk factors for postoperative bronchopleural fistula following pulmonary resection?**

Diabetes mellitus, malnutrition, radiation therapy, infection, inflammation or devascularization of the bronchial stump and residual tumor at the site of bronchial closure.

○   **What is the initial bedside therapy for an acute bronchopleural fistula following pneumonectomy?**

Turn the patient operated side down to prevent the aspiration of pleural fluid into the contralateral lung and perform a tube thoracostomy.

❍   **T/F: Pre-thoracotomy diagnosis of ipsilateral mediastinal lymph node metastases from non-small cell lung cancer precludes curative resection of the primary tumor.**

True. Five-year survival after resection of a stage IIIA (N2) lung cancer is less than 10% and warrants consideration of non-surgical therapy or multi-modality therapy with induction chemotherapy and radiation followed by surgical resection.

❍   **What are the possible complications of mediastinoscopy?**

Bleeding, injury to the left recurrent laryngeal nerve, esophageal perforation, pneumothorax and infection.

❍   **What is the clinical significance of ipsilateral supraclavicular lymph node metastases from non-small cell lung cancer?**

These are considered N3 nodal metastases (stage IIIB) and preclude curative resection of the primary lung tumor.

❍   **What is the etiology of Hamman's sign, a crunching sound heard with cardiac auscultation?**

Pneumomediastinum.

❍   **Through what interspace should a chest tube be inserted for treatment of a pneumothorax?**

Fourth or fifth intercostal space, mid axillary line.

❍   **What complications are seen from chest tubes placed too low on the chest wall?**

Injury to the diaphragm or abdominal viscera.

❍   **What are the indications for the surgical treatment of a spontaneous pneumothorax?**

1) Massive air leak preventing lung re-expansion, 2) air leak persisting longer than 5-7 days, 3) ipsilateral recurrence, 4) simultaneous bilateral pneumothoraces, 5) presentation with tension pneumothorax, 6) associated empyema or hemothorax and 7) lifestyle indications (airline pilot, scuba diver, resides in remote area).

❍   **What technique should be combined with bleb resection during the surgical treatment of a pneumothorax?**

Mechanical pleurodesis or pleurectomy.

❍   **What potential advantages might thoracoscopic surgery have over conventional surgical techniques in treating spontaneous pneumothoraces?**

Easier examination of all lung surfaces, less postoperative pain, shorter hospital stay and earlier return to work.

❍   **What opportunistic organism produces pneumonia with diffuse subpleural blebs in immunocompromised patients?**

Pneumocystis carinii.

❍   **What are the indications for surgical treatment of a chylothorax?**

Failure of non-operative therapy after 7 to 14 days, continued drainage of more that 1500 ml per day in adults, persistent electrolyte abnormalities and /or malnutrition.

❍   **Why can ligation of the thoracic duct at the diaphragmatic hiatus be performed without significant side effects?**

This is due to the existence of minor lymphatic - venous anastamoses between the thoracic duct system and the azygous, intercostal and lumbar veins.

○   **If during the operative treatment of a chylothorax the site of leakage cannot be identified, what definitive procedures should be performed?**

Ligation of the thoracic duct at the diaphragm.

○   **What is the most common location of the thoracic duct at the level of the diaphragm?**

It usually enters the chest via the aortic hiatus to the right of the aorta between the aorta and vertebral bodies.

○   **What technique is 90% successful in identifying the etiology of pleural effusions undiagnosed after thoracentesis and pleural biopsy?**

Thoracoscopy.

○   **What is the initial management of refractory malignant pleural effusions not relieved by chemotherapy and radiation therapy of the primary tumor?**

Thoracostomy tube drainage followed by talc or chemical pleurodesis.

○   **T/F: Most pleuroperitoneal shunts occlude soon after placement precluding successful palliation in patients with malignant pleural effusions.**

False. Occlusion of the shunt device can be a significant problem. However, most remain patent for the relatively short remainder of the patient's life.

○   **What type of pulmonary resection is most frequently associated with postoperative empyema?**

Pneumonectomy (2-12%).

○   **When is lung decortication indicated in the treatment of an empyema?**

When a residual undrained space prevents complete lung reexpansion in spite of less invasive measures of tube thoracostomy with or without fibrinolytic enzymes or thoracoscopic debridement.

○   **What is an Eloesser flap procedure?**

Open drainage of an empyema cavity.

○   **What options remain for a persistent empyema cavity that cannot be sterilized by open drainage or irrigation?**

Expansion of the lung by decortication, obliteration of the pleural space using muscle flaps or omentum, thoracoplasty, or filling of the carefully prepared pleural cavity with antibiotic solution followed by chest closure (Claggett Procedure).

○   **What compensatory measures obliterate the intrathoracic space left by pulmonary resection?**

Mediastinal shift, elevation of ipsilateral hemidiaphragm, contraction of intercostal spaces and expansion of remaining ipsilateral pulmonary parenchyma.

○ **T/F: Pleural pneumonectomy for malignant mesothelioma has been shown to increase overall patient survival when compared to chemotherapy or radiation therapy.**

False. It has been shown to increase recurrence free survival significantly longer than other therapy but has no effect on overall survival.

○ **What is the generally accepted etiology of pectus excavatum?**

Misdirected rapid growth of the lower costal cartilages in a concave manner creating a depressed sternum.

○ **What conditions are consistently associated with pectus excavatum?**

Marfan's syndrome (65%), mitral valve prolapse (40-65%) and scoliosis (21.5%).

○ **T/F: Pectus carinatum repair has been shown to significantly improve patients' pulmonary function and progressive work exercise performance.**

False.

○ **What are the two most common primary malignant tumors of the chest wall?**

Myeloma (33%) and chondrosarcoma (30%).

○ **What is the most common benign tumor of the chest wall?**

Osteochondroma.

○ **What is the most common indication for pectus carinatum repair?**

Cosmetic improvement.

○ **T/F: Following chest wall resection, skeletal defects located near the tip of scapula should always be reconstructed.**

True. To avoid entrapment of the tip of the scapula in the defect during arm movement.

○ **T/F: Skeletal defects larger that 5 cm rarely need to be reconstructed following chest wall resection.**

False. Although 5 cm defects that are covered by large posterior chest wall muscles or the scapula and do not routinely require reconstruction, defects larger than 5 cm elsewhere on the chest wall should be reconstructed to provide structural support, prevent a flail segment and improve cosmetic outcome.

○ **What are considered adequate margins when resecting a primary chest wall malignancy?**

4 cm circumferential margins of chest wall including any involved lung, pericardium, diaphragm, chest wall muscles, or skin.

○ **What are the goals of decortication in the setting of a hemothorax refractory to tube thoracostomy drainage?**

Relieve pulmonary entrapment, preserve pulmonary function and prevent empyema formation.

○ **When should decortication be considered in treating hemothorax that is refractory to chest tube drainage?**

When a significant collection persists in spite of tube thoracostomy, intrapleural fibrinolytic enzymes and thoracoscopic debridement.

○   **What are the anatomic boundaries of the mediastinum?**

1.   Superior - thoracic inlet   Posterior - vertebral bodies
2.   Inferior - diaphragm   Lateral - mediastinal pleura
3.   Anterior - sternum

○   **What is acute descending necrotizing mediastinitis?**

A necrotizing inflammatory process resulting from the extension of an oropharyngeal infection. It is often accompanied by thoracic empyema and /or acute pericarditis.

○   **When postoperative infection is excluded, what etiology is responsible for approximately 90% of cases of acute mediastinitis?**

Esophageal perforation.

○   **What is the treatment for descending necrotizing mediastinitis?**

Broad spectrum antibiotics (aerobes and anaerobes) and wide surgical drainage usually requiring neck and transthoracic drainage with frequent reevaluation for possible undrained collections.

○   **Why is it important to obtain a tissue diagnosis prior to treating superior vena cava syndrome in all patients?**

High dose radiation therapy may alter the tumor's histology and prevent a subsequent accurate diagnosis and to differentiate between benign conditions and tumors that may respond to chemotherapy or radiation therapy.

○   **What is the most common origin of an anterior mediastinal mass in an adult?**

The thymus, which is the origin of thymic cyst, thymic hyperplasia and thymoma.

○   **What is the most common posterior mediastinal tumor?**

A neurogenic tumor.

○   **What diagnostic study is most useful for defining a mediastinal mass identified on chest radiograph?**

CT scan of the chest with oral and intravenous contrast.

○   **What important serum studies should be obtained in male patients with a mediastinal mass?**

Alpha fetoprotein and human chorionic gonadotropin are usually elevated in germ cell tumors and may be diagnostic precluding need for a tissue diagnosis to initiate treatment.

○   **What are the most common mediastinal tumors in children < 2 years old and children 4-18 years of age?**

Neurogenic and lymphoma, respectively.

○   **What incision provides the best exposure for resecting a mass located in the anterior mediastinum?**

Median sternotomy.

О   **Masses located in the middle or posterior mediastinum are best resected through what type of incision?**

Posterolateral thoracotomy.

О   **What surgical technique is useful in evaluating and biopsying a mass of the middle mediastinum?**

Mediastinoscopy if the mass is cephalad to the main branch pulmonary arteries.

О   **T/F: Asymptomatic substernal goiters harbor malignancy more often than cervical goiters.**

False.

О   **What special anesthetic and surgical considerations are necessary before anesthetic induction in patients with large anterior or middle mediastinal masses?**

Airway compression from the mass could result in airway occlusion during the induction of anesthesia and vascular collapse from a compromised venous return to the heart.

О   **What should be immediately available during the induction of anesthesia in patients with large mediastinal masses?**

Rigid bronchoscopy. It can be used to establish an airway and ventilate the patient if airway occlusion occurs.

О   **How should neurogenic mediastinal tumors involving the spinal cord be resected?**

One stage removal with neurosurgical resection of the intraspinal portion and resection of the thoracic component. This prevents spinal cord hemorrhage/hematoma with manipulation of the intrathoracic tumor.

О   **Why should asymptomatic mediastinal tumors of neurogenic origin be resected?**

To provide histologic confirmation of benignancy, prevent the local effects of progressive enlargement and prevent malignant degeneration of the tumor.

О   **What percentage of patients with a thymoma have myasthenia gravis?**

50%

О   **What percentage of thymic masses are malignant?**

33%.

О   **What percentage of patients with myasthenia gravis are found to have a thymoma on chest CT scan or MRI?**

10 to 42%.

О   **What percentage of patients with myasthenia gravis will show clinical improvement following the resection of a thymoma?**

85 to 95%.

О   **What is the standard therapy for a patient with a thymoma?**

Complete surgical excision of the thymus with postoperative radiation therapy for invasive tumors (stage II or III).

O   **Modern differentiation between benign and malignant thymic tumors is based on what factors?**

Presence of gross invasion of adjacent structures at the time of surgery, presence of metastases and microscopic evidence of capsular invasion in the specimen.

O   **T/F: Posterior mediastinal masses in adults are most often malignant.**

False (16%).

O   **What treatment is required for a bronchogenic cyst?**

Surgical excision to alleviate symptoms, establish a histologic diagnosis and prevent possible malignant degeneration.

O   **T/F: Pericardial cysts often occur in the right pericardiophrenic angle, can usually be diagnosed by CT scan and infrequently require surgical excision.**

True.

O   **T/F: Enteric mediastinal cysts are not routinely excised.**

False. Standard therapy is excision to provide a histologic diagnosis and alleviate or prevent the development of symptoms.

O   **What conditions are found in the anterior mediastinum?**

Germ cells tumors (teratoma, seminoma, choriocarcinoma, embryonal cell carcinoma), lymphomas, Hodgkin's disease, thymus-related (thymoma, thymolipoma, thymic cyst), substernal goiter, Castleman's disease and sarcoidosis.

O   **What conditions are found in the middle mediastinum?**

Cysts (bronchogenic, esophageal, neuroenteric, pericardial), lymphomas and myxomas.

O   **What conditions are found in the posterior mediastinum?**

Neurogenic tumors (schwannoma, ganglioneuroma, pheochromocytoma), lymphomas and sarcomas.

O   **T/F: In adults, most mediastinal masses are malignant.**

False. Only 25% are malignant.

O   **T/F: In children, most mediastinal masses are malignant.**

Trick question! About 50% are malignant.

O   **What are causes of the most common mediastinal masses in adults?**

Neurogenic tumor, thymoma, lymphoma and germ cell tumor.

O   **What are the causes of the most common mediastinal masses in children?**

Neurogenic tumor, lymphoma and germ cell tumor.

❍   **What is the treatment for benign teratomas?**

Surgical resection is curative.

❍   **What is the treatment for malignant teratomas?**

Chemotherapy and surgical resection.

MYCOBACTERIAL INFECTIONS

"All the infections that the sun sucks up"
The Tempest, Shakespeare

○ **A positive TB (mycobacterium tuberculosis) test is which type of hypersensitivity reaction?**

Type 4. Hypersensitivity is delayed and neither complements nor antibodies are involved.

○ **What is the most common side effect of rifampin?**

Orange discoloration of urine and tears.

○ **What negative outcome can be avoided by supplementing pyridoxine in patients receiving isoniazid?**

Peripheral neuritis and convulsions.

○ **Which factors have contributed to the increase in TB cases in the early 1990s?**

HIV epidemic, increased immigration from high-prevalence countries, transmission of TB in congregate settings and deterioration of the health care infrastructure.

○ **Which factors may contribute to a false-negative TST (TB skin test)?**

1. Viral infections (measles, mumps, chickenpox, HIV) and live virus vaccination.
2. Bacterial (typhoid fever, typhus, overwhelming TB).
3. Advanced renal disease.
4. Severe malnutrition.
5. Decreased immunity (steroids, sarcoidosis, Hodgkin's, lymphoma and chronic lymphatic leukemia).
6. Advanced age.
7. Errors in application, reading and documentation.

○ **Describe TB positivity based on size of induration and risk groups.**

5 mm or more: persons known to have or suspected to have HIV infection, close contacts of a person with infectious TB, persons who have a chest radiograph suggestive of previous TB, persons who inject drugs (if HIV status unknown).

10 mm or more: persons with certain medical conditions (excluding conditions that satisfy the 5 mm criteria; see below), persons who inject drugs (if HIV negative), foreign-born persons from areas where TB is common, medically underserved, low-income populations, including high-risk racial and ethnic groups, residents of long-term care facilities, children younger than 4 years of age, locally identified high-prevalence groups (e.g. migrant farm workers or homeless persons).

15 mm or more: all persons with no known risk factors for TB.

○ **Which medical conditions increase the risk of TB disease?**

1. HIV infection.
2. Substance abuse.
3. CXR findings suggestive of previous TB (in a person inadequately treated).
4. Diabetes mellitus.
5. Silicosis.

6. Low body weight (10% or more below the ideal).
7. Cancer of the head and neck.
8. Hematologic and reticuloendothelial diseases.
9. End-stage renal disease.
10. Intestinal bypass or gastrectomy.
11. Chronic malabsorption syndromes.
12. Prolonged corticosteroid therapy.
13. Other immunosuppressive therapy.

O   **Who are high priority candidates for preventive therapy regardless of age?**

1. Persons known to have or suspected of having HIV infection (5 mm or more of induration).
2. Close contacts of a person with infectious TB (5 mm or more).
3. Persons who have a CXR suggestive of previous TB and who have received inadequate treatment (5 mm or more).
4. Persons who inject drugs and who are known to be HIV negative (10 mm or more).
5. Persons with certain medical conditions (excluding those conditions that meet the 5 mm criteria; 10 mm or more, see above).
6. Persons whose TST reaction converted from negative to positive within the past 2 years (10 mm or more if younger than 35 years of age; 15 mm or more if 35 years of age or older).

O   **Who are high priority candidates for preventive therapy and younger than 35 years of age?**

1. Foreign born persons from areas where TB is common.
2. Medically underserved, low-income populations, including high risk racial and ethnic groups.
3. Residents of long-term care facilities.
4. Children younger than 4 years of age.
5. Locally identified high prevalence groups (e.g., migrant farm workers or homeless persons).

O   **Who should receive two step skin testing?**

Adults who will be tested periodically, such as health care workers. If the first test is negative, give second test 1 to 3 weeks later. If this test is positive, consider the person infected.

O   **T/F: It is appropriate to substitute rifampin (RIF) for isoniazid (INH) in preventive therapy if INH is not tolerated.**

True. RIF is an accepted alternative.

O   **May the TST be repeated in persons with a previously positive TST?**

Yes. It is never contraindicated. It is useful with an unclear history, a borderline TST, a questionable reading, or recent transmission.

O   **T/F: Isoniazid (INH) is indicated in a 3-year-old child with a 0 mm TST and a normal chest radiograph who is a close contact to a patient with smear-positive pulmonary TB.**

True. INH is indicated for a "window period" of 3 months. If the TST remains below 5 mm after a repeat TST at 3 months, INH can be discontinued.

O   **What is the usual length of INH preventive treatment?**

6 months for adults, 9 months for patients < 18 years, 12 months with HIV-infection, silicosis, or "fibrotic" CXR.

O   **In which patients with a 5 mm tuberculin skin test (TST) is INH indicated?**

Close contacts, patients with HIV-infection, injection drug users with unknown HIV status and CXR suggestive of old tuberculosis (TB).

○   **T/F: INH is contraindicated in women who are breast feeding.**

False.

○   **What is the booster effect?**

The initial TST may be falsely negative because of waning immunity. A reaction is "boosted" if the repeat TST is positive (not a conversion). Boosting occurs in people with BCG or in the elderly.

○   **Which interventions are useful in preventing TB transmission in the hospital?**

1.   Triage.
2.   Isolation.
3.   Airflow > 6 air exchanges/hour, air filtration.
4.   UV light.
5.   Covering the mouth of a sneezing patient (mask or hand kerchief).
6.   Respirator masks.

○   **What CXR findings are associated with primary versus reactivated TB.**

Primary: normal, air space consolidation in any segment of the lung (more often in middle or lower lung zone), hilar or paratracheal lymph node enlargement, most often seen in infants and children.

Reactivated: focal air space consolidation, linear densities connecting to the ipsilateral hilum and cavitation. Most often seen in apical or posterior segment of the upper lobes or in the superior segment of the lower lobes.

○   **What CXR findings are associated with HIV infected patients.**

Early in HIV infection TB presents radiographically as typical reactivation disease. In advanced HIV disease, lower lung zone or diffuse infiltrates and adenopathy are more frequent while cavitation is less often seen.

○   **T/F: The CXR pattern of "fibrosis" in the upper lobes is adequate to rule out active disease.**

False. Disease activity is determined by microbiological studies.

○   **T/F: A negative TST "rules-out" TB in an HIV-negative patient.**

False. In miliary disease 50% are TST negative and in pulmonary TB probably <10%.

○   **What is the difference between unilateral and bilateral pleural effusions in TB?**

A unilateral pleural effusion often indicates localized disease. Bilateral effusions often indicate disseminated extrapulmonary disease.

○   **Which occupational group has the highest risk for TB?**

Hospital housekeepers who go to many different patients rooms.

○   **T/F: TB can involve any organ of the body.**

True.

❍   **What should be considered in an asymptomatic patient with a normal CXR and ONE culture-positive smear-negative sputum?**

Laboratory cross-contamination, especially with repeatedly smear and culture negative sputum samples (false-positive result). RFLP is helpful.

❍   **Which diseases can mimic TB?**

1.   Nocardiosis, meliodosis, paragonimiasis.
2.   Ankylosing spondylitis.
3.   Sarcoidosis, berylliosis.
4.   Lymphoma, cancer.
5.   Klebsiella, aspergillus.

❍   **T/F: HIV counseling and testing is important in every person with a positive TST.**

True. A positive HIV test is an indication for INH regardless of age. Treatment time is always longer.

❍   **How is neonatal TB diagnosed?**

By examination of the placenta (or occasionally bacteremia of the newborn).

❍   **T/F: Hyponatremia correlates with severity of TB.**

True.

❍   What is the significance of an air-fluid level in the pleural space of TB patients?

It suggests a bronchopleural fistula. Surgical intervention is often indicated.

❍   **What is lupus vulgaris?**

Cutaneous TB.

❍   **What is Pott's disease?**

TB of the skeletal spine. 50% of patients have a normal CXR.

❍   **What is empyema necessitans?**

A late manifestation of TB empyema. The exudate invades tissue layers and may cause skin bulging. Surgical intervention is often required to relieve pressure.

❍   **What is Poncet's disease?**

"Immune-mediated" arthritis associated with TB. However, the most common cause of joint pain is PZA-induced.

❍   **What is erythema nodosum?**

Inflammation in subcutaneous fat of both anterior lower legs (tender painful erythematous nodules, ESR often elevated). It is associated with TB and other diseases as sarcoidosis.

❍   **T/F: CD4+ lymphopenia is common in TB and does not prove HIV infection.**

True.

○   **What should you do next in a patient with clinical TB and smear positive sputum?**

Call the lab and request the plating of the specimen on standard susceptibility agar. Results occur in about 3 weeks without having to wait for the culture to grow first.

○   **Which form of extrapulmonary TB is considered the most infectious?**

Laryngeal TB produces the highest number of contacts. It probably reflects extensive pulmonary cavitary TB with spillover to the larynx.

○   **T/F: HIV-positive patients can have culture positive pulmonary TB with a normal CXR.**

True, about 10%.

○   **T/F: PCR gives increased false-positive results in patients with previously treated TB.**

True.

○   **What is the difference between miliary TB, disseminated TB and TB mycobacteremia?**

1.   Miliae are small foci of TB all over the body.
2.   Dissemination is disease in at least 2 different sites (e.g., lung and liver).
3.   Mycobacteremia refers to bacilli detected in the blood (more common in HIV-positive patients) but may reflect only pulmonary "spillage."

○   **T/F: Histoplasmosis may mimic miliary TB.**

True.

○   **Why is the difference between calcified and noncalcified TB granuloma important?**

1.   A calcified granuloma requires only INH prevention (similar to a normal CXR).
2.   Noncalcified granulomas (tuberculomas) represent active disease and require treatment with 4 drugs.

○   **T/F: RFLP (restriction fragment length polymorphism = "DNA fingerprinting") is used to examine potential lab problems with cross-contamination.**

True. It is occasionally used to investigate transmission within a community.

○   **What biochemical abnormalities can be seen in active TB?**

Anemia, leukocytosis with neutrophilia, lymphopenia, monocytopenia, thrombocytosis, increased ESR, ferritin, or B12, abnormal RBC folic acid, increased LFTs, hyponatremia and hypoalbuminemia.

○   **What are the intrathoracic complications of TB?**

Pneumothorax, endobronchial stenosis, bronchiectasis, empyema, mycetoma, hemorrhage, Rasmussen's aneursym (dilated vessel in the wall of an old TB cavity) and broncholithiasis.

○   **What are the extrapulmonary manifestations of TB?**

Miliary, genitourinary, skeletal, CNS tuberculoma, meningitis, abdominal (any intra-abdominal organ), pericardial and pleural disease.

○   **What are the treatment options for pulmonary TB?**

6 month regimen: INH, RIF (rifampin), PZA (pyrazinamide), EMB (ethambutol) or SM (streptomycin) daily for 2 months followed by 4 months of INH and RIF. If low prevalence (<4%) of INH resistance, then can drop EMB or SM from regimen. Alternatively, the initial 4 drugs can be given daily for 2 weeks followed by 6 weeks of direct observation of the same drugs twice per week. Subsequently, complete the course with twice weekly INH and RIF for 4 months. The third 6 month regimen is the same four drugs three times weekly for 6 months.

9 month regimen: nine months of daily INH and RIF or 1-2 months of daily INH and RIF followed by 7-8 months of twice-weekly dosing. EMB or SM should be given in the first 2 months if INH resistance is not known to be < 4%.

HIV-related disease: the six month regimen may be used for a total of 9 months or at least 6 months after culture conversion.

○ **What is the therapy for extrapulmonary TB?**

Generally, the same regimen as for pulmonary TB with the following exception. Bone and joint TB, miliary TB, or TB meningitis in children should be treated for 12 months. Corticosteroids are beneficial in pericarditis, CNS tuberculomas and meningitis.

○ **What is the regimen for TB resistant to INH only?**

Discontinue INH and continue three other drugs for entire 6 months in the 6 month regimen. In the 9 month therapy INH should be discontinued. If ETH was in the initial regimen, treat with RIF and ETH for 12 months. If ETH was not included initially, two new drugs should be added (ETH and PZA) while discontinuing INH.

○ **Which drug allows anti-TB treatment time to be reduced to 6 months?**

PZA for the first 2 months; treatment without PZA during the first 2 months must be at least 9 months.

○ **Why is ethambutol (EMB) used for TB treatment?**

To prevent development of resistance.

○ **How frequent is the "wild type" of resistance in TB (no prior treatment)?**

1 out of every 10^6 organisms has naturally occurring resistance to INH, 10^{6-7} for streptomycin, 10^8 for RIF, 10^{4-5} for EMB.

○ **When should steroids be considered for TB?**

1. Meningitis or tuberculomas (focal deficits, cerebral edema, highly elevated CSF protein).
2. Pericarditis.
3. Shock related to adrenal insufficiency.

○ **T/F: A tuberculous effusion requires chest tube drainage.**

False. Often it is a hypersensitivity reaction and will usually resolve with adequate medical treatment.

○ **What are surgical indications for TB treatment?**

1. Decortication for "trapped lung"/fibrothorax.
2. Lobectomy/pneumonectomy for cavitary multidrug resistant TB on a weak or failing regimen.
3. Drainage for empyema or pericardial effusion.
4. Drainage for a large pleural effusion with midline shift or symptoms.
5. Mycobacteria other than tuberculosis cervical lymph node resection (95% cure rate).

○ **Which anti-TB drug should usually not be used in hemodialysis patients?**

EMB. It can accumulate. Serum levels should be obtained if it has to be used.

○   **T/F: Hyperuricemia of 18 mg/dL in a patient without arthritis is a sufficient reason to discontinue PZA.**

False. Asymptomatic hyperuricemia can be left untreated.

○   **How long is the treatment duration in patients with silico-TB?**

9 months. The relapse rate is 20% with only 6 months.

○   **Which anti-TB drugs may be used in a pregnant woman?**

INH, RIF and ETH.   PZA is probably safe but this has not yet been established in the U.S. STM should not be used.

○   **Which organisms other than TB are AFB stain positive?**

1.   Mycobacteria other than tuberculosis
2.   Nocardia
3.   Cryptosporidium, Isospora belli
4.   Corynebacterium
5.   Legionella (some subspecies)
6.   Rhodococcus equi

○   **What are treatment options for multidrug resistant TB contacts with a positive TST?**

1.   2 drugs to which the source case isolate is susceptible for 6-12 months.
     E.g., cycloserine, ethionamide.
     E.g., quinolone, PZA.
2.   3-months observations (with CXR) for the next 2 years.

○   **What is the most important next step with a failing TB treatment regimen?**

Add at least new 2 drugs.

○   **What is the fastest way to decide whether a sputum smear positive for AFB is TB or MAC (Mycobacterium avium complex)?**

Polymerase chain reaction (PCR) takes only a few hours.

○   **In which TB patients has paradoxical enlargement been observed (and does not indicate treatment failure)?**

Cerebral tuberculoma and rarely TB lymph nodes.

○   **Which 3 drugs can cause hepatitis?**

INH, RIF and PZA.

○   **Which anti-TB drug may cause optic neuritis?**

Ethambutol.

○   **Which anti-TB drug may cause depression, psychosis and even suicide?**

Cycloserine ("psychoserine").

○   **T/F: INH can increase phenytoin serum levels.**

True.

○   **Which anti-TB drugs may cause hypothyroidism, especially in combination?**

Ethionamide and p-amino-salicylic acid (PAS).

○   **Which anti-TB drug causes a cholestatic pattern of liver dysfunction (increased bilirubin and alkaline phosphatase)?**

Rifampin.

○   **Which anti-TB drug most likely causes thrombocytopenia?**

Rifampin.

○   **Rifampin accelerates the clearance of which drugs?**

Methadone, coumadin, steroids, estrogens, oral hypoglycemics, digitalis, anticonvulsants, ketoconazole, fluconazole and cyclosporine.

○   **Which anti-TB drug most likely causes transaminitis (elevation of AST, ALT)?**

Isoniazid.

○   **What is the most common side effect of ethionamide?**

Gastrointestinal disturbance.

○   **What is the most important side effect of clofazimine?**

Hyperpigmentation.

○   **Which anti-TB drug causes the most pruritus and skin rash?**

Pyrazinamide.

○   **What are the risk factors for pulmonary MAC disease?**

1.   COPD, bronchiectasis.
2.   History of pulmonary TB.
3.   Pulmonary fibrosis.
4.   Pectus excavatum, asthenia.
5.   Mitral valve prolapse, cyanotic heart disease.
6.   Nonsmoking elderly woman with chronic cough.
7.   Immune deficiencies (e.g., CVID, HIV).

○   **What are the clinical scenarios of M. avium complex (MAC)?**

1.   Colonization of the oral cavity and upper respiratory tract (without disease).
2.   Upper lobe cavities (mostly in male smokers with COPD).
3.   Bronchiectasis and small reticulonodular infiltrates in elderly women.
4.   Disseminated disease and mycobacteremia in HIV-patients.

O   **Which non-tuberculosis mycobacteria (NTMs) are commonly implicated in pulmonary disease?**

MAC, M. kansasii, M. abscessus, M. xenopi and M. malmoense.

O   **Which NTMs are commonly implicated in lymphadenitis?**

MAC, M. scrofulaceum and M. malmoense.

O   **Which NTMs are commonly implicated in cutaneous disease?**

M. marinum, rapidly growing NTMs and M. ulcerans.

O   **Which NTMs are commonly implicated in disseminated disease?**

MAC, M. kansasii, M. chelonae and M. haemophilum.

O   **T/F: Isoniazid is active against rapidly growing NTMs (M. fortuitum, M. abscessus, M. chelonae).**

False.

O   **Which NTM is most commonly a contaminant/saprophyte/colonizer?**

M. gordonae.

O   **T/F: M. gordonae may be a pathogen in AIDS patients.**

True. It has been found in bronchoalveolar lavage fluid, blood cultures and bone marrow.

O   **Which 3 NTMs have been best studied?**

MAC, M. kansasii and M. abscessus. Too little is known of other NTMs to formulate established guidelines.

O   **What is the treatment for M. kansasii pulmonary disease?**

INH, RIF and ETH for 18 months because of a high relapse rate.

O   **What is MAC associated with in elderly women who have never smoked?**

Bathing in poorly ventilated shower stalls.

O   **What is the "Lady Windermere's syndrome" (adapted from a play by Oscar Wilde)?**

MAC pulmonary disease in elderly woman with isolated nodular infiltrates of the middle lobe or the lingula.

O   **T/F: Routine susceptibility testing with rifabutin and clarithromycin is recommended for MAC disease.**

False. Testing against clarithromycin should only be performed on patients who failed prior macrolide therapy.

O   **T/F: Susceptibility testing of rapidly growing mycobacteria should not be performed with anti-TB drugs.**

True. They should be tested against drugs such as amikacin, doxycycline, imipenem, fluoroquinolones, sulfonamide, cefoxitin and clarithromycin.

❍   **Which NTM is associated with water exposure and swimming pools?**

M. marinum.

❍   **What is the most common clinical presentation of tuberculous meningitis?**

Rupture of a chronic tuberculous focus into the subarachnoid space is the most common precipitating cause of tuberculous meningitis. Tubercles may lie dormant for long periods of time and reactivate related to a decline in health, alcohol abuse, or head trauma.

Symptoms are generally chronic or subacute in nature, although the occasional patient may present with fulminant meningitis. Typically, intermittent headaches and low-grade fevers progress to persistent headache, lethargy, nausea and vomiting and altered mental status. A gelatinous mass may ultimately extend to encase the base of the brain, optic chiasm, floor of the third ventricle and may surround the spinal cord. Invasion of vessels may result in cerebral infection. Obstructive hydrocephalus may also occur. The majority of patients will have an extrameningeal site of tuberculosis present. The propensity for tuberculosis to involve the basilar aspects of the subarachnoid space accounts for the cranial nerve palsies seen in some patients.

❍   **What are the diagnostic tests in tuberculous meningitis?**

CT or MRI may reveal tuberculomas or basilar enhancement. Traditional teaching is that the CSF will show hypoglycorrhachia, with the glucose being less than 45 mg/dl. In fact, this was shown to be present in only a minority of cases. Cell counts may range from 0 to 1500, usually with a lymphocytic predominance. Earlier on, polymorphonuclear leukocytes may predominate. CSF protein is usually moderately elevated. AFB stains are positive on average only one third of the time with a single lumbar puncture, but the yield increases to 87% after four lumbar punctures.

❍   **What is the treatment for tuberculous meningitis?**

Four drug therapy with INH, rifampin, pyrazinamide and ethambutol should be initiated. Steroids have been recommended.

❍   **What organisms constitute the M. avium complex?**

M. avium, M. intracellulare and M scrofulaceum.

❍   **What condition does the M. fortuitum complex cause?**

The M. fortuitum complex consists of M. chelonei and M. abscessus. It causes soft tissue abscesses related to trauma or surgery. The organisms are resistant to anti-TB drugs.

❍   **T/F: TB may mimic the atypical pneumonia syndrome (as stereotyped by a Mycoplasma pneumoniae infection).**

True.

❍   **T/F: The presence of a cavity in active TB decreases the risk of infection to other people.**

False. A 2 cm cavity contains 10^8 organisms.

❍   **T/F: Most patients who present with hemoptysis have TB.**

False. Less than 19% of patients with hemoptysis will ultimately have TB.

❍   **TB is a leading cause of severe hemoptysis.**

True.

○   **The mycobacterium most commonly isolated in an HIV infected patient is MAC.**

True.

○   **What is the histological appearance of all mycobacteria?**

Necrotizing (caseous) granulomatous inflammation.

○   **T/F: Finding mycobacteria on histological slides is, in general, very easy.**

False. The organisms are often not seen on histology but later grow out in culture.

PULMONARY EMBOLISM AND DEEP VENOUS THROMBOSIS

"Constant in spirit, not swerving with the blood"
King Henry V, Shakespeare

○ **What are the three syndromes of pulmonary embolism?**

1. Acute cor pulmonale: occurs with massive embolism that obstructs a large fraction of the pulmonary circulation.
2. Pulmonary infarction: occurs with embolization to the distal branches of the pulmonary circulation.
3. Acute dyspnea: milder obstruction not enough to warrant infarction.

○ **What is the equation for the A-a gradient?**

A-a $= ((713 \text{ mmHg} \times FIO2) - pCO2 / .8 - pO_2)$

The normal A-a gradient is 5 to 15 mmHg. The A-a gradient increases with PE.

○ **Most pulmonary emboli arise from what veins?**

The iliac and femoral veins.

○ **What does normal ventilation with mismatched decreased lung perfusion suggest?**

Pulmonary embolus.

○ **Can a patient with a PE have a pO_2 greater than 90 mmHg?**

Yes, but rarely (5%).

○ **What are two relatively specific CXR findings in PE?**

Hampton's hump: a wedge shaped infiltrate abutting the pleura.
Westermark's sign: decreased lung vasculature markings on the side with a PE.

○ **What test is considered the gold standard for the diagnosis of DVT? For the diagnosis of PE?**

The gold standard test for the diagnosis of DVT is venography. The gold standard for the diagnosis of PE is pulmonary angiography.

○ **When treating DVT/PE, when should warfarin therapy be initiated?**

On the first day after initiation of therapeutic levels of heparin.

○ **How long should chronic warfarin therapy for DVT be given?**

Warfarin should be administered for at least 3 to 6 months after a DVT

○ **How is a thrombus distinguished from an embolus on arteriography?**

195

A thrombus appears as a tapering lumen. An embolus has a sharp cutoff.

O   **What is the risk of PE in a patient with an axillary or subclavian vein thrombus?**

About 15%.

O   **What is Virchow's triad?**

1. Injury to the endothelium of the vessels.
2. Hypercoagulable state.
3. Stasis.

O   **What is the therapy of choice to neutralize heparin in a patient who was inadvertently been administered too much?**

Protamine sulfate. 1 mg of protamine will neutralize about 100 units of heparin.

O   **What are the most common symptoms of a PE?**

Chest pain and dyspnea.

O   **What are the most common signs of a PE?**

Tachypnea and rales.

O   **Of patients with a PE, what percentage of ECGs show the classic $S_1Q_3T_3$ pattern?**

7%.

O   **A 48 year old woman is transferred from another hospital a week and a half after sustaining a left upper extremity fracture, a complex pelvic fracture, bilateral lower extremity femur fractures and a left tibial fracture. While sitting in bed, she experiences severe dyspnea, tachypnea and tachycardia. Pulse oximetry reveals an oxygen saturation of 88% on room air. She is given supplemental oxygen and transferred to the ICU. What is your diagnosis?**

Pulmonary embolism secondary to deep vein thrombosis.

O   **What risk factors for deep vein thrombosis did she have?**

Trauma or surgery of pelvis or lower extremities, indwelling vascular catheters and prolonged immobility.

O   **What preventative measures can be taken in patients at risk for developing DVTs?**

Early ambulation, elastic stockings that provide graded compression from ankle to thigh, low-dose heparin, intermittent pneumatic compression and prophylactic inferior vena cava filters.

O   **What tests can be used to diagnosis pulmonary embolism?**

Pulmonary angiogram is the gold standard. V/Q (ventilation/perfusion) scans are the best non-invasive tests to establish or exclude the diagnosis of PE. A high probability scan in a clinical scenario of high likelihood for PE is an indication to treat. An intermediate or low probability scan necessitates further studies. Duplex ultrasound is used to detect DVT not to diagnose PE. However, if the duplex ultrasound is positive, then therapy for DVT will also treat PE.

O   **What patients are at high risk for complications during pulmonary angiography?**

Patients with recent myocardial infarct, severe pulmonary hypertension and arrhythmias. Safety can be improved with selective injections.

○ **What are the indications for pulmonary angiography?**

Non-diagnostic non-invasive venous study with a non-diagnostic ventilation-perfusion scan and anticipated embolectomy.

○ **What are the indications for vena cava filter placement?**

Contraindication to anticoagulation, hemorrhage after anticoagulation, failure of anticoagulation to prevent recurrent pulmonary embolism and prophylaxis for extremely high-risk patients.

○ **What is the diagnostic test of choice for documenting DVT?**

Duplex ultrasound. The accuracy of physical examination for DVT is generally quoted to be 50%.

○ **What are the risk factors for DVT?**

1. Surgery (knee and hip greater than abdominal and urological)
2. Pregnancy
3. Cardiac disease, especially post-MI
4. Age greater than 50 years
5. Prior DVT
6. Immobilizaton
7. Acute paraplegia (but not chronic paraplegia)
8. Oral contraceptives (but not hormonal replacement therapy)
9. Major trauma
10. Malignancy, especially adenocarcinoma
11. Factor deficiency state
12. Antiphospholipid antibodies
13. Nephrotic syndrome
14. Paroxysmal nocturnal hemoglobinuria
15. Protein losing enteropathy

○ **Which factor deficiency states predispose to DVT?**

1. Activated protein C resistance
2. Protein C deficiency
3. Protein S deficiency
4. Plasminogen deficiency
5. Antithrombin III deficiency

○ **What is activated protein C deficiency?**

A point mutation in factor V results in resistance of factor V to the natural anticoagulant effects of protein C. This is the most common deficiency state known to predispose to DVT.

○ **T/F: The more risk factors a patient has, the greater the chances of developing a DVT.**

True.

○ **T/F: Only patients with known risk factors develop DVTs.**

False.

❍   **What are the symptoms of a PE?**

Dyspnea, pleurisy, cough, hemoptysis and syncope.

❍   **Which symptom is more common in massive PE than submassive PE?**

Syncope.

❍   **What are the signs of PE?**

Crackles, increased P2, thrombophlebitis, heart gallop, peripheral edema, cardiac murmur and cyanosis.

❍   **What is the most common CXR finding in PE?**

Atelectasis or pulmonary parenchymal defect.

❍   **What are other CXR findings in PE?**

Pleural effusion, pleural based opacity, elevated diaphragm, Westermark's sign and normal.

❍   **Is a normal CXR the most common finding in a PE?**

No. It occurred 16% of the time in the PIOPED database.

❍   **What is the most common ECG finding in PE?**

Nonspecific ST-T wave changes.

❍   **What are other ECG findings in PE?**

Sinus tachycardia, normal, left axis deviation, RBBB, atrial fibrillation and pseudo-infarction pattern.

❍   **T/F: A patient can have a pO2 greater than 100 or an A-a gradient less than 10 and still have a PE.**

True.

❍   **T/F: The pO2 or A-a gradient differentiates between a patient with a PE and a patient without a PE.**

False.

❍   **T/F: A blood gas is indicated in every patient suspected of having a PE.**

False.

❍   **What is the primary utility in getting an ECG and CXR in a patient suspected of have a PE?**

To rule out other causes for their respiratory symptoms.

❍   **In a patient with a high probability V/Q scan and a high clinical risk for PE, are any other studies needed?**

No.

❍   **In a patient with a normal V/Q scan and a low clinical risk for PE, are any other studies needed?**

No.

❍ **What is the probability of a PE in all patients with a low probability V/Q scan?**

14%. This varies from 4% to 40%, depending on the clinical likelihood of a PE.

❍ **In a patient with high clinical and V/Q scan probabilities for pulmonary embolism and being considered for thrombolysis, is an angiogram necessary prior to thrombolysis?**

No. The prevalence of PE in patients with high clinical and V/Q scan probabilities for PE is 96%.

❍ **What can be performed in a patient whose post V/Q test probability is still uncertain?**

A lower extremity ultrasound can be performed. If positive, the patient will be treated the same as for a PE. If negative, a pulmonary angiogram can be performed.

Some support the use of serial lower extremity ultrasounds in patients with adequate cardiopulmonary reserve. For those with limited reserve, an angiogram is recommended. The use of serial lower extremity ultrasound in such a setting has not been commonly practiced in the United States.

The role of D-dimers in the setting of suspected PE has yet to be clarified.

❍ **What is the difference between D-dimer ELISA and latex assays?**

The ELISA is thought to be more accurate.

❍ **What are the accepted indications for the use of thrombolytics in PE?**

Definitely accepted: hemodynamic instability.
Controversial: 40% or more of pulmonary vasculature involved with PE, obstruction of blood flow to one lobe or multiple pulmonary segments, severe hypoxia and right heart failure seen echocardiographically.

❍ **What is the advantage of using thrombolytic agents for PE?**

The only proven benefits have been short-term hemodynamic parameters. No randomized study has been performed with a large enough sample size to assess the impact on mortality.

❍ **Which drugs prolong the effect of coumadin?**

Alcohol (with liver disease), amiodarone, cimetidine, erythromycin, fluconazole, INH, metronidazole, omeprazole, phenylbutazone, propafanone and propranolol.

❍ **Which drugs shorten the effect of coumadin?**

Barbiturates, carbamazepine, griseofulvin, nafcillin, rifampin, sucralfate and vitamin K.

❍ **What are the modified PIOPED criteria for a high probability V/Q scan?**

1. 2 large V/Q mismatches
2. 1 large and 2 or more moderate mismatches
3. 4 or more moderate mismatches
    (Large = >75% of a segment)

❍ **What are the modified PIOPED criteria for an intermediate probability V/Q scan?**

1. 1 large V/Q mismatch, with or without 1 moderate mismatch

2. 1-3 moderate mismatches
3. 1 matched defect with a normal CXR
    (Moderate = 25% to 75% of a segment)

○   **What are the modified PIOPED criteria for a low probability V/Q scan?**

1. 1 or more perfusion defect that is smaller than the CXR defect
2. 2 or more matches with a normal CXR and some areas of normal perfusion in lung
3. 1 or more small perfusion defect with a normal CXR
4. Perfusion defects thought to be caused by effusions, cardiomegaly, aortic dilatation, hila, mediastinum and
    elevated hemidiaphragms
    (Small = <25% of a segment)

○   **Has one type of IVC filter been proven to be superior to the other types?**

No.

○   **What is the goal for heparin therapy?**

To maintain a PTT between 1.5 and 2.5 times control.

○   **What is the goal for coumadin therapy?**

To maintain the INR between 2-3.

○   **Is coumadin safe for the fetus in pregnancy? What about heparin?**

Coumadin is not. Heparin is safe (from a teratogenic perspective) in pregnancy.

○   **In a bedridden patient with the sudden onset of chest tightness, shortness of breath and tachycardia,
the diagnosis of acute pulmonary embolus is made by nuclear scanning. Due to hemodynamic instability a
pulmonary artery catheter is inserted and the right atrial pressure is 24 mmHg and pulmonary artery
occlusion pressure measured at end-expiration is 20 mmHg with a low cardiac output. What is the most
likely diagnosis?**

Cor pulmonale. The increase in right atrial pressure over pulmonary artery occlusion pressure means the right
ventricle is likely to be overdistended, decreasing LV diastolic compliance.

○   **What is the treatment for chronic thromboembolic pulmonary hypertension?**

Pulmonary thromboendarterectomy.

○   **What is the in-hospital mortality rate of pulmonary thromboendarterectomy?**

5.4%.

○   **What is the pathophysiology of chronic thromboembolic pulmonary hypertension?**

A pulmonary embolism that results in symptoms secondary to obstruction or stenosis of the pulmonary arteries due
to unresolved clot. Typically pulmonary emboli are naturally lysed by the fibrinolytic system resulting in no or
minimal residual clot.

○   **Do calf vein thrombi embolize to the lung?**

Generally no, but they may propagate to the popliteal vein. Popliteal vein thrombi can embolize to the lung.

○   **How is a subclavian vein thrombosis usually diagnosed?**

With ultrasonography.

○   **What is the histopathological pattern of a pulmonary infarct?**

Classically, it is a wedge-shaped peripheral lesion.   Fibrinous pleuritis is common. Coagulation necrosis is present in different stages of resorption.

○   **What are the ultrasonographic findings in acute DVT?**

Presence of echogenic material in vein lumen, noncompressibility of vein, venous distention, free-floating thrombus and absence of Doppler tracing.

○   **What is a weakness of using helical CT scanning to diagnose PE?**

This device tends to miss peripheral emboli. Its use in diagnosing PE is currently under investigation.

○   **Is coagulation monitoring necessary when using low molecular weight heparin for prophylaxis?**

No.

○   **T/F: The incidence of thrombocytopenia is greater with low molecular weight heparin compared to unfractionated heparin.**

False. Some studies suggest that thrombocytopenia is less common with low molecular weight heparin.

○   **What is the rate of PE in patients who have had IVC filters placed?**

2 to 3%.

PULMONARY FUNCTION TESTING AND PHYSIOLOGY

"Are melted into air, into thin air"
The Tempest, Shakespeare

○ **Name several indications for Pulmonary Function Testing (PFT).**

1. Screen patients at risk for lung
2. Evaluate signs and symptoms of pulmonary disease
3. Follow response to therapy for lung disease
4. Assess preoperative risk
5. Assess prognosis

○ **What is spirometry?**

A test that measures the volume of air a patient inhales or exhales as a function of time. It can also measure flow or the rate at which these volumes change as a function of time.

○ **What is required for spirometry results to be valid?**

Valid spirometry requires at least three acceptable trials that are reproducible by American Thoracic Society (ATS) criteria.

○ **What is the Vital Capacity (VC)?**

It is the maximal volume of air expired from a maximal inspiratory level. It can be measured during a forced expiratory effort (FVC) or a more relaxed expiration (usually denoted as VC or SVC). The VC and FVC should be equal in a normal, non-obstructed patient. In patients with obstructive diseases the FVC is generally lower than the VC/SVC.

○ **What is the FEV_1?**

The FEV_1 is perhaps the single most important spirometric value. It is the volume of air expired in the first second of an FVC maneuver. It can be expressed as an absolute value or as a percentage of the FVC (FEV_1/FVC ratio).

○ **What is a normal FEV_1?**

It is usually interpreted in the context of established predicted normal mean values. A normal FEV_1 is a value greater than 80% of predicted normal.

○ **What is maximal voluntary ventilation (MVV)?**

This is a maneuver where the patient is asked to breathe as rapidly and deeply as possible over a 12-second period. Exhaled volume is measured and extrapolated over a minute and is expressed in liters per minute. This test provides an overall assessment of pulmonary function, including respiratory muscle strength.

○ **What is the relationship between FEV_1 and MVV?**

The MVV is usually 35 to 40 times the FEV_1.

○ **What are three causes of an MVV reduced out of proportion to the FEV_1?**

Poor patient effort, respiratory muscle weakness or fatigue and upper airway obstruction.

○ **Which spirometric value distinguishes between obstructive and non-obstructive patterns?**

The FEV_1/ FVC ratio. It is reduced in obstructive diseases and normal in non-obstructive diseases.

○ **What are the most common causes of obstructive pulmonary physiology?**

Asthma, COPD (emphysema and chronic bronchitis), small airways disease, bronchiectasis and upper airway obstruction.

○ **What criteria define a positive response to bronchodilators by spirometry?**

A 12% increase and an absolute increase of 200cc or greater in either FEV_1 or FVC.

○ **What is "small airways disease"?**

This term refers to obstructive disease localized to peripheral airways with diameters 2 mm or smaller. Small airway disease may be characterized by decrement in $FEF_{25-75\%}$, which correlates with airflow in the middle 50% of VC maneuver and is effort independent.

○ **What tests are used to assess small airway function?**

Helium-oxygen flow-volume curves and measurement of closing volumes.

○ **What is SGaw?**

This refers to specific airway conductance and is the reciprocal of airway resistance. It can be measured by body plethysmography. Decrements in SGaw are most commonly seen in obstructive lung diseases such as asthma.

○ **What are the most common causes of restrictive pulmonary physiology?**

Parenchymal lung disease (e.g. pulmonary fibrosis), pleural disease (e.g. fibrothorax), neuromuscular disease and thoracic cage abnormalities (e.g. kyphoscoliosis).

○ **What methods are available for lung volume measurements?**

Closed-circuit helium dilution, nitrogen washout and body plethysmography.

○ **What is the functional residual capacity (FRC)?**

The volume of air remaining in the lungs after a normal expiration. It is measured with the patient's glottis open to atmosphere.

○ **What is total lung lapacity (TLC)?**

The volume of air in the lungs after a maximal inspiration. It represents the sum of all volume compartments in the lungs.

○ **What is a normal TLC?**

Values between 80 and 120% of established predicted normal mean values.

○ **What is the residual volume (RV)?**

The volume of air remaining in the lungs after a maximal expiration. It represents the difference between FRC and expiratory reserve volume (ERV), or the maximal volume of air expired from a resting end-expiratory level.

○ **What is a normal RV?**

Values between 80 and 120% of established predicted normal mean values.

○ **The diagnosis of a restrictive pattern requires a decrement in which lung volume?**

Total lung capacity (TLC). While a reduction in FEV1 and FVC, with a normal FEV_1/FVC ratio may suggest restriction, the diagnosis of restriction is based on a decreased TLC. The assessment of the severity of restriction is also based on the TLC.

○ **What is the difference between hyperinflation and air-trapping?**

Hyperinflation refers to a significant increase in TLC or RV, while air-trapping refers to a significant increase in slow VC compared to FVC.

○ **Which PFT data is useful for the clinical assessment of upper airway obstruction?**

The flow-volume loop.

○ **What are the three types of upper airway obstruction (UAO)?**

1. Fixed: flattening of both inspiratory and expiratory limbs of the flow-volume loop.
2. Variable intrathoracic: flattening of the expiratory limb of the flow-volume loop.
3. Variable extrathoracic: flattening of the inspiratory limb of the flow-volume loop.

○ **What may cause a fixed UAO?**

Tracheal stenosis after prolonged endotracheal intubation, goiter and tumor.

○ **What may cause a variable extrathoracic UAO.**

Vocal cord paralysis and tumor.

○ **What is the diffusing capacity?**

It provides a measure of volume of gas transferred across the alveolar-capillary membrane. Diffusing capacity is defined as the rate of gas flow across the lung divided by the pressure gradient for flow. Carbon monoxide (CO) is a useful gas for determining diffusing capacity as its uptake is diffusion limited. The diffusing capacity is designated as D_{LCO}.

○ **What are three factors, other than a true diffusion defect, that can reduce the diffusing capacity?**

Anemia, elevated carboxyhemoglobin level and reduced lung volume

○ **What are three causes of an abnormally elevated diffusing capacity?**

Polycythemia, alveolar hemorrhage and left to right shunt.

○ **What are two common causes of an isolated reduction in diffusing capacity?**

Interstitial lung disease and occlusive pulmonary vascular disorders.

○ **Which pulmonary function test may be useful in distinguishing emphysema from chronic bronchitis in a smoker with airflow obstruction?**

The diffusing capacity. It is reduced in emphysema due to the loss of alveolar surface area for gas exchange, but should be normal in chronic bronchitis. It should also be normal in asthma.

○ **Which pulmonary function value best predicts prognosis/mortality in COPD?**

The FEV_1.

○ **What is a methacholine challenge test?**

A bronchoprovocation test. It is generally used to document the presence of airways hyperreactivity in patients with clinical history suggesting bronchospasm but otherwise normal pulmonary function tests. Methacholine itself is a parasympathomimetic agent. Spirometry is first performed at baseline and after a challenge with an aerosolized diluent and then after increasing concentrations of methacholine. A test is considered positive if there is a 20% or greater drop in FEV_1 from baseline.

○ **What is a contraindication to methacholine challenge testing?**

Abnormal baseline spirometry

○ **What are maximal inspiratory and expiratory pressures (MIP, MEP)?**

Specific tests of respiratory muscle function. Pressures generated by maximal inspiratory and expiratory efforts are measured by a pressure gauge.

○ **What are three causes of decrements in maximal inspiratory and expiratory pressures (MIP, MEP)?**

Poor patient effort, respiratory muscle fatigue and respiratory muscle weakness.

○ **Interpret the following PFT data:**

FEV_1	1.2L (42% pred)
FVC	2.1L (51% pred)
FEV_1/FVC	57%
TLC	115% pred
RV	240% pred
D_{LCO}	48% pred

Severe obstruction with hyperinflation and a gas transfer abnormality. This is consistent with emphysema.

○ **Interpret the following PFT data:**

FEV_1	1.1L (38% pred)
FVC	2.6L (66% pred)
FEV_1/FVC	42%
TLC	60% pred
RV	66% pred
D_{LCO}	40% pred

Severe obstruction with accompanying restriction and a gas transfer abnormality. There are a number of scenarios where this pattern could be seen: emphysema with concomitant pulmonary fibrosis, emphysema s/p lung resection and sarcoidosis.

○ **Interpret the following PFT data:**

FEV_1	2.4L (74% pred)
FVC	2.9L (62% pred)
FEV_1/FVC	83%
MVV	84L

Restriction is suggested by the reduced FEV1 and FVC. There is no evidence of obstruction as the FEV1/FVC ratio is normal. The MVV is normal. Lung volume measurements are necessary to establish restriction.

○ **Interpret the following PFT data:**

FEV_1 (pre-BD)	2.6L (80% pred)
FEV_1(post-BD)	3.1L (95% pred)
% change in FEV_1	19%
FVC (pre-BD)	4.2 (105% pred)
FVC (post-BD)	4.4 (108% pred)
% change in FVC	4%
FEV_1/FVC (pre-BD)	62%
FEV_1/FVC (post-BD)	70%

BD = bronchodilator

Obstruction with positive response to bronchodilator, indicating a significant reversible component to the obstruction. This is compatible with asthma.

○ **Interpret the following PFT data:**

FEV_1	1.7L (70% pred)
FVC	2.1L (64% pred)
FEV_1/FVC	81%
MVV	50L
MIP	45% pred
MEP	40% pred

Restriction is suggested by reduction in FEV_1 and FVC with an otherwise normal FEV_1/FVC ratio. The MIP, MEP and MVV are all reduced, suggesting respiratory muscle weakness or fatigue.

○ **What is the definition of normal pulmonary function?**

Normal pH, PCO2 and PO_2, without excessive pulmonary or cardiac work.

○ **What is the definition of restrictive lung disease?**

Decreased total lung capacity.

○ **How are the lung volumes altered in patients with severe obstructive disease?**

The RV and TLC are increased, indicating hyperinflation.

○ **What are the main functions of the respiratory muscles?**

Inspiratory:
Principal - external intercostals (elevate ribs) and diaphragm (descend and increase chest longitudinal dimension).

Accessory - sternocleidomastoid and scalenii (elevate and fix ribs).
Expiratory:
Passive - results from passive recoil of lungs.
Active - internal intercostals (depress ribs) and abdominal muscles (compress abdominal contents).

○   **What are the four lung volumes and the four lung capacities?**

Lung volumes:
1.   Tidal volume (TV)
2.   Inspiratory reserve volume (IRV)
3.   Expiratory reserve volume (ERV)
4.   Residual volume (RV)

Lung capacities:
1.   Functional residual capacity (FRC = ERV + RV)
2.   Inspiratory capacity (IC = IRV + TV)
3.   Vital capacity (IC + ERV)
4.   Total lung capacity (VC + RV)

○   **What is the most important input in control of breathing?**

Arterial PCO2 (while awake the PCO2 is held within 3 mmHg).

○   **What are the ways to measure FRC (functional residual capacity)?**

Helium dilution and plethysmography.

○   **T/F: The difference between chronic bronchitis and emphysema when measuring PFTs is that the DLCO is decreased in chronic bronchitis and is normal in emphysema.**

False. The DLCO is decreased in emphysema and it is normal in chronic bronchitis.

○   **T/F: Lung volumes are increased in COPD, chronic bronchitis, emphysema and asthma.**

True.

○   **T/F: Restrictive ventilatory defects can be broadly categorized into intraparenchymal and extraparenchymal.**

True. Any process which significantly floods the alveoli, as with blood, serum, or pus, causes a restrictive ventilatory defect. Any process which restricts the expansion of the chest wall, either by increased load or decreased neuromuscular strength, causes an extraparenchymal restrictive ventilatory defect.

○   **What happens to the airflow and the lung volumes in restrictive ventilatory defects?**

The airflow, as measured by the FEV1/FVC ratio, is unchanged or increased. The lung volumes are decreased.

○   **What is the change in shape of the flow-volume loop in a patient with obstructive lung disease?**

The expiratory flow is reduced, the vital capacity is reduced, the shape of the expiratory flow curve is scooped out giving the appearance of a ski slope.

○   **What is the change in shape of the flow-volume loop in a patient with restrictive lung disease?**

The expiratory and inspiratory flows are generally preserved. The vital capacity is reduced. This results in a shape reminiscent of pinching a normal flow-volume curve at both ends inwards.

❍   **What causes a decrease in the maximal inspiratory pressure?**

Neuromuscular disease, poor effort and increased lung volumes.

❍   **What causes a decrease in the maximal expiratory pressure?**

Neuromuscular disease, poor effort and decreased lung volumes.

❍   **What percentage increase in FEV1 or FVC is necessary to consider a positive response to bronchodilators?**

12%.

❍   **What percentage of predicted values for VC, FEV1, TLC and DLCO must a subject have to be considered as normal lung physiology?**

80%.

❍   **What is the value of FEV1/FVC above which subjects are considered to have normal lung physiology?**

0.70.

❍   **What will happen to the DLCO and DLCO/VA (KCO) in a patient with a pneumonectomy?**

The DLCO will be reduced. When corrected for lung volume (KCO), the value will be normal provided there is no underlying lung disease.

❍   **What happens to the DLCO in patients with COPD, IPF and PE?**

They are all decreased.

❍   **A patient presents with a history of CHF and COPD, related to cigarette smoking. His lung exam reveals rhonchi and crackles with a prolonged expiratory phase. CXR shows pulmonary edema. What is this patients pulmonary physiology?**

A mixed obstructive and restrictive ventilatory defect. This patient will require diuretics as well as bronchodilators.

❍   **There are two fundamental differences between spontaneous and positive pressure ventilation that impact cardiovascular status. The first difference is that spontaneous ventilation requires effort, what is the second?**

The directional change in intrathoracic pressure. It decreases during spontaneous inspiration and increases during positive-pressure inspiration.

❍   **Which factor is more important in determining the hemodynamic effects of positive pressure ventilation, the increase in airway pressure or the increase in lung volume?**

The increase in lung volume. Increasing lung volume, not airway pressure, determines the increase in pleural pressure, pulmonary vascular resistance and cardiac compression.

❍   **What determines the relationship between changes in airway pressure and lung volume during positive pressure ventilation?**

Lung and chest wall compliance combine to define the relation between airway pressure and lung volume. Increased stiffness of the lungs (pulmonary fibrosis or overdistention) or the chest wall (tense ascites) will decrease the amount to which lung volume will increase for a given increase in airway pressure.

○   **Does acute lung injury of the entire lung, as may be induced by smoke inhalation, cause lung compliance to decrease similarly in each region of the lung?**

No. Marked regional differences in the degree of lung consolidation and compliance characterize all forms of acute lung injury.

○   **Can one assume a constant proportion of the increase in airway pressure induced by positive pressure ventilation will be transmitted to the pleural surface?**

Definitely not. Differences in lung or chest wall compliance can profoundly alter the degree to which increases in airway pressure are felt within the chest and thus the degree to which they alter hemodynamics.

○   **Esophageal pressure recordings are more accurate for spontaneous or positive pressure breathing?**

Spontaneous breathing, where they have been shown to be highly accurate, especially in the patient stand ing or sitting upright.

○   **A young male patient awaiting general anesthesia is found to have a heart rate of 60 beats per minute which increases up to about 80 beats per minute with each spontaneous inspiration. What is this patient's condition?**

He is normal. Healthy young adults normally have a relative bradycardia and normal inspiration induces an in-phase vagal withdrawal that causes heart rate to increase during inspiration and decrease during expiration. This phenomenon is referred to as respiratory sinus arrhythmia.

○   **In a diabetic patient breathing spontaneously prior to induction of general anesthesia, the physician noted that the baseline heart rate was 88 beats per minute but that there was no discernable heart rate variability on the cardiac monitor, suggesting the absence of respiratory sinus arrhythmia. Is this a problem?**

Potentially yes. Absence of normal respiratory sinus arrhythmia infers severe dysautonomia. Thus, the patient is at increased risk of systemic hypotension following induction of general anesthesia because the normal adaptive autonomic responses may also be absent.

○   **Acute elevations in pulmonary arterial pressure do what to left ventricular diastolic compliance?**

It is decreased because of interventricular dependence of the left and right ventricles.

○   **How does spontaneous ventilation, by inducing negative swings in intrathoracic pressure, affect myocardial oxygen demand ?**

It will increase by increasing left ventricular afterload.

○   **Under normal conditions at rest, what percentage of the cardiac output goes to the respiratory muscles?**

Less than 3%.

○   **In patients with COPD, what percentage of the total cardiac output can be directed to the muscles of respiration?**

25 to 30%

○   **Positive end-expiratory pressure (PEEP) primarily impairs cardiac output by what mechanism?**

Decrease in LV preload.

○   **To the extent that LV preload is maintained, positive pressure ventilation has what effect on cardiac output in patients with normal cardiovascular function?**

No measurable effect as compared to spontaneous ventilation.

○   **When two different modes of ventilation, such as pressure-support and inverse ratio ventilation, have similar changes in intrathoracic pressure and ventilatory effort, their hemodynamic effects are likely to be what?**

Similar.

○   **Can the hemodynamic effects of mechanical ventilation be seen in non-intubated patients during non-invasive ventilatory support?**

Yes. Identical effects should be seen for the same changes in lung volume and intrathoracic pressure.

○   **Is there any hemodynamic difference between increasing airway pressure to generate a breath and decreasing extrathoracic pressure (iron lung-negative pressure ventilation) to generate a similar tidal volume?**

None, if the iron lung encompasses the entire body. However, if it surrounds only the chest and abdomen, it may have less detrimental effects due to the sparing of venous return.

○   **T/F: Total lung volume (TLC) is equal to the sum of functional residual capacity (FRC) and vital capacity (VC).**

False. TLC = VC + RV.

○   **What causes an oxygen saturation curve to shift to the right?**

A shift to the right delivers more O_2 to the tissue.
Remember: CADET! Right face!

Hyper   Carbia
          Acidemia
2,3   DPG
          Exercise
Increased Temperature
          Release to tissues

○   **What is a normal tidal volume?**

500 cc.

○   **What is a normal amount of anatomic dead space?**

150 cc.

○   **What is a normal minute ventilation?**

7,500 cc/min.

O   **In which zone is the Pa > Pv > Palveolar?**

Zone 3.

O   **What is Laplace's law?**

P = 4 x wall tension / radius.

O   **What is Poiseuille's law?**

Flow rate = $P\pi r^4/8nL$ where P is the difference in pressure, r is the radius, n is the viscosity, and L is the length.

O   **How are airway conductance and resistance related?**

They are the inverse of one another: Conductance = 1/resistance.

O   **What is the Fick equation for cardiac output?**

Cardiac output = VO2 / (CaO2 – CvO2)
Where VO2 is the oxygen consumption, CaO2 is the arterial content of oxygen and CvO2 is the venous content of oxygen.

O   **What happens to the V/Q relationship when moving from the top of the lung to the bottom of the lung?**

It decreases. At the top of the lung, the ventilation exceeds flow, so the V/Q relationship is greater than one. At the bottom of the lung, the flow exceeds ventilation, so the V/Q relationship is less than one. Both flow and ventilation are greater in the bottom of the lung than the top. The reason the V/Q changes while moving from top to bottom of the lung is that the change of flow with vertical distance is different than the change of ventilation with vertical distance.

O   **Why does ventilation increase when moving from the top to bottom of the lung?**

The weight of lung causes the intrapleural pressure to be greater at the top of the lung than the bottom. Ths causes the lung units at the bottom of the lung to be relatively compressed and able to open and accept incoming gas. The lung units at the top of the lung are relatively more open, thus less able to accept incoming gas.

O   What is the normal pressure around the lung (intrapleural pressure)?

It is just subatmospheric. This is necessary to keep the lung and chest wall in close proximity.

O   **What is the intrapleural pressure in the case of a pneumothorax?**

It is zero in a non-tension pneumothorax at end expiration. The lung collapses because of the intrinsic elastic properties of the lung. The intrapleural pressure is positive in the case of a tension pneumothorax.

PLEURAL CONDITIONS

"When clouds appear, wise men put on their cloaks"
King Richard III, Shakespeare

○ **Why is supplemental oxygen recommended in the conservative treatment of pneumothorax?**

Absorption of a loculated pneumothorax is hastened by oxygen inhalation, which increases the pressure gradient of gases between the pleura and the venous blood.

○ **What are the treatment goals for patients with an empyema?**

Control of local infection with drainage and systemic antibiotics and re-expansion of the lung with obliteration of the pleural space.

○ **T/F: Sympathetic pleural effusions resulting from subphrenic abscesses are usually sterile.**

True.

○ **What is the most common cause of a large pleural effusion?**

Malignancy.

○ **What is the most common cause of a malignant pleural effusion?**

Carcinoma of the lung.

○ **What is the most common metastatic tumor to produce a malignant pleural effusion?**

Breast cancer.

○ **What is the volume of pleural fluid needed to obliterate the costophrenic angle on chest radiograph?**

Approximately 250 – 500 cc.

○ **What type of chest radiograph is helpful in distinguishing a pleural effusion from other intrathoracic densities?**

Lateral decubitus chest radiograph.

○ **When trauma and pulmonary infarction are excluded, what etiology is responsible for 90% of bloody pleural effusions?**

Malignancy.

○ **What laboratory values suggest a pleural effusion is an exudate?**

Pleural fluid/serum protein ratio > 0.5, pleural fluid/serum LDH ratio > 0.6.

○ **What two causes of persistent pleural effusions are diagnosed by pleural biopsy?**

Tuberculosis and malignancy involving the pleura.

O   **What is the most common type of pleural effusion in infants?**

Chylothorax.

O   **What are the complications of a prolonged chylothorax?**

Protein malnutrition, intravascular volume loss and decreased cellular immunity secondary to the loss of circulating T cells.

O   **What is the initial management of a chylothorax?**

Thoracostomy tube drainage, maintenance of fluid and electrolytes and bowel rest with parenteral nutrition.

O   **What is the best way to distinguish a pneumothorax from large lung bullae?**

CT scan which can show septae of bullae filling hyperlucent areas.

O   **What is the most common etiology of a spontaneous pneumothorax?**

Rupture of a pulmonary bleb.

O   **What are the recurrence rates of an ipsilateral spontaneous pneumothorax following a first, second, or third episode?**

30%, 50% and 80% respectively.

O   **What is the most common underlying lung disease in elderly patients who are diagnosed with a spontaneous pneumothorax?**

Chronic obstructive pulmonary disease.

O   **At what rate will the intrapleural air of a pneumothorax be reabsorbed if left untreated?**

1.25% per day.

O   **What are the disadvantages associated with treating a pneumothorax with catheter aspiration alone?**

It is difficult to evacuate the entire pneumothorax in order to re-expand the lung and it is not applicable in patients with an active air leak.

O   **Why can a large pneumothorax produce arterial hypoxemia?**

Shunt. Poorly ventilated areas of the lung continue to be perfused.

O   **Which diseases are associated with pneumothorax?**

COPD, asthma, IPF, eosinophilic granuloma and lymphangioleiomyomatosis.

O   **Which types of pneumonia are commonly associated with pneumothorax?**

Staphylococcal, TB, klebsiella and PCP.

O   **What is the indication for a tube thoracostomy in patients with a pneumothorax?**

Over 20 % pneumothorax or a clinical indication such as respiratory distress or enlarging pneumothorax.

O   **What therapy may increase the body's absorption of a pneumothorax or pneumomediastinum?**

A high FIO2.

O   **What is the profile of a classic patient with a spontaneous pneumothorax?**

Male, athletic, tall, slim and 15 to 35 years of age.

O   **What is the recurrence rate of spontaneous pneumothorax?**

30 to 50%.

O   **What special chest x-ray may be useful for diagnosing pneumothorax?**

An expiratory film.

O   **What is a catamenial pneumothorax?**

That which occurs during menses. It is usually recurrent and women often have coincidental endometriosis.

O   **What agents are used for pleurodesis?**

Monocycline, doxycycline and talc. Tetracycline is no longer available for this.

O   **Which tumors metastasize to the pleura?**

Bronchogenic, breast, lymphoma, ovarian, sarcoma and melanoma.

O   **What is a benign fibrous mesothelioma?**

It is a localized pleural tumor arising from either the visceral or parietal pleura.

O   **What is the typical clinical presentation in patients with a benign fibrous mesothelioma?**

Presenting symptoms include cough, chest pain and dyspnea. Hypertrophic pulmonary osteoarthropathy and symptomatic hypoglycemia may occur. Local invasion occasionally occurs. Surgery is curative. This tumor is not related to prior asbestos exposure.

O   **What is a chylothorax?**

It is a fluid collection in the pleural space due to disruption of the thoracic duct. Common causes include trauma related to cardiovascular surgery, lymphoma, Kaposi's sarcoma and other tumors. The fluid is milky and remains cloudy after centrifugation. The presence of chylomicrons verifies the diagnosis. If the fluid triglyceride level exceeds 110, then it is highly likely that a chylothorax is present. Treatment consists of spontaneous repair, pleuroperitoneal shunt, pleurodesis and duct ligation.

O   **What is a pseudochylothorax?**

It is a long standing pleural fluid collection in which the fluid has become chyliform. The presence of cholesterol crystals verifies the diagnosis. A fluid cholesterol level above 250 suggests the diagnosis. The most common causes of this effusion are TB and RA.

O   **What is a hemothorax?**

It is when the pleural fluid hematocrit is at least 50 % of that in the blood. All traumatic hemothoraces should have chest tube drainage. Thoracotomy is necessary for ongoing bleeding. Nontraumatic hemothorax is usually due to metastatic disease or as a complication of anticoagulation.

O   **What is a fibrothorax?**

It is a layer of fibrous connective tissue in the pleural space. Usual causes include empyema, hemothorax, TB and collagen vascular diseases. Calcification may occur. Decortication is the only treatment.

O   **What are the main characteristics of a transudate?**

Protein <3 g/dl, pleural fluid protein/plasma protein ratio <0.5, pleural fluid LDH <2/3 upper level of serum LDH (<200 IU) and pleural fluid LDH/plasma LDH ratio <0.6.

O   **What are the main characteristics of an exudate?**

Protein >3 g/dl, pleural fluid protein/plasma protein ratio > 0.5, pleural fluid LDH >2/3 of upper level of serum LDH (>200 IU) and pleural fluid LDH/plasma LDH ratio >0.6.

O   **What is the usual specific gravity of an exudate?**

1.020 or greater on a refractometer.

O   **What are some clinical disorders associated with increased capillary permeability causing exudative pleural effusion?**

Pleuripulmonary infections, circulating toxins, systemic lupus erythematosus, rheumatoid arthritis, sarcoidosis, tumor, pulmonary infarction and viral hepatitis.

O   **What are the clinical features associated with pleural effusion?**

A pleural rub (may be the only finding in the early stages), pleuritic chest pain due to inflammation of parietal pleura, cough (distortion of lung), dyspnea (mechanical inefficiency of respiratory muscles), diminished chest wall movements, dull percussion, decreased tactile and vocal fremitus, decreased breath sounds and whispered pectoriloquy. With large amounts, there may be contralateral shift of the mediastinum.

O   **Is there a role of a lateral decubitus film with the suspected side being superior?**

In this position the fluid gravitates towards the mediastinum. This facilitates the evaluation of the underlying lung for infiltrates or atelectasis.

O   **What is the most common cause of an exudative effusion?**

Parapneumonic effusions are the most common cause of exudative effusion.

O   **What is a parapneumonic effusion?**

 A pleural effusion associated with pneumonia, lung abscess and bronchiectasis.

O   **What are the common organisms causing empyema?**

Anaerobes are the most common organisms found in culture positive empyema, followed by staphylococcus, gram negative aerobes and pneumococcus.

O   **What are the clinical features of parapneumonic pleural effusion?**

When associated with aerobic organisms, it presents with acute illness, such as fever, chest pain, sputum production and leukocytosis. Those effusions due anaerobes usually present as a subacute illness over 7-10 days.

○   **What features indicate development of complicated parapneumonic effusion?**

Presence of persistent fever or chest pain on appropriate antibiotics. On CXR, a complicated effusion is seen as a moderate to large ipsilateral loculated effusion or a reverse D-sign on lateral view.

○   **How does the presence or absence of a complicated parapneumonic effusion affect the treatment strategies?**

An uncomplicated parapneumonic effusion responds to the antibiotics directed at the pneumonia. A complicated effusion must be treated with antibiotics and a drainage procedure with or without a fibrinolytic agent.

○   **What are the surgical strategies for complicated parapneumonic effusions?**

The surgical approach varies with the stage of complicated effusion and it may involve tube thoracostomy or a radiologically guided catheter, with or without fibrinolytic agents, empyemectomy and decortication, thoracoscopy or thoracotomy, or open drainage.

○   **What are the indications for the chest tube placement in parapneumonic effusion?**

Presence of a complicated parapneumonic effusion indicates the need for a chest tube. This is demonstrable by the gross appearance of purulent fluid (pus), low glucose (usually <40 mg/dl), low pH (less than 7.0 or 0.15 less than the arterial pH) and elevated LDH (>1000 IU/L).

○   **What are the fibrinolytic agents used in the treatment of complicated effusions?**

Streptokinase and urokinase.

○   **What is the treatment of choice for multi-loculated empyema in children?**

Early decortication.

○   **How long should a chest tube be left in after it has been placed for the treatment of parapneumonic pleural effusion?**

The chest tube should be left in place until the volume of the pleural drainage per 24 hours is under 50 ml and the draining fluid becomes serous.

○   **What factors predict whether closed tube drainage will not be sufficient for the treatment of a complicated parapneumonic effusion?**

The presence of multiple loculations or trapped lung usually necessitates thoracotomy instead of chest tube drainage alone.

○   **What are the typical roentgenographic features of a tuberculous pleural effusion?**

These are usually unilateral, small to moderate and more commonly on the right side. Two thirds are associated with coexisting parenchymal disease. The incidence of loculations may be up to 30%.

○   **What are the biochemical features of a tuberculous pleural effusion?**

Pleural fluid is exudative with a protein content > 0.5 g/L and > 90-95% lymphocytes (in the acute phase, there may be a polymorphonuclear response).

O   **What is the typical eosinophil count of a tuberculous pleural effusion?**

An eosinophil count of greater than 10% usually excludes a tuberculous effusion.

O   **What common conditions may cause an increased pleural fluid eosinophil count?**

The eosinophil count in pleural fluid can be elevated after a pneumothorax and thoracentesis.

O   **How is a tuberculous pleural effusion diagnosed?**

A combination of histology and culture of pleural biopsy tissue can diagnose 90-95% of cases. Pleural fluid culture, sputum culture and AFB smear of pleural fluid can provide additional diagnostic yield. Measurement of adenosine deaminase, lysozyme and gamma interferon may be helpful, but are not diagnostic.

O   **What kinds of tuberculous effusions may occur?**

The first kind is a hypersensitivity reaction to a small number of organisms that entered the pleural space. This is associated with a positive pleural biopsy culture or AFB stain. The second kind is a true empyema where the fluid is thick and cloudy. AFB staining and cultures are usually positive, obviating the need for pleural biopsy.

O   **What is the typical response to treatment in a case with hypersensitivity type of tuberculous pleural effusion?**

The patient usually becomes afebrile in 2 weeks, the effusion usually resolves in 4-6 weeks and resorption will occur with or without treatment.

O   **What is the treatment for patients with a tuberculous pleural effusion?**

The same antibiotics are used as for treating parenchymal TB. Occasionally repeat thoracentesis is necessary in the hypersensitivity type of tuberculous effusion (to relieve symptoms). Tuberculous empyema requires tube thoracostomy.

O   **What is the incidence of pleural involvement in patients with thoracic actinomycosis?**

Fifty percent.

O   **What is the most common cause of a transudative pleural effusion?**

Congestive heart failure.

O   **What are the common features of pleural effusion associated with congestive heart failure?**

Bilateral effusions, more commonly right-sided, are associated with cardiomegaly. The fluid is transudative and serous with <1000 mononuclear cells, the pH greater than or equal to 7.4 and pleural fluid glucose levels equal to serum.

O   **What are the radiological features of a pleural effusion associated with cirrhosis?**

Small to massive right sided effusion in 70%, left sided in 15% and bilateral in 15%. The heart size is normal.

O   **What is the mechanism of a pleural effusion associated with atelectasis?**

Atelectasis leads to decreased perimicrovascular pressure, resulting in a pressure gradient. Fluid moves from the parietal pleural interstitium into the pleural space due to decreased perimicrovascular pressure.

O   **What conditions are associated with atelectatic induced pleural effusions?**

Atelectasis is a common cause of pleural effusions in the ICU. Pleural effusions are seen in postoperative atelectasis associated with thoraco-abdominal surgery including upper abdominal surgery, thoracotomy and open heart surgery (phrenic nerve injury). These effusions are seen after pulmonary embolism and with other abdominal conditions such as pancreatitis, splenic infarction, subphrenic and hepatic abscess.

O   **What is the mainstay of treatment for pleural effusions associated with atelectasis?**

Treatment of the underlying condition and chest physiotherapy.

O   **What is the incidence pleural effusion associated with nephrotic syndrome?**

Approximately 20%.

O   **What is the primary mechanism of pleural effusions in the nephrotic syndrome?**

Decreased plasma oncotic pressure due to hypoalbuminemia.

O   **What are the roentgenographic features of pleural effusions seen with the nephrotic syndrome?**

Small, bilateral effusions, frequently sub-pulmonic.

O   **What are the characteristics of an effusion associated with pulmonary embolism?**

These may be transudative, exudative or hemorrhagic. The predominate cell type may be polymorphonuclear or mononuclear.

O   **What is the incidence of pleural effusion associated with malignancy?**

Malignant pleural effusions are the second most common exudative effusions after parapneumonic effusions. The most common underlying malignancies are lung and breast cancer.

O   **What conditions are associated with malignant transudative effusions?**

Lymphatic obstruction, endobronchial obstruction and hypoalbuminemia due to the primary malignancy.

O   **What are the typical chest x-ray findings in pleural effusion associated with lung cancer?**

Ipsilateral massive effusion with a mass, with or without adenopathy.

O   **When do you suspect malignancy?**

Massive effusion, large effusion without contralateral mediastinal shift and bilateral effusions with normal heart size.

O   **In a case with malignant effusion, what is the yield of various diagnostic procedures?**

Positive cytology in 60-95%, positive pleural biopsy in 50% and positive thoracoscopy in 95% cases.

O   **What type of pleural effusion is associated with malignant mesothelioma?**

A large unilateral effusion. Contralateral pleural plaques are present in 20% of the cases. Loculated pleural masses may be evident after thoracentesis.

O   **What factors play a role in the pathogenesis of pleural effusion associated with pulmonary embolism?**

Increased capillary permeability, due to ischemia and leak of protein rich fluid into pleural space, are the main factors. Atelectasis may contribute to a transudate and lung necrosis can lead to hemorrhage.

O   **What are the conditions causing amylase rich pleural effusion?**

Acute and chronic pancreatitis, adenocarcinoma of lung and ovary, lymphoma, esophageal rupture, chronic lymphatic leukemia, pneumonia and ruptured ectopic pregnancy.

O   **What are the characteristics of a pleural effusion associated with chronic pancreatitis?**

A large or massive unilateral effusion that recurs rapidly after thoracentesis. The pleural fluid may have a very high amylase content (>200,000 IU/L). Direct fistulous communications from the pancreatic bed are responsible. Failure of conservative treatment is an indication for the surgical intervention, such as drainage (up to 50%)

O   **What factors differentiate acute pancreatitis associated pleural effusion from that associated with chronic pancreatitis?**

Pleural effusion is more commonly associated with acute pancreatitis. The reported incidence is 15%. This is usually a small, left sided pleural effusion formed due to increased capillary permeability and usually does not require specific treatment.

O   **What is the incidence of pleural involvement in systemic lupus erythematosus?**

50% to 75% of patients with systemic lupus erythematosus develop pleural effusion or pleuritic pain during the course of their disease.

O   **What are the clinical features of lupus pleuritis?**

Pleuritic chest pain is the most common presentation. Other features include cough, dyspnea, pleural rub and fever. An episode of pleuritis usually indicates an exacerbation of lupus.

O   **What are the radiological features of lupus pleuritis?**

Small to moderate bilateral effusions are most common. Unilateral and massive effusion can occur. Other radiographic abnormalities such as alveolar infiltrates, atelectasis and increasing cardiac silhouette can occur.

O   **What are the characteristic features of pleural fluid in patients with lupus?**

LE cells in the pleural fluid. A ratio of pleural fluid/serum ANA of >1.0 is suggestive of lupus.

O   **What type of pleural effusion is associated with lymphangiomyomatosis?**

Chylothorax.

O   **What is the usual size of pleural effusion associated with uremia?**

Usually unilateral, small to moderate effusion, but bilateral and massive effusions can occur.

O   **What is the most common type of pleural effusion in patients with AIDS?**

Parapneumonic effusion.

O   **What is the usual clinical presentation of a pleural effusion in a patient with AIDS?**

The pleural effusion is small and unilateral or bilateral and the patient is without respiratory complaints. Tuberculosis, Kaposi's sarcoma and lymphoma are associated with large pleural effusions. These patients tend to have respiratory complaints.

○   **What are the common causes of drug-associated pleural effusion?**

Pleural effusions are common in drug-induced lupus and acute nitrofurantoin reaction.

○   **What drugs are associated with pleural effusion?**

Procainamide, nitrofurantoin, dantrolene, methysergide, procarbazine, methotrexate, amiodarone, mitomycin and bleomycin.

○   **Differentiate between transudate and exudate.**

Transudate: effusion to serum protein ratio is < 0.5 and LDH is < 0.6. Most commonly occurs with CHF, renal disease and liver disease.
Exudate: effusion to serum protein ratio is > 0.5 and LDH > 0.6. Most commonly occurs with infections, malignancy and trauma.

○   **How does a patient present with Boerhaave's syndrome?**

Boerhaave's syndrome is spontaneous esophageal perforation. It usually occurs after forceful vomiting. The patient suffers an acute collapse with chest and abdominal pain. A left pleural effusion is seen on chest x-ray in 90% of patients. Most have mediastinal emphysema.

○   **A transudative pleural effusion can be associated with congestive failure, atelectasis and hypoalbuminemia. What mechanism(s) play a role in each of these situations?**

Increased microvascular pressure is the mechanism in congestive failure, increased perimicrovascular pressure in atelectasis and decreased oncotic pressure is the mechanism in hypoalbuminemia.

○   **How can a lateral decubitus chest radiograph help before a diagnostic thoracentesis.**

The amount of pleural fluid can be semiquantitated, in a lateral decubitus chest radiograph, by measuring the distance between the inner border of the chest wall and the outer border of the lung (measuring the thickness of the fluid layer). When the distance is less than 10 mm, the amount of pleural fluid is small and a diagnostic thoracentesis is unlikely to be successful.

○   **What are the stages of a complicated parapneumonic effusion?**

There are three stages of parapneumonic effusion: exudative, fibrinopurulent and organizational. The exudative stage is associated with increased capillary leak during first three days. The fibrinopurulent stage is associated with bacterial invasion, usually from days 3 to 7. The organizational stage is characterized by fibroblast growth into the exudate, occurs at 2 to 3 weeks and leads to formation of a pleural peel that encases the lung resulting in loss of function.

○   **What does decortication involve and when is this procedure indicated?**

Decortication involves evacuation of pus and removal of fibrous tissue from the pleural surface thereby permitting the lung to re-expand. Decortication is considered in complicated parapneumonic effusions when chest tube drainage and topical instillation of fibrinolytic agents have not been successful and the lung is trapped in a thick fibrous peel.

○   **What are the features of yellow nail syndrome?**

Nail abnormalities (slow growing, discolored), lymphedema, chronic recurrent pleural effusions are typical. Other pulmonary problems such as bronchiectasis, chronic bronchitis, pneumonia and sinusitis can occur.

O   **Name two possible factors active in the pathogenesis of pleural effusions in patients with AIDS?**

Increased capillary permeability from infectious causes and hypoalbuminemia leading to decreased oncotic pressure.

O   **T/F: Pleural effusions do not occur in mycoplasma pneumonia.**

False. Effusions occur in 30% of cases. They tend to be small.

O   **T/F: In cases of undiagnosed exudative pleural effusions (routine labs, negative cytology and pleural biopsy), carcinoma is an unlikely cause.**

False.

PNEUMOCONIOSIS AND INHALED TOXINS

"Sir, I am a true laborer: I earn that I eat, get that
I wear, owe no man hate, envy no man's happiness, glad of
Other men's good, content with my harm and the
Greatest of my pride is to see my ewes graze and my
Lambs suck."
As You Like It, Shakespeare

○ **At what concentration is ozone damaging to your health?**

10 ppm. Initial effects are tearing, pulmonary edema and pain in the trachea.

○ **A 14 year-old boy was exposed to asbestos for three days and has a non-productive cough and chest pain. Does this boy have asbestosis?**

No. Although a non-productive cough and pleurisy are symptoms of asbestosis, other signs, such as exertional dyspnea, malaise, clubbed fingers, crackles, cyanosis, pleural effusion and pulmonary hypertension should be displayed before making a diagnosis of asbestosis. In addition, asbestosis does not develop until 10 to 15 years after the beginning of consistent, regular exposure to asbestos.

○ **Asbestosis increases the risk of what diseases?**

Lung cancer and malignant mesothelioma.

○ **Upper lobe nodules and eggshell hilar node calcification are displayed on x-rays of an individual with what disease?**

Silicosis (may rarely occur in sarcoidosis).

○ **What occupations are most commonly associated with silicosis?**

Sand blasting and mining.

○ **Is there a higher risk of lung cancer for patients with silicosis?**

No, although this has not been firmly established.

○ **What is the average exposure time necessary for the development of silicosis following silicon dioxide inhalation?**

20 to 30 years. Employees in mining, pottery, soap production and granite quarrying are at risk.

○ **What are the clinical types of silicosis?**

Acute: exposure occurs over months, alveoloproteinosis is seen histopathologically, CXR demonstrates air space disease predominantly in the lower lung zones and TB is a complication.

Accelerated: exposure occurs over 5-15 years, silicotic islets are seen on histopathology, upper lung zone fibrosis is seen on CXR and cavitation with superinfection by mycobacteria may occur.

Chronic: exposure occurs over 20 years, silicotic islets are seen histopathologically and the rounded opacities seen in upper lobes are due to the summation of superimposed silicotic nodules.

Progressive massive fibrosis: occurs when numerous silicotic lesions combine to form lesions greater than 10 mm. These occasionally cavitate.

Silicoma: single coin lesion.

❍   **What are the CXR findings of silicosis?**

Small rounded opacities in the upper lung zones that occasionally calcify. Eggshell calcifications can be seen in the lymph nodes. The acute form involves infiltrates in the lower lung zone.

❍   **Describe the histopathology of a silicotic lesion.**

Central cell-free area of collagen fibers surrounded by cellular connective tissue. Birefringent particles are seen in the periphery under a polarized light.

❍   **What is the typical presentation of a patient with silicosis?**

Asymptomatic, dyspnea on exertion and cough. Hemoptysis or weight loss suggests tuberculosis or cancer.

❍   **What are the physiological defects seen with silicosis?**

Obstruction, restriction, or mixed. Obstruction is due to small airway involvement. Hypoxemia at rest or with exercise may occur. The DLCO is decreased.

❍   **How is silicosis diagnosed?**

In most cases a clear history, physical exam and characteristic CXR findings are sufficient. Lung biopsy is occasionally necessary. PFTs provide supporting evidence.

❍   **What is the treatment for silicosis?**

Avoidance. No specific treatment is available, except possibly for the acute variant (alveoloproteinosis) in which steroids and bronchoalveolar lavage have been used. The management strategy is to treat complications as mycobacterial infection and to prevent other lung disease from developing. Patients with a positive PPD (and no active TB) should be given INH preventive therapy if the degree of induration exceeds 10 mm, regardless of age.

❍   **Which organisms may complicate silicosis?**

Tuberculosis, non-tuberculous mycobacteria and nocardia.

❍   **In which type of silicosis may tuberculosis be involved?**

Any: acute, accelerated, or chronic. TB is more common in the first two.

❍   **Can one person have histopathological changes of both silicosis and coal workers pneumoconiosis (CWP)?**

Yes.

❍   **What are the histopathological changes of CWP?**

The coal macule consists of dust containing macrophages with fibroblasts, surrounding a respiratory bronchiole. These lesions tend to accumulate in the upper lobes. Centriacinar emphysema is seen as well.

O   **What are the clinical types of CWP?**

Simple CWP is occasionally asymptomatic. Progressive massive fibrosis is characterized by one or more lesion being 1 cm or more in size.

O   **What are the clinical features of CWP?**

Asymptomatic, cough, dyspnea on exertion and melanoptysis (coughing up black sputum is more often seen in progressive massive fibrosis). Clubbing is not seen. Cor pulmonale is the end stage result of PMF.

O   **What are the radiographic findings of CWP?**

Small rounded opacities in the upper lung zones. Progressive massive fibrosis has one or more lesions greater than 1 cm, occasional calcification and more involvement of the mid and lower lung zones.

O   **How is CWP diagnosed?**

By history of exposure (usually at least 5-10 years), exam findings, PFTs and characteristic CXR.

O   **What physiological defects are seen in CWP?**

Obstructive and restrictive ventilatory defects. Decreased DLCO and hypoxemia occurs in advanced disease.

O   **What are potential complicatons of CWP?**

Cor pulmonale, tuberculosis and atypical mycobacteria (less then for silicosis) and hypoxemia.

O   **What is the treatment for CWP?**

Avoidance of continued exposure and management of complications.

O   **What is the most common form of asbestos exposure?**

Pleural plaques.

O   **Describe pleural plaques.**

They are found on the parietal pleura, are irregular, raised, white lesions that may calcify. They may be seen en face or on edge. The plaques may enter the lobar fissures.

O   **What is the significance of these plaques?**

Generally none, other than they have been associated with a propensity for the development of asbestosis.

O   **What other conditions may cause pleural plaques?**

Trauma, TB and collagen vascular disease.

O   **What is a benign pleural effusion associated with asbestos exposure?**

It refers to an effusion with an absence of malignant cells. These patients are not at risk for development of malignant mesothelioma. However, as the latter condition may be clinically occult, careful follow up is necessary. A benign pleural effusion is a risk factor for the development of pleural thickening and pleural fibrosis.

○   **What is the latency time for development of benign pleural effusions?**

12 to 15 years. Patients typically are 20 to 40 years of age.

○   **What are the biochemical characteristics of a benign pleural effusion?**

Exudative, frequently bloody, mesothelial cells are often seen and occasionally eosinophilic cells are present. Asbestos bodies are rarely isolated.

○   **How is a benign pleural effusion diagnosed?**

The diagnosis is by exclusion. Pleural fluid must be evaluated cytologically. Pleural biopsy should be performed to rule out malignancy.

○   **What is the natural history of these effusions?**

They often spontaneously resolve and they may recur, even to the contralateral pleural space.

○   **Can patients with this condition be symptomatic?**

Yes. Patients have symptoms of pleurisy, fever and dyspnea.

○   **What radiological findings are seen in diffuse pleural thickening?**

Pleural fibrosis, unilateral or bilateral, forming a thick white peel that may encase part of the lung. If this peel folds in on itself, it forms an opacity called a pseudotumor or rounded atelectasis.

○   **What ventilatory defect is seen in severe diffuse pleural thickening?**

Restrictive.

○   **What is the treatment for diffuse pleural thickening?**

Supportive. If severe enough, pleurectomy may be necessary.

○   **What is asbestosis?**

Parenchymal fibrosis resultant from asbestos exposure.

○   **What are the histopathological features of asbestosis?**

Parenchymal fibrosis with asbestos bodies and uncoated asbestos fibers. Early on, peribronchiolar fibrosis is seen in the lower lobes and subpleural location. Progressive massive fibrosis does not occur.

○   **What are the clinical features of asbestosis?**

Dyspnea, cough, chest tightness, wheezing and clubbing.

○   **What are the PFT findings in asbestosis?**

A restrictive ventilatory defect predominates, especially in severe cases. Mild airway obstruction may be seen as well.

○   **What is the radiographic feature of asbestosis?**

A fine reticular pattern, classically known as "small irregular opacities."

○ How is asbestosis diagnosed?

By exposure history, physical findings, PFT results and characteristic CXR. Exposure may be as short as several months if there was high intensity exposure. It is typically more on the magnitude of 10-20 years. Occasionally, lung biopsy is necessary. Asbestos bodies are visible with light microscopy. Asbestos fibers are visible only with electron microscopy.

Bronchoalveolar lavage has been used to identify asbestos bodies. The limitation is that the presence of asbestos bodies signifies exposure, not necessarily disease. Some have attempted to correlate the number of asbestos bodies with the presence of disease and not exposure. This method requires further elucidation.

○ What is the treatment for asbestosis?

No specific treatment. Surveillance for the development of lung cancer and malignant mesothelioma is necessary.

○ What are the clinical findings of malignant mesothelioma?

Age between 50 and 70 years, significant exposure to asbestos fibers, chest pain, dyspnea, pleural effusion (which is exudative, may be large, bloody and have high levels of hyaluronic acid), fever and hypertrophic pulmonary osteoarthropathy may occur.

○ What are the radiographic findings of malignant mesothelioma?

Pleural effusion, thick pleural peel, multiple pleural nodules or masses, plaques and local invasion.

○ What is more common, local invasion or metastases?

Local invasion.

○ What is the average duration of survival of this condition?

8 to 12 months.

○ How is malignant mesothelioma diagnosed?

By cytologic or histologic exam. The latter is preferred, as malignant mesothelioma can be confused with other tumors and with reactive mesothelial cells. The biopsy needle tract is often a site for the tumor to invade, so open biopsy is preferred.

○ What are the clinical types of beryllium lung disease?

Acute beryllium disease: no longer seen since environmental control. Acute inflammation of airways and lung parenchyma.
Chronic beryllium disease: multisystem disorder with granuloma formation throughout the body but mostly in the lungs. Clinically this disease is similar to sarcoidosis.

○ What are the clinical features of chronic beryllium lung disease?

Primarily respiratory symptoms, including dyspnea, cough, chest pain, weight loss, hypoxemia and rarely fevers.

○ What are the radiological features of this disease?

Diffuse round and reticular abnormalities with hilar adenopathy. Radiographically beryllium lung disease cannot be distinguished from sarcoidosis.

○   **How is this disease diagnosed?**

Biopsy demonstrating a granulomatous reaction and either BAL fluid or blood that is positive for the lymphocyte transformation test. History, physical exam, CXR and PFTs must support the diagnosis as well.

○   **What are the PFT findings in this disease?**

Obstructive, restrictive, or both.

○   **What is the treatment for chronic beryllium lung disease?**

Corticosteroids.

○   **What are the respiratory manifestations of inhaled toxins?**

Upper airway mucosal injury, bronchitis, reactive airway disease, pneumonitis, ARDS, obliterative bronchiolitis, COPD and BOOP.

○   **Which clinical syndromes may result from inhalation of sulfur dioxide, ammonia, or nitrogen oxides?**

All of the above.

○   **What is reactive airway dysfunction syndrome (RADS)?**

It is bronchospasm that does not temporally resolve after a single exposure to an inhaled toxin. Implicated toxins include sulfuric acid, chlorine, ammonia and smoke. Treatment consists of environmental control, bronchodilators and corticosteroids.

○   **What is metal fume fever?**

It is a flu-like syndrome that begins several hours after exposure to certain metals. Symptoms are self-limited, usually resolving in one to two days.

○   **Why is acute smoke inhalation difficult to study?**

Because there are many components, including particulates, carbon monoxide, hydrogen cyanide, aldehydes and others.

○   **What is the most common cause of death in smoke inhalation victims?**

Carbon monoxide exposure.

○   **How does carbon monoxide exposure present?**

With a spectrum of CNS symptoms, as severe as coma and seizures. Respiratory arrest and myocardial dysfunction may occur as well.

○   **How is carbon monoxide exposure treated?**

With 100% oxygen and hyperbaric oxygen.

○   **How does cyanide toxicity present?**

With a history of an odor of bitter almonds, pink skin, tachycardia, bright red venous blood, altered mental status, hypotension and anion gap acidosis (due to lactic acid accumulation).

❍ **How is cyanide toxicity treated?**

With a combination of nitrates and sodium thiosulfate.

❍ **What are the respiratory complications of acute smoke inhalation?**

Edema of the upper airways, bronchospasm, bronchitis and ARDS.

PO2, PCO2 AND pH

"Angels and ministers of grace defend us!
Be thou a spirit of health or goblin damn'd,
Bring with thee airs from heaven or blasts from hell,
Be thy intents wicked or charitable,
Thou comest in such a questionable shape
That I well speak to thee: I'll call thee Hamlet"
Hamlet, Shakespeare

○ **What are the clinical signs of hypercarbia?**

Flushed hot hands and feet, bounding pulses, confusion or drowsiness, muscular twitching and engorged retinal veins (all secondary to vasodilatation).

○ **Under normal conditions (pH 7.4, PCO2 40 mmHg, T 37°C) what are the corresponding PO_2 values to oxygen saturations of 60%, 90% and 95%?**

PO_2 of 30, 60 and 85, respectively.

○ **What is the primary cause of hypercapnia?**

Hypoventilation (due to central depression, neuromuscular disease, upper/ lower airway obstruction).

○ **A 50 year-old woman presents with pneumonia in the right lower and middle lobes. On 50% oxygen by face mask, her PaO_2 is 75 mmHg. Should the patient be positioned right side down or up?**

From an oxygenation perspective, right side up. Blood flow is gravity dependent. If the patient is positioned right side down, blood flow will preferentially go to the right side. However, because of the pneumonia, this will increase the amount of shunt, lowering the PaO_2 further.

From a pulmonary hygiene perspective, right side down. The infected material may move with gravity from the infected lung to the uninfected lung.

○ **A 65 year-old male presents with dyspnea and a dry cough. Chest x-ray reveals bilateral interstitial infiltrates and biopsy reveals idiopathic pulmonary fibrosis. Room air PaO_2 is 60 mmHg. What is the mechanism of hypoxemia?**

Ventilation-perfusion inequality. It is a common mistake to attribute the hypoxemia as secondary to diffusion impairment because of the pulmonary fibrosis. Diffusion impairment is a rare cause of hypoxemia.

○ **T/F: If a patient presents with a $PaCO_2$ of 75, he/she should be emergently intubated.**

False. There is no $PaCO_2$ level at which a patient must be intubated. Intubation is based upon the total clinical condition of a patient, not just upon a blood gas result.

○ **A 45 year old presents to the ER after being rescued from a fire. He is dyspneic and cyanotic. SaO_2 on 50% mask is 84%. The blood gas, however, reveals a PaO_2 of 125 mmHg. Why the discrepancy?**

A fire victim is likely to have carbon monoxide poisoning. The carbon monoxide has converted the hemoglobin to carboxyhemoglobin, which decreases the binding of oxygen to hemoglobin and prevents an accurate pulse oximetry reading. However, carbon monoxide does not affect dissolved oxygen, which is what is measured in the arterial blood gas.

O   **What is the treatment for carbon monoxide poisoning?**

100% oxygen, which increases carbon monoxide clearance by competing for binding to hemoglobin. Hyperbaric oxygen (oxygen provided at higher than atmospheric pressure) is recommended in more severe cases.

O   **T/F: A normal $PaCO_2$ in a patient with an asthma exacerbation is a good sign.**

Maybe. A normal $PaCO_2$ in an asthmatic is good if the patient is feeling improved and less dyspneic. However, it can be a sign of impending respiratory failure if the patient continues to feel dyspneic and is working hard to breathe.

O   **T/F: Oxygen should never be given to a hypoxemic patient with COPD who has chronic CO_2 retention.**

False. Oxygen should always be given to a patient who is hypoxemic.

O   **But I was taught that patients with chronic CO_2 retention given oxygen will have their drive to breathe blunted. Why should I give them oxygen?**

It has been shown that giving oxygen to a chronic CO_2 retainer usually does not result in a significant decrease in minute ventilation. The $PaCO_2$ will go up, but the rise is probably a result of changes in the ventilation-perfusion inequalities.

It is important to give these patients oxygen because a patient is more likely to die of hypoxemia than of hypercapnia. However, oxygen should be given judiciously with repeat $PaCO_2$ determinations to ensure that the $PaCO_2$ does not rise precipitously.

O   **What are the indications for chronic oxygen therapy?**

1.   Resting $PaO_2 < 55$ mmHg or $SaO_2 < 88\%$.
2.   Resting PaO_2 56-59 mmHg or SaO_2 89% in the presence of evidence of cor pulmonale and /or polycythemia.
3.   During exercise if the PaO_2 falls below 55 mmHg or the SaO_2 below 88% with a low level of exertion.

O   **What are the major mechanisms of hypoventilation and what clinical conditions are associated with each?**

1.   Failure of the central nervous system ventilatory centers - drugs (narcotics, barbiturates) and stroke.
2.   Failure of the chest bellows - chest wall diseases (kyphoscoliosis), neuromuscular diseases (amyotrophic lateral sclerosis) and diaphragm weakness.
3.   Obstruction of the airways – asthma and chronic obstructive pulmonary disease.

O   **How can hypoxemia secondary to hypoventilation alone be distinguished from other causes of hypoxemia?**

If the hypoxemia is from hypoventilation alone, the A-a O_2 gradient is normal. It is elevated in all other causes.

O   **What are the most common clinical conditions in which shunt is the primary mechanism for hypoxemia?**

Alveolar filling with fluid (pulmonary edema) and pus (pneumonia) are the most commonly seen clinically. Any condition that fills or closes the alveoli preventing gas exchange can lead to a shunt

O   **How can shunt be distinguished from the other causes of hypoxemia?**

If given 100% oxygen, the hypoxemic patient with a shunt will not have a significant increase in their PaO_2. There will be a significant increase in PaO_2 when 100% oxygen is given to patients with hypoventilation or ventilation-perfusion inequality.

○   **T/F: A leftward shift in the oxyhemoglobin dissociation curve indicates an increased hemoglobin affinity for oxygen.**

True.

○   **Changes in temperature, $PaCO_2$ or pH, or the level of 2,3-diphosphoglycerate (2,3-DPG) cause a shift in the oxyhemoglobin dissociation curve. To cause a rightward shift, what are the changes that must occur?**

Increased temperature, increased $PaCO_2$, decreased pH and increased 2,3-DPG level. An easy way to remember this is that these conditions are often associated with decreased tissue oxygen levels. By right-shifting the curve, more oxygen is released from the hemoglobin to the tissues.

○   **Which types of hemoglobin are associated with a leftward shift of the oxyhemoglobin dissociation curve?**

Hemoglobin F (fetal hemoglobin), carboxyhemoglobin and methemoglobin.

○   **What drugs cause methemoglobinemia?**

Oxidant drugs, such as antimalarials, dapsone, nitrites/nitrates (nitroprusside) and local anesthetics (lidocaine). Methemoglobinemia occurs when the iron moiety of hemoglobin is oxidated from the ferrous to the ferric state.

○   **Which common enzyme deficiency predisposes to the development of methemoglobinemia in the presence of the above drugs?**

G-6-PD deficiency.

○   **What is the treatment of methemoglobinemia?**

Methylene blue.

○   **What are the determinants of the oxygen content of blood?**

Hemoglobin concentration, PaO_2 and SaO2. The equation to determine the oxygen content of blood is: $CaO_2 = (1.34 \times [Hgb] \times SaO_2) + (PaO_2 \times 0.003)$. The first term is the hemoglobin bound oxygen and the second is the dissolved oxygen. Dissolved oxygen content is a minor portion of total oxygen content unless PaO_2 is very high.

○   **How does the shape of the oxyhemoglobin dissociation curve effect the oxygen content of blood?**

Since SaO_2 does not increase significantly if the $PaO_2 > 60$ mmHg, the oxygen content of blood will increase significantly above this level only by increasing the hemoglobin concentration.

○   **What are the determinants of oxygen delivery to the peripheral tissues?**

The oxygen content of the blood (CaO_2) and cardiac output. An increase in either will increase oxygen delivery to the tissues.

○   **What are some common causes of respiratory alkalosis?**

Respiratory alkalosis is defined as a pH above 7.45 and a pCO2 less than 35. Common causes of respiratory alkalosis include any process that may induce hyperventilation: shock, sepsis, trauma, asthma, PE, anemia, hepatic failure, heat stroke, exhaustion, emotion, salicylate poisoning, hypoxemia, pregnancy and inadequate mechanical ventilation.

○   **Calculate the alveolar-arterial oxygen (A-aO$_2$) gradient given the following arterial blood gas obtained at sea level: pH 7.24, PaCO$_2$ 60 and PaO$_2$ 45.**

30 mmHg.

To calculate the alveolar-arterial oxygen gradient, you must first calculate the expected alveolar partial pressure of oxygen (PAO$_2$) using the alveolar gas equation. The alveolar gas equation is commonly written: PAO$_2$ = PIO$_2$ - PaCO$_2$/R, where PIO$_2$ is the partial pressure of oxygen in the inspired gas and R is the respiratory exchange ratio, commonly estimated at 0.8. PIO$_2$ is calculated as follows: PIO$_2$ = FIO2 (P$_B$-P$_{H2O}$) where FIO2 is the inspired concentration of oxygen (0.21 at sea level), P$_B$ is the atmospheric pressure (760 mmHg at sea level) and P$_{H2O}$ is the partial pressure of water (47 mmHg). At sea level, PIO$_2$ is equal to 150 mmHg. Thus, for this example, PAO$_2$ = 150 - 60/0.8 or 75 mmHg.

The A-aO2 gradient is PAO$_2$ - PaO$_2$. Therefore, in this example, the A-aO$_2$ gradient is 75 - 45 or 30 mmHg.

○   **What is the normal A-aO$_2$ gradient?**

10 mmHg in a 20 year old.

○   **What is the age related decline in PaO$_2$?**

The PaO$_2$ declines by 2.5 mmHg per decade. Given that a PaO$_2$ of 95-100 mmHg is normal for a 20 year old, a PaO$_2$ of 75-80 would be normal for an 80 year old. This decline is secondary to an increase in the A-aO$_2$ gradient, which increases from about 10 mmHg in a 20 year old to 20-25 mmHg in an 80 year old.

○   **What are the principal mechanisms that lead to hypoxemia?**

Hypoventilation, diffusion limitation, shunt, ventilation-perfusion inequality, low inspired oxygen concentration and low mixed venous oxygen in the presence of V/Q mismatch.

○   **Which of the above mechanisms is the most common?**

Ventilation-perfusion inequality.

○   **Why does hypoventilation lead to hypoxemia?**

Hypoventilation results in an increase in PaCO$_2$, which in turn decreases the PAO$_2$ (see the alveolar gas equation above).

○   **Can shunt be seen in patients without alveolar abnormalities?**

Yes. Shunt can also occur if venous blood enters the left atrium without being oxygenated. This can occur in pulmonary arteriovenous malformations and intracardiac shunts.

○   **T/F: Diffusion limitation is an important cause of hypoxemia clinically.**

False. Diffusion limitation is rarely a cause of hypoxemia.

○   **Does oxygen or carbon monoxide bind to hemoglobin with more affinity?**

Carbon monoxide has a 240-fold greater affinity for hemoglobin than oxygen.

○   **What are the effects of carbon monoxide on hemoglobin?**

Carbon monoxide bound to hemoglobin, carboxyhemoglobin, impairs tissue oxygenation by two mechanisms:
1. It decreases oxygen carrying capacity by decreasing the amount of hemoglobin available for oxygen binding.
2. It shifts the oxyhemoglobin dissociation curve to the left.

O   **What is platypnea?**

Difficulty breathing in the upright position which is relieved by the recumbent position. It is the opposite of orthopnea.

O   **What is orthodeoxia?**

A decrease in PaO_2 that occurs when the patient changes from the supine to the upright position.

O   **Which conditions are associated with platypnea and orthodeoxia?**

Conditions in which there is right-to-left shunt. Most commonly the right-to-left shunt is associated with intracardiac disease (especially atrial septal defect) or intrapulmonary arteriovenous malformations.

O   **What are the common clinical signs and symptoms of acute hypoxia?**

1. Respiratory: tachypnea, dyspnea and cyanosis.
2. Cardiovascular: tachycardia, palpitations, arrhythmias and angina.
3. Central nervous system: headache, impaired judgment, inappropriate behavior, confusion and seizures.

O   **What is the normal tidal volume and minute ventilation in an average 70 kg subject?**

The normal tidal volume (V_T) is 500 to 600 ml and the normal minute ventilation (V_E) is 5 to 6 L/min.

O   **What is the difference between anatomic and physiologic dead space?**

Dead space refers to areas of lung that are ventilated but not perfused. Anatomic dead space refers to the conducting airways (trachea, bronchi and bronchioles) where there is no gas exchange because there are no alveoli. Physiologic dead space includes the anatomic dead space and any diseased lung in which there is ventilation but no perfusion.

O   **What is the normal dead space in an average 70-kg subject?**

150 ml.

O   **What is the effect of rapid, shallow breathing on the ratio of dead space volume to tidal volume (V_D/V_T)?**

The V_D/V_T increases with rapid, shallow breathing. This is because the anatomic dead space (V_D) is a fixed volume. Thus, if tidal volume (V_T) decreases secondary to rapid breathing, the dead space is a larger proportion of the tidal volume.

O   **Which pulmonary diseases are most associated with an increased physiologic dead space?**

Asthma and chronic obstructive pulmonary disease (COPD).

O   **How is the minute ventilation related to alveolar and dead space ventilation?**

Minute ventilation (V_E) is the product of tidal volume times breathing frequency ($V_E = V_T * f$). Alveolar ventilation (V_A) is that portion of the minute ventilation that contributes to gas exchange while dead space ventilation (V_D) is that portion that does not contribute to gas exchange. Thus, $V_E = V_A + V_D$.

○ **What is the effect of increased carbon dioxide production (VCO$_2$) on the PaCO$_2$?**

PaCO$_2$ will increase as VCO$_2$ increases.

○ **What common clinical conditions increase the VCO$_2$?**

Any condition in which there is increased oxygen consumption will increase CO$_2$ production. Common conditions include exercise, increased work of breathing, fever and shivering.

○ **What is the effect of increased alveolar ventilation (V$_A$) on PaCO$_2$?**

PaCO$_2$ will decrease as V$_A$ increases.

○ **What is relationship between PaCO$_2$ and V$_D$/V$_T$?**

PaCO$_2$ is inversely related to the term (1-V$_D$/V$_T$). Thus, any process that increases the dead space will increase the PaCO$_2$.

○ **Why do most asthmatics present with a decreased PCO2?**

First, the increased PaCO$_2$ associated with the increased dead space stimulates the central nervous system chemoreceptors to increase minute ventilation, which in turn decreases PaCO$_2$. Also, the associated hypoxemia and sensation of dyspnea causes the patient to hyperventilate, which lowers the PaCO$_2$.

○ **Why do asthmatics eventually have an increased PaCO$_2$ if untreated?**

As the asthma attack continues untreated, the work of breathing will continue to increase. Eventually, the diaphragm fatigues and the patient hypoventilates. The hypoventilation, in association with the increased dead space and increased CO$_2$ production, increases the PaCO$_2$.

○ **What is the normal PaCO$_2$ and does it vary with age?**

The normal PaCO$_2$ is 35 to 45 mmHg and does not vary with age.

○ **What is the normal expected change in pH if there is an acute change in the PaCO$_2$?**

The pH will increase or decrease 0.8 units for every 10 mmHg decrease or increase (respectively) in PaCO$_2$.

○ **In chronic respiratory acidosis or alkalosis, what is the expected change in pH?**

The pH will increase or decrease 0.3 units for every 10 mmHg decrease or increase (respectively) in PaCO$_2$.

○ **What is the expected change in serum bicarbonate in chronic respiratory acidosis or alkalosis?**

Bicarbonate increases by approximately 3 mEq/L for each 10 mmHg increase in PaCO$_2$ in chronic respiratory acidosis. Bicarbonate decreases by 4 to 5 mEq/L for each 10 mmHg decrease in PaCO$_2$ in chronic respiratory alkalosis.

○ **What are the consequences of hypercapnia?**

Acute hypercapnia has physiologic consequences due to the increased PaCO$_2$ itself and due to the decreased pH.

Physiologic effects of the PaCO$_2$ increase include:
1. Increases in cerebral blood flow.
2. Confusion, headache (PaCO$_2$ > 60mmHg), obtundation and seizures (PaCO$_2$ > 70mmHg).
3. Depression of diaphragmatic contractility.

The primary consequences of the decreased pH are on the cardiovascular system with changes in cardiac contractility (decreased), the fibrillation threshold (decreased) and vascular tone (predominantly vasodilatation).

○   **What are the consequences of hypocapnia?**

Acute hypocapnia has physiologic consequences due to the decreased $PaCO_2$ itself and secondary to the increased pH.

Physiologic effects of the $PaCO_2$ decrease include:
1.   Decreases in cerebral blood flow (this reflex is used in the management of neurologic disorders with high intracranial pressures).
2.   Confusion, myoclonus, asterixis, loss of consciousness and seizures.

The primary consequences of the increased pH are again primarily on the cardiovascular system with increased cardiac contractility and vasodilatation.

○   **A 32 year old male presents to the emergency room obtunded. Examination is significant for a respiratory rate of 8 and pinpoint pupils. An arterial blood gas reveals pH 7.28, $PaCO_2$ 55 and PaO_2 60. What is the cause of the hypercapnia?**

Acute narcotic overdose leading to hypoventilation.

○   **T/F: A chest x-ray in the above patient would most likely show signs of aspiration pneumonia.**

True. The $A\text{-}aO_2$ gradient is 19 (PAO_2 is 150 - 55/0.8 or 81), which is high, indicating that there are two reasons for the hypoxemia.

○   **A 30 year old female presents with dyspnea and signs of right-sided heart failure. The PaO_2 on room air is 55 mmHg and on 100% oxygen is 70 mmHg. What is the cause of the hypoxemia?**

Shunt, as there is no significant increase in the PaO_2 on 100% oxygen.

○   **The chest x-ray reveals no pulmonary parenchymal lesions but does show prominent hila and an enlarged right ventricle. What diagnostic test should be performed?**

The patient has no pulmonary parenchymal lesions to cause a shunt; therefore, she most likely has an intracardiac right-to-left shunt (most likely a previously undiagnosed atrial septal defect). An echocardiogram should be performed.

○   **A 45 year old obese male presents with dyspnea, peripheral edema, snoring and excessive daytime sleepiness. A room air arterial blood gas shows the pH is 7.34, $PaCO_2$ 60 mmHg, PaO_2 58 mmHg and the calculated HCO_3^- is 28 mEq/L. What is the acid-base disturbance?**

Chronic, compensated respiratory acidosis. If this were acute, the pH would be 7.28 with a normal HCO_3^-.

○   **What is the cause of the hypoxemia in the above patient?**

Hypoventilation is one cause. However, since the $A\text{-}a\ O_2$ gradient is elevated, there is another cause in addition to the hypoventilation. In an obese patient, both ventilation-perfusion inequality and shunt (secondary to atelectasis) can contribute to the development of hypoxemia.

○   **What is the cause of the hypoventilation?**

Obesity-hypoventilation syndrome.

O   **A 25 year old woman with a history of mitral valve prolapse presents with anxiety, chest tightness, hand numbness and mild confusion. Arterial blood gas reveals: pH 7.52, $PaCO_2$ 25 mmHg, and PaO2 108 mmHg. What is the most likely diagnosis?**

An acute anxiety attack.

O   **Why is the PaO_2 elevated in the above patient?**

Because the lower $PaCO_2$ means a higher PAO_2 (see alveolar gas equation above).

O   **What is the treatment?**

Having the patient breathe in and out of a bag can terminate the acute hyperventilation. Anxiolytics can also be provided.

O   **In which pulmonary disease has long term continuous oxygen therapy been proven to be of clinical benefit?**

Studies in both the United States and Great Britain have shown that mortality is reduced in patients with chronic obstructive pulmonary disease and hypoxemia who use long-term oxygen.

O   **What are the maximal oxygen concentrations that can be achieved by nasal cannula and face mask?**

6 L/min of nasal cannula oxygen can achieve an FIO2 of ~44%. A simple face mask can achieve an FIO2 of ~60%.

O   **What is a nonrebreather mask?**

A nonrebreather mask has a one-way valve between the mask and a reservoir bag, such that the patient can only inhale from the reservoir bag (which contains 100% oxygen) and exhale through separate valves on the side.

O   **What is a Venturi mask?**

An oxygen delivery device in which room air and 100% oxygen are mixed in a fixed ratio allowing for the delivery of an accurate FIO2 up to 50%.

O   **Why is a Venturi mask clinically useful?**

The Venturi mask is mostly commonly used for patients with chronic CO_2 retention and acute hypoxemia, where precise titration of the FIO2 is necessary to prevent a precipitous increase in the $PaCO_2$.

O   **What is the effect of pregnancy on $PaCO_2$?**

Pregnancy is characterized by a chronic, compensated respiratory alkalosis. The pH is typically 7.40 to 7.45, $PaCO_2$ 28 to 32 mmHg and serum HCO_3^- 18 to 21 mEq/L.

O   **What is the effect of pregnancy on the A-a O_2 gradient?**

In the upright position, pregnancy is associated with a normal $A-aO_2$ gradient. However, in the supine position, the A-a gradient increases secondary to increased ventilation-perfusion inequality because of the enlarged uterus impinging upon the lungs.

O   **As pCO2 increases, pH will decrease. Acutely, how much is the pH expected to decrease for every 10 mmHg increase in pCO_2?**

pH decreases by 0.08 units for each 10 mmHg increase in pCO_2.

○   **What is the equation that describes the relation between pH and [H⁺] and what are normal values for each?**

pH is defined as -Log [H⁺]. The normal plasma pH is 7.4 and the normal [H⁺] = 40 nEq/L = 40 nM/L.

The intracellular pH is lower and values depend on the specific region/organelle of the cell, but typical cytoplasmic pH values are: muscle pH = 6.8-6.9, hepatocyte pH = 7.1 and erythrocyte pH = 7.3.

○   **What is a buffer?**

Buffers are weak acids or bases (proton donor/acceptor) that resist changes in solution pH with addition of acid or base. Buffers are most effective within 1 pH unit above and below their pK (isoelectric point).

○   **What is the equation that describes the relation between pH, HCO_3^- and PCO2?**

The Henderson-Hasselbach equation describes the biologic acid-base relation by examining the CO_2-bicarbonate system, which describes the overall reaction:

$$CO_2 + H_2O \rightarrow H_2CO_3 \rightarrow H^+ + HCO_3^-$$

When CO_2 dissolves in water, formation of H_2CO_3 (carbonic acid) occurs very slowly. Carbonic anhydrase, an enzyme found in erythrocytes and the renal tubules, greatly accelerates the rate of this reaction.

The law of mass action states:

$$Ka = \frac{[H^+][HCO_3^-]}{[H_2CO_3]}$$

The [H⁺] in solution can be derived to give the following:

$$[H^+](nEq/L) = \frac{24 * PCO2}{[HCO_3^-]}$$

○   **What happens to the pH if the [H+] increases from 40 to 80 nEq/L?**

The pH falls from 7.40 to 7.10. Each doubling/halving of the [H⁺] causes the pH to decrease/increase by 0.3, respectively. Similarly, a change in proton ion concentration of 1 nEq/L causes a change in pH of 0.015 units in the opposite direction.

○   **What is an open buffer system?**

An open buffer system describes a state where one member of the buffer pair can exchange with the environment. For example, the bicarbonate system results in the formation of carbon dioxide gas, which is rapidly eliminated by pulmonary ventilation. The advantage of this system is that it allows for rapid adjustment to moment-to-moment changes in acid production (for example, a large increase in carbon dioxide production with exercise).

○   **Why does the kidney excrete fixed acids?**

To regenerate HCO_3^-.

○   **What are the major body buffer systems?**

In the intravascular space, bicarbonate, hemoglobin, phosphate and plasma proteins are the major buffer systems. The bicarbonate system functions as the proton shuttle carrying carbon dioxide from tissue to lung using the erythrocyte as the transporter and it is the major way in which the body eliminates volatile acid.
In the extravascular space, the major buffers are bicarbonate, phosphate, cellular proteins and bone hydroxyapatite.

○   **What determines the level of PCO2 in body fluids?**

CO_2 homeostasis is determined by relative rates of CO_2 production and removal. The rate of CO_2 production is determined by tissue metabolism. The rate of CO_2 elimination is determined by alveolar ventilation. During a cardiac arrest, no CO_2 is eliminated even if ventilation is adequate.

$$PaCO2 = \frac{0.86 * VCO_2}{F * (Vt - Vd)}$$

Where VCO_2 is the rate of CO_2 production (ml/min), Vt is the tidal volume (ml), Vd is the dead space and F is the breathing frequency (breaths/min).

○   **Regarding CO_2 blood transport, what are the forms of CO_2 carriage and what contribution do they make to the total CO_2 transport?**

81% is transported as bicarbonate, 11% as carbamino grouped bound directly to hemoglobin and 8% is dissolved in the plasma.

○   **What are normal and abnormal blood gas values?**

VALUE	NORMAL	DECREASED	INCREASED
ARTERIAL BLOOD			
pH	7.35-7.45	<7.35 acidemia	>7.45 alkalemia
$PaCO_2$, mmHg	40	<36 respiratory alkalosis, hyperventilation	>44 respiratory acidosis, hypoventilation
HCO_3^-a, mEq/L	24	<24 metabolic acidosis	>24 metabolic alkalosis
VENOUS BLOOD			
PHv, units	7.30-7.35		
$PvCO_2$, mmHg	45		
HCO_3v, mEq/L	20-22		

○   **What are the normal compensatory responses to alkalosis and acidosis?**

The goal of homeostasis is to maintain constancy of the blood pH by maintaining a constant ratio between PCO2 and HCO_3^-, which is accomplished as follows:

PRIMARY ACID/BASE DISORDER	COMPENSATORY RESPONSE
Increased PCO2 (respiratory acidosis)	Increased HCO_3^- (metabolic alkalosis)
Decreased PCO2 (respiratory alkalosis)	Decreased HCO_3^- (metabolic acidosis)
Increased HCO_3^- (metabolic alkalosis)	Increased PCO2 (respiratory acidosis)
Decreased HCO_3^- (metabolic acidosis)	Decreased PCO2 (respiratory alkalosis)

○   **How does alteration of arterial CO_2 correspond to changes in arterial pH?**

Disorder	Primary Disorder	Secondary Compensation
Metabolic Acidosis	Decreased HCO_3^-	Expected $PCO2 = 1.5 * HCO3^- + 8 (\pm 2)$ $PCO2 =$ last 2 digits of pH * 100
Metabolic Alkalosis	Increased HCO_3^-	Expected $PCO2 = 0.7 * HCO3^- + 20 (\pm 1.5)$
Respiratory Acidosis Acute (1-2 hr)	Increased $CO2$	$pH = 0.005$ to $0.008 * PCO2$ and $HCO3 = 0.1 * PCO2$
Chronic (<12-24 hr)	Increased $CO2$	$pH = 0.003 * PCO2$ and $HCO3 = 0.35 * PCO2$
Respiratory Alkalosis Acute (1-2 hr)	Decrease $CO2$	$pH = 0.008$ to $0.01 * PCO2$ and $HCO3 = 0.2 * PCO2$
Chronic (<12-24 hr)	Decrease $CO2$	$pH = 0.002 * PCO2$ and $HCO3 = 0.5 * PCO2$

○   **What is a better index of tissue CO2, arterial or venous CO2?**

Venous CO_2.

○   **Is it possible to have the identical PCO2 in arterial and mixed venous blood?**

During respiratory arrest, pulmonary arterial blood and systemic arterial blood have the same PCO2. However, at the tissue level, the arteriolar PCO2 is less than that of the tissue venous PCO2.

○   **What is the normal arterial-venous PCO2 gradient and how would this gradient be affected by decreased cardiac output?**

The normal arterial-venous PCO2 gradient is 4 to 6 mmHg. The arterial-venous PCO2 gradient is increased by low cardiac output.

○   **What is the affect of decreased cardiac output on the arterial PO_2?**

In most circumstances, cardiac output has no/minimal influence on arterial blood gas tensions.

Low cardiac output may decrease PaO_2 when there is a high pulmonary shunt fraction (Qs/Qt > 20%). In this case, the decreased cardiac output causes a sufficient reduction in mixed venous saturation such that the venous blood cannot be fully oxygenated during passage through the alveolar capillaries because of the presence of shunting.

○   **What are the indications for $NaHCO_3$ administration?**

1.   To replace gastroenteric bicarbonate losses, e.g. chronic treatment after pancreas transplant, duodenal fistula, diarrhea (e.g. after bowel preparation).
2.   To replace renal bicarbonate losses: e.g. renal tubular acidosis, chronic treatment after kidney transplant.
3.   Treatment of acute hyperkalemia.
4.   Treatment of tricyclic antidepressant overdose.
5.   To correct metabolic acidosis ONLY in the presence of adequate tissue perfusion and pulmonary ventilation.

○   **For every ampule of $NaHCO_3$, how much CO_2 is generated?**

One 50 ml ampule of adult $NaHCO_3$ solution has the following properties, pH = 7.8, pK = 6.1, PCO2 = 85, 1800 mOsm/L, Na = 892 mmol/L and it contains 44.6 mEq of bicarbonate.

Acutely about 10 to 15% of the administered $NaHCO_3$ is converted to CO_2 gas. Thus, a 44.6 mEq dose of bicarbonate generates 4.5 to 6.7 mEq of CO_2 and assuming ideal gas properties, this corresponds to about 100 to 150 mL of CO_2 gas. To prevent hypercapnia, the drug should be given slowly and it necessitates a transient doubling of alveolar ventilation (for about one to two minutes).

Eventually, most/all of the HCO_3^- is converted to CO_2 and 44.6 mEq of CO_2 corresponds to 1,000 ml of CO_2 gas.

○ How much sodium bicarbonate would you administer to correct a respiratory acidosis with the pH=7.21 and PCO2 =90?

None, its a (partially compensated) respiratory acidosis.

○ What are treatments for respiratory acidosis?

1. Intubation
2. Increase minute ventilation
3. Decrease dead space ventilation
4. Correct auto-PEEP (air-trapping), e.g. bronchospasm, endotracheal tube obstruction.
5. Treat (prevent) embolism
6. Reverse muscle weakness
7. Reverse sedatives and narcotics
8. Decrease CO_2 production (shivering, hyperthermia and excess glucose load due to hyperalimentation)
9. Nasal CPAP or BiPAP

○ What are the causes of high anion gap metabolic acidosis?

Addition of strong acids to the ECF, with the exception of HCl, increases the number of unmeasured anions. Frequent causes can be remembered by the mnemonic:
M: methanol, congenital errors of metabolism
U: uremic acidosis
D: diabetic ketoacidosis
P: paraldehyde, phenformin
I: iron, isoniazid
L: lactic acidosis, D-lactic acidosis
E: ethanol, ethylene glycol
S: salicylate poisoning, solvents

○ What are the causes of normal anion gap metabolic acidosis?

A normal anion gap acidosis is associated with a relatively high chloride, i.e. hyperchloremic metabolic acidosis.

Gastrointestinal
Diarrhea
Following a bowel preparation
High-output ileal fistula or external pancreatic fistula
Ingestion of substances that bind $NaHCO_3$, e.g. cholestyramine

Renal
Proximal (Type II) renal tubular acidosis: bicarbonate wasting due to impaired HCO_3^- reabsorption.
Distal (Type I) renal tubular acidosis: failure of distal nephron urinary acidification (Urine pH > 5.5).
Distal (Type IV) hyperkalemic renal tubular acidosis: major problem is hyperkalemia.

Other
Mineralocorticoid deficiency, i.e. hypoaldosteronism
Addition of HCl acid or one of its precursors, e.g. NH_4Cl
Post-hyperventilation metabolic acidosis

Dilutional acidosis, i.e. volume infusion with high chloride containing fluids (normal saline)

❍   **How are ketones detected?**

Ketones in urine can be assayed with the Acetest (employs the nitroprusside colorimetric reaction). This test, however, only detects acetoacetate (AcAc) and acetone. If beta-hydroxybutyrate is the predominate species (e.g. alcoholic ketoacidosis) the level of AcAc may be too low to be detected by the Acetest.

❍   **What is the treatment of alcoholic ketoacidosis?**

NaCl, glucose and thiamine.

❍   **What are the different kinds of metabolic alkalosis, how are they diagnosed and treated?**

Chloride responsive, urine chloride < 10 mmol/L
Volume contraction, e.g. diuretic use
Loss of gastric acid, e.g. due to nasogastric suction (can treat with H_2 blockers)
Post-hypercapnia

Chloride resistant, urine chloride > 20 mmol/L
High blood pressure: renovascular hypertension, renin-producing tumor, hyperaldoserosnism (tumor, licorice), Cushing syndrome and exogenous steroid use.
Normal blood pressure: laxative abuse, Bartter's syndrome, severe hypokalemia, (impairs renal HCO_3^- excretion) and magnesium deficiency (impairs renal HCO_3^- excretion)

❍   **What are the causes of respiratory alkalosis (hyperventilation)?**

Hypoxemia or tissue hypoxia
Pulmonary edema
Heart failure
Pulmonary embolism (air, fat, thromboembolism, amniotic fluid, etc).
Shock
Cyanide toxicity
Carboxyhemoglobin
Methemoglobin
Stimulation of chest wall dyspnea receptors
Patients with pulmonary disease

Central
Agitation, anxiety, pain
CNS infection
Central hyperventilation associated with injury to midbrain and upper pons

Metabolic acidosis
DKA
Lactic acidosis
Ingestion of acids, aspirin and alcohol

Other
Sepsis
Pregnancy
Hepatic failure
Respiratory stimulants: doxepram, progesterone and nicotine

❍   **What is permissive hypercapnia?**

Permissive hypercapnia is the use of deliberate hypoventilation by using reduced tidal volumes to prevent lung injury from barotrauma and volutrauma.

PULMONARY HYPERTENSION, VASCULITIS AND OTHER VASCULAR CONDITIONS

"A bawbling vessel was he captain of"
Twelfth Night, Shakespeare

○ **What are the pulmonary manifestations of Paget's Disease?**

High output cardiac failure with pulmonary edema, impaired respiratory control from bony involvement at base of skull, vertebral fractures leading to kyphosis and restrictive lung disease.

○ **Describe Kerley B lines.**

Horizontal, non-branching lines at the periphery of the lower lung fields.

○ **T/F: Pulmonary arteriovenous malformations should undergo resection or embolization because of their associated complications.**

True. Embolic stroke occurs in 36% of patients.

○ **Up to 50% of pulmonary arteriovenous malformations are associated with what inherited disorder?**

Hereditary hemorrhagic telangiectasia (Osler-Weber-Rendu Disease).

○ **What is the histopathology of primary pulmonary hypertension?**

A combination of plexiform lesions, thrombosis in situ, medial hypertrophy and intimal hypertrophy.

○ **What are the symptoms of primary pulmonary hypertension (PPH)?**

Progressive dyspnea, fatigue, chest pain, syncope and eventually cor pulmonale.

○ **What are the physical exam findings of PPH?**

Initially peripheral cyanosis due to decreased cardiac output, later central cyanosis due right to left shunting through a patent foramen ovale. A pulmonary insufficiency murmur may be heard. Right heart failure results in peripheral edema and ascites. Raynaud's discoloration of the digits may occur.

○ **How is PPH diagnosed?**

It is diagnosed after ruling out cardiac, pulmonary and other causes of pulmonary hypertension. A right heart catheterization confirms the presence of pulmonary hypertension. Echocardiography is useful to noninvasively follow the disease progression. A V/Q scan is useful to rule out pulmonary embolism as a cause for the elevated pulmonary arterial pressures.

○ **What is the treatment for PPH?**

Oxygen, calcium channel blockers, prostacyclin (which can only be given intravenously) and anticoagulation. Inhaled nitric oxide is being studied.

O   **What are the causes of secondary pulmonary hypertension?**

Cardiac disease, interstitial lung disease, COPD, hypoventilation syndromes, collagen-vascular diseases, pulmonary emboli that went undetected, HIV infection and drugs as fenfluramine and aminorex.

O   **What is pulmonary veno-occlusive disease?**

It is characterized by pulmonary hypertension resulting from inflammation and thrombosis of the pulmonary veins and venules. The wedge pressure is often normal. The CXR may show signs of pulmonary edema without the pulmonary artery pruning seen in PPH. The diagnosis is made by catheterization and lung biopsy.

O   **Which systemic vasculitides are associated with cANCA?**

Wegener's granulomatosis and microscopic polyangiitis.

O   **Which vasculitides are associated with pANCA?**

Churg-Strauss, microscopic polyangiitis, rheumatoid arthritis, ulcerative colitis, Crohn's disease and primary biliary cirrhosis.

O   **What is the antibody target in pANCA?**

Myeloperoxidase.

O   **What is Wegener's granulomatosis?**

It is a multisystemic disease characterized by necrotizing granulomas of the upper and/or lower respiratory tract, necrotizing vasculitis of the lung and other organs and glomerulonephritis. Limited Wegener's granulomatosis excludes renal involvement and a systemic vasculitis.

O   **What are the clinical findings in Wegener's granulomatosis?**

ENT findings include nasal obstruction, saddle nose deformity, rhinorrhea, purulent or bloody nasal discharge, nasal septal perforation and ulceration of the vomer. Lung involvement includes cough, hemoptysis, diffuse alveolar hemorrhage, inflammation or scarring in the bronchi, ulceration of the larynx and trachea and subglottic stenosis.

The CXR shows infiltrates, cavitation and nodules. Renal involvement includes proteinuria, hematuria, RBC casts and glomerulonephritis on biopsy. The PNS is involved with mononeuritis multiplex, occasionally involving the cranial nerves. Skin involvement includes palpable purpura, ulcerations, papules and nodules and pyoderma gangrenosum. Eye involvement includes scleritis, conjunctivis and episcleritis. Arthritis is mono- or polyarticular and symmetric or asymmetric.

O   **What is the treatment of Wegener's granulomatosis?**

Corticosteroids and cyclophosphamides are the mainstay. In the early granulomatous phase, trimethoprim/sulfamethoxasole is beneficial. Gamma globulin is under investigation.

O   **A 30 year old patient presents with progressive destruction and ulcerations of the upper respiratory tract and associated arthritis and acute glomerulitis. The presumptive diagnosis of Wegener's granulomatosis is made. What are the therapeutic options?**

Corticosteroids and cyclophosphamide.

O   **What rare vasculitis should be considered in an 18 year-old African-American girl with obscure hypertension, increased ESR and fever?**

Takayasu's arteritis.

O   **The presence of antineutrophil cytoplasmic antibodies (c-ANCA) with a diffuse staining pattern in serum immunofluorescence is most commonly associated with what disease?**

Wegener's granulomatosis.

O   **What are the characteristics of Churg-Strauss (allergic granulomatosis and angiitis) syndrome?**

Asthma, hypereosinophilia, necrotizing vasculitis and extravascular granulomas.

O   **What are the clinical features of Churg-Strauss syndrome?**

Allergic manifestations including asthma occur initially. The CXR may show transient and patchy infiltrates due to eosinophil infiltration. Nodules and diffuse alveolar hemorrhage are also seen. Nasal obstruction, polyps, rhinorrhea and perforation occur. Neurologic involvement includes mononeuritis multiplex, symmetric polyneuropathy, cerebral infarction and ischemic optic neuropathy. CHF, renal failure and GI bleeding may also occur.

O   **What is the treatment for Churg-Strauss syndrome?**

Steroids. In sicker patients the steroids are given intravenously.

O   **What is microscopic polyangiitis?**

A vasculitides of the small vessels involving multiple organs. It is usually pANCA positive but can also be cANCA positive. Pulmonary involvement is usually with alveolar hemorrhage. Pleurisy, pleural effusions and pulmonary edema occur as well. This condition is treated with steroids and immunosuppressive agents.

O   **What is Behcet's disease?**

A multisystemic disease that presents with aphthous ulcers, genital ulcers and uveitis. Pulmonary manifestations include pulmonary artery aneurysms, DVT/PE, hemoptysis, pulmonary infiltrates and pleural effusions. Treatment includes steroids and immunosuppressive agents.

O   **What is Takayasu's arteritis?**

A vasculitides affecting the aorta and its branches, typically seen in Asians, North Africans and women. The pulmonary artery is often involved. Steroids and immunosuppressive agents are the treatment modalities.

O   **What is necrotizing sarcoid granulomatosis?**

A rare syndrome consisting of a combination of granulomatous involvement of the lung parenchyma but without significant hilar adenopathy, a vasculitis of the pulmonary arteries and veins and a benign clinic course. Thrombosis and aneursym formation do not occur. Steroids are the treatment of choice.

O   **What is bronchogenic granulomatosis?**

A disease that affects the lower airways by invasion of lymphocytes and plasma cells causing ulcerations. It is often associated with evidence of aspergillus involvement.

O   **Primary pulmonary hypertension is most common in what population?**

Young females. PPH is rapidly fatal within a few years.

❍   **What heart sounds accompany pulmonary hypertension?**

A narrowed second heart sound split and a louder P2.

❍   **What is the major etiology of pulmonary hypertension?**

Chronic hypoxia.

❍   **What CXR findings occur with a dissecting thoracic aortic aneurysm?**

Tortuosity of the proximal aorta with an enlarged aortic knob, mediastinal widening, pleural effusion (most common on the left), extension of the aortic shadow, displaced trachea to the right and a separation of the intimal calcification from the outer contour that is greater than 5 mm.

❍   **What triad of findings confirms the diagnosis of pericarditis?**

Chest pain, pericardial friction rub and ECG abnormalities.

❍   **What are the ECG changes associated with pericarditis?**

Concave upward ST elevation in multiple leads, except V1 and AVR. PR segment depression may also be present.

❍   **What is the treatment for acute pericarditis?**

Treatment of the underlying problem. Anti-inflammatory agents such as non-steroidal anti-inflammatory agents help pain and inflammation. Patients not responding to the above treatment may require steroids. Narcotic analgesics may be needed for pain control.

❍   **Postpericardiotomy syndrome, occasionally confused with infectious pericarditis, occurs in what percentage of patients who have undergone pericardotomy?**

10 to 30%.

❍   **Are aortic aneurysms more common in men or women?**

Men (10:1). Other risk factors are hypertension, atherosclerosis, diabetes, hyperlipidemia, smoking, syphilis, Marfan's disease and Ehlers-Danlos disease.

❍   **What is a true aortic aneurysm?**

True aortic aneurysms involve a dilation of all layers of the aorta.

❍   **Why are true aortic aneurysms more likely to occur in the abdominal aorta?**

The abdominal aorta has less elastin, less vasa vasorum and fluid dynamics that contribute to increased wall stress.

❍   **A patient presents with sudden onset chest and back pain. Further work-up reveals an ischemic right leg. What is the most likely diagnosis?**

An acute aortic dissection should be suspected when chest or back pain is associated with ischemic or neurologic deficits.

❍   **What physical findings suggest an acute aortic dissection?**

Blood pressure differences between arms and/or legs and an aortic insufficiency murmur.

O   **Where do aortic dissections most often occur?**

In the proximal ascending aorta (60%). Twenty percent of aortic dissections are found between the origin of the left subclavian and the ligamentum arteriosum in the descending aorta and 10% are found in the aortic arch or the abdominal aorta. Dissection involves intimal tears propagated by hematoma formation.

O   **Describe Debakey's classification of aortic dissections.**

Type I: dissection of the aortic root, arch and descending aorta.
Type II: ascending aorta only.
Type III: distal aorta only.

O   **Describe the Stanford classification of aortic dissections.**

Stanford Type A: involve the ascending aorta.
Stanford Type B: do not involve the ascending aorta.

O   **What dissections can be treated medically?**

Patients with Type B (and Debakey's Type III) are eligible for medical, rather than, surgical treatment. Surgical treatment may be required for those with uncontrollable pain, aortic bleeding, hemodynamic instability, increasing hematoma size, or an impending rupture.

O   **Describe the stages of CXR findings in CHF.**

Stage I: pulmonary arterial wedge pressure (PAWP) of 12 to 18 mmHg. Blood flow increases in the upper lung
        fields (cephalization of pulmonary vessels).
Stage II: PAWP of 18 to 25 mmHg. Interstitial edema is evident with blurred edges of blood vessels and Kerley B
        lines.
Stage III: PAWP > 25 mmHg. Fluid exudes into alveoli with the generation of the classic butterfly pattern of
        perihilar infiltrates.

O   **What is the most common manifestation of Goodpasture's disease?**

Hemoptysis. These patients usually develop pulmonary hemorrhage before any signs of renal failure develop.

O   **How are the diffuse alveolar hemorrhage syndromes usually categorized?**

Whether they produce a capillaritis or not.

O   **Can one have diffuse alveolar hemorrhage without hemoptysis?**

Yes.

O   **What is Goodpasture's syndrome?**

A multisystemic disease in which patients present with alveolar hemorrhage and rapidly progressive glomerulonephritis. A circulating antibody, anti-GBM is present. The urinalysis contains RBC, casts and proteinuria. The CXR demonstrates bilateral alveolar infiltrates. Renal biopsy shows a proliferative or necrotizing glomerulonephritis.

O   **What is the pattern of IgG deposition in the kidneys?**

Linear.

○   **What is the treatment for Goodpasture's syndrome?**

Plasmapheresis, steroids and cyclophosphamide.

○   **What happens to the DLCO in active Goodpasture's syndrome?**

It rises.

○   **What conditions cause diffuse alveolar hemorrhage due to capillaritis?**

Wegener's granulomatosis, Goodpasture's syndrome, microscopic polyarteritis, connective tissue diseases, Behcet's syndrome, Henoch-Schonlein purpura and lupus.

○   **What diseases cause diffuse alveolar hemorrhage without capillaritis?**

Idiopathic pulmonary hemosiderosis, lupus, Goodpasture's, coagulopathies and pulmonary veno-occlusive disease.

○   **What is idiopathic pulmonary hemosiderosis?**

This condition usually presents in children with hemoptysis, which can be life threatening. CXR demonstrates patchy or diffuse air space disease. The treatment consists of blood transfusion, iron and immunosuppressive agents. Steroids, azathioprine and plasmapheresis have been tried in this uncommon disease.

○   **What is Henoch-Schonlein Purpura?**

A multisystemic disease presenting with palpable purpura, glomerulonephritis, arthritis and GI tract involvement. It rarely causes alveolar hemorrhage. Steroids are the treatment of choice.

○   **What are the clinical features of fat embolism syndrome?**

It is characterized by hypoxemia, diffuse infiltrates, neurological abnormalities (confusion, seizures, coma, focal defects) and petechiae that appear on the head, neck and axillae. The syndrome usually occurs 24 to 72 hours after the inciting event.

○   **How is the fat embolism syndrome diagnosed?**

Clinically. There are no specific tests available. The presence of fat globules in the serum is neither sensitive nor specific.

○   **How is fat embolism syndrome treated?**

Supportively. There is no specific treatment. Some have suggested that corticosteroids are effective in preventing the occurance of the syndrome.

○   **What is lymphomatoid granulomatosis?**

It is a destructive inflammatory granulomatous angiitis affecting the skin, CNS, lungs and rarely, the kidneys. Radiographic presentation includes multiple lower and peripheral nodules, which can cavitate. This condition has been associated with severe hemoptysis, severe cavitary disease and development of an aggressive lymphoma. Occasionally the course is benign. Chemotherapy and radiation therapy are treatment options, the latter for localized disease.

PULMONARY EOSINOPHILIC SYNDROMES

"Most smiling, smooth, detested parasites"
Timon of Athens, Shakespeare

○ **What are the clinical findings of Löffler's syndrome (simple pulmonary eosinophilia)?**

Pulmonary infiltrates, peripheral eosinophilia and minimal symptoms that may include cough, wheezing, myalgia and low grade fever.

○ **What are the known causes of Löffler's syndrome (simple pulmonary eosinophilia).**

Nitrofurantoin, sulfonamides and para-aminosalicyclic acid. Forty drugs have been found to cause it. Parasites including ascaris and strongyloides can also cause it. However, no cause is found in up to 30% of cases.

○ **What are the classical chest x-ray findings in patients with Löffler's syndrome?**

Transient, migratory, pleural based infiltrates.

○ **What is the usual range of peripheral blood eosinophilia in Löffler's syndrome (simple pulmonary eosinophilia)?**

10 to 30%.

○ **What is the pathophysiology of Löffler's syndrome due to Ascaris lumbricoides?**

Ingested eggs hatch into larvae that enter the mesenteric lymphatics and portal-hepatic venules, traverse into the pulmonary capillaries, then penetrate from the pulmonary capillaries into the alveoli and ascend through the airways to the epiglottis where they enter the GI tract. In the intestine the adult form matures and develops eggs, which completes the life cycle.

○ **What is the long term prognosis for patients with Löffler's syndrome?**

Excellent. The disease resolves within four weeks with or without treatment.

○ **What is the treatment for patients with Löffler's syndrome?**

Discontinuing the drug responsible, treatment of parasites identified and in severe cases, a brief tapering course of prednisone. Some patients require no treatment.

○ **What are the chemotactic factors responsible for eosinophil migration into tissues?**

IL-5, platelet activating factor, histamine, the C5a fragment of complement, eosinophil chemotactic factor of anaphylaxis (ECF-A), leukotriene B_4 (LTB_4), lymphokines and tumor associated factors.

○ **What are functions of the eosinophils?**

Host defense against parasites and modulation of inflammation.

○ **What are the enzymes and cationic polypeptides found in eosinophils?**

Eosinophil peroxidase (EPO), histaminase, lysophopholipase (Charcot-Leyden crystal protein), major basic protein (MBP), eosinophil cationic proteins, eosinophil-derived neurotoxin and eosinophil protein X.

○ **What disease has chest x-ray findings described as the "photographic negative of pulmonary edema" with central lung sparing.**

Chronic eosinophilic pneumonia.

○ **What are the laboratory findings in patients with chronic eosinophilic pneumonia?**

Peripheral eosinophilia (present in two-thirds), elevated IgE level, high ESR and iron deficiency anemia.

○ **Is chronic eosinophilic pneumonia more common in men or women?**

Women 2:1.

○ **What do pulmonary function tests show in chronic eosinophilic pneumonia?**

A restrictive pulmonary defect with reduced diffusing capacity, hypoxemia and an increased A-a gradient. An obstructive pulmonary defect can be seen in patients with asthma. Small airway obstruction may be due to a component of bronchiolitis.

○ **What symptoms do patients with chronic eosinophilic pneumonia complain of?**

Insidious onset of dyspnea, cough, fever, weight loss and less commonly, sputum production, wheezing, sweats and malaise.

○ **What are the histologic findings in chronic eosinophilia pneumonia?**

Bronchoalveolar lavage shows a high percentage of eosinophils (usually > 25%). Pathology shows eosinophil accumulation in alveoli and the interstitium, with thickened alveolar walls. Interstitial fibrosis occurs in about one half of cases. One-fourth of cases will show evidence of bronchiolitis obliterans. Low grade vasculitis may also be seen.

○ **What is the standard treatment for chronic eosinophilic pneumonia?**

Corticosteroids. Most references state that corticosteroids should be continued for six months, even though symptoms and x-ray abnormalities usually resolve within two weeks. The longer course prevents relapse.

○ **Wheezing and peripheral eosinophilia are seen in what diseases?**

Allergic bronchopulmonary aspergillosis, Churg-Strauss syndrome (allergic angiitis and granulomatosis), Löffler's syndrome (simple pulmonary eosinophilia), asthma and chronic eosinophilic pneumonia.

○ **What interstitial lung diseases can have increased BAL eosinophils (> 5%) without significant peripheral eosinophilia?**

Idiopathic pulmonary fibrosis, sarcoidosis, systemic lupus erythematosus, acute eosinophilic pneumonia and eosinophilic granuloma.

○ **What is the prognostic significance of finding BAL eosinophilia in a patient with idiopathic pulmonary fibrosis?**
The presence of BAL eosinophilia correlates with clinical deterioration and a poor response to corticosteroid treatment.

O   **What are the extrapulmonary clinical manifestations of Churg-Strauss syndrome (allergic angiitis and granulomatosis)?**

Fever, weight loss, skin rash (nodules, purpura, urticaria), arthritis, mononeuritis multiplex, central nervous system involvement, sinusitis, abdominal symptoms (pain, diarrhea, GI bleeding), heart failure and pericarditis.

O   **What are the laboratory findings of Churg-Strauss Syndrome (allergic angiitis and granulomatosis)?**

Peripheral eosinophilia, microscopic hematuria, elevated IgE levels, anemia, elevated erythrocyte sedimentation rate and BAL eosinophilia.

O   **Which antineutrophil cytoplasmic antibody (ANCA) pattern is seen in patients with Churg-Strauss syndrome (allergic angiitis and granulomatosis)?**

p-ANCA (perinuclear).

O   **What are the pathological features in the lung in Churg-Strauss syndrome (allergic angiitis and granulomatosis)?**

A necrotizing giant cell vasculitis, especially of small arteries and veins, with interstitial and perivascular granulomas. Eosinophils may also accumulate in blood vessels, the interstitium and in alveoli.

O   **What is the treatment for Churg-Strauss syndrome (allergic angiitis and granulomatosis)?**

Corticosteroids are the mainstay of therapy.

O   **What disease other than Churg-Strauss syndrome (allergic angiitis and granulomatosis) can have similar angiographic findings in the renal and abdominal vasculature?**

Polyarteritis nodosa.

O   **Eosinophilia-myalgia syndrome was described in the late 1980's in people who took what compound to treat insomnia?**

L-tryptophan.

O   **What parasites can cause pulmonary infiltrates with peripheral eosinophilia.**

Most common in the U.S. are strongyloides, ascaris, toxocara and ancylostoma. It is important to get a travel history especially to areas endemic with the filarial worms Wuchereria bancrofti and Brugia malayi. Other parasites include clonorchis, Dirofilaria immitis, echinococcus, opisthorchiasis, Paragonimus westermani, schistosoma and trichinella.

O   **What are specific diagnostic criteria of hypereosinophilic syndrome?**

1.   Blood eosinophilia of > 1500 for more than six months
2.   Absence of parasitic, allergic, vasculitic or other causes of secondary eosinophilia.
3.   Multisystem involvement.

O   **What are the cardiac manifestations of hypereosinophilic syndrome?**

Endocardial fibrosis, restrictive cardiomyopathy, valvular damage, especially the mitral valve and mural thrombi
.

O   **What are the chest x-ray findings in idiopathic hypereosinophilic syndrome?**

Pulmonary edema pattern, interstitial and nonlobar infiltrates. Fifty percent have pleural effusions. Long standing findings include pulmonary fibrosis.

O   **What organ is the major cause of morbidity and mortality in hyperosinophilic syndrome?**

The heart.

O   **Is the prevalence of hypereosinophilic syndrome higher in men or women?**

Men (men 7: women 1).

O   **What eosinophilia syndrome, often involving the lungs, is associated with arterial and venous thromboembolic disease?**

Hypereosinophilic syndrome.

O   **What are the diagnostic criteria for allergic bronchopulmonary aspergillosis?**

Asthma, peripheral blood eosinophilia, increased serum IgE levels, serum precipitating antibodies against aspergillus antigen, immediate skin prick test for aspergillus antigen and chest x-ray infiltrates.

O   **What lung disease is associated with peripheral eosinophilia and central bronchiectasis?**

Allergic bronchopulmonary aspergillosis.

O   **In which eosinophilic lung disease does the patient classically expectorate brown plugs?**

Allergic bronchopulmonary aspergillosis.

O   **What are the classic x-ray findings in a patient with allergic bronchopulmonary aspergillosis?**

Central bronchiectasis, especially of the upper lobes, with a "gloved finger" appearance, "tram lines" and consolidation secondary to airway obstruction. Occasionally a transient pulmonary infiltrate may be seen.

O   **What serum test correlates with disease activity and if a normal level is found, excludes the diagnosis of allergic bronchopulmonary aspergillosis?**

Serum IgE level. In active cases it is usually > 2000 ng/ml or > 1000 IU/ml.

O   **What is the treatment of choice for patients with allergic bronchopulmonary aspergillosis?**

Prednisone for two weeks or until the chest x-ray clears, followed by a tapering dose of prednisone and bronchodilators.

O   **Which connective tissue diseases and vasculitides are associated with eosinophilic lung disease?**

Rheumatoid arthritis, Wegener's granulomatosis, allergic granulomatosis and angiitis, polyarteritis nodosa and necrotizing sarcoid granulomatosis.

O   **What treatment may be successful in hypereosinophilic syndrome?**

Corticosteroids are tried first. A variety of immunosuppressive agents have been used.

○ **What malignancies may be associated with peripheral blood eosinophilia and eosinophilic pulmonary infiltrates?**

Non-small cell bronchogenic carcinoma, Hodgkin's disease, non-Hodgkin's lymphoma, lymphocytic leukemia and malignancies that metastasize to the lungs.

○ **What pulmonary infection in AIDS patients may be associated with BAL eosinophilia?**

Pneumocystis carinii.

○ **Which fungal disease affecting the lung is associated with peripheral eosinophilia?**

Primary coccidiomycosis.

○ **Which eosinophilic lung disease is seen in smokers and does not have peripheral eosinophilia?**

Eosinophilic granuloma (Langerhan's cell granulomatosis).

○ **What stain is specific for identifying Langerhan's cells in lung tissue?**

Stains for S-100 protein.

○ **What are the chest x-ray findings associated with eosinophilic granuloma?**

Increased interstitial markings which predominate in the mid and upper lung zones with sparing of the costophrenic angles. Stellate nodules, cysts, honeycombing and pneumothorax may also be found.

○ **What clinical findings outside of the lung may also be found in patients with eosinophilic granuloma?**

Diabetes insipidus, fever, skin rash, lymphadenopathy, enlarged spleen and bone granuloma.

○ **Which patients with eosinophilic granuloma have a poor prognosis?**

Those having an initial low diffusing capacity, presenting at a relatively young or old age, having multiple organ involvement and a history of recurrent pneumothoraces.

○ **Clinically, patients with bronchocentric granulomatosis fall into what two rather distinct groups?**

Patients with asthma and those without. Asthmatics are generally younger, have striking eosinophilia and almost always have non-invasive fungal hyphae within mucous plugs.

○ **What are the major pathologic changes seen in bronchocentric granulomatosis?**

Major changes occur in the small bronchi and bronchioles which are filled with yellow-white cheesy material associated with necrotic granulomata surrounded by pallisaded epithelioid cells.

○ **What are the major symptoms of bronchocentric granulomatosis?**

Dyspnea, cough, hemoptysis, malaise and fever.

○ **What are the roentgenographic manifestations of bronchocentric granulomatosis?**

Findings are similar to those of bronchopulmonary aspergillosis and mucoid impaction except that the findings are more peripherally located. Segmental consolidation and atelectasis, irregular masses, linear opacities and shadows are also found. Findings are unilateral in 75% and may how upper lobe predominance.

❍   **What is the presentation of a patient with acute eosinophilic pneumonia?**

It presents with fever, myalgias, cough, pleurisy, hypoxemia often requiring mechanical ventilation and a leukocystosis without an eosinophilia.

❍   **What is the prognosis of a patient with acute eosinophilic pneumonia?**

Generally good, although fatalities have occurred.

❍   **What is the treatment for a patient with acute eosinophilic pneumonia?**

Corticosteroids.

SLEEP APNEA SYNDROMES

"That, if I then had waked after long sleep,
Will make me sleep again"
The Tempest, Shakespeare

○   **Is obstructive sleep apnea common in hypothyroidism?**

Yes. Contributing factors include enlarged tongue and myopathy. Hypothyroidism should be excluded in most patients with sleep apnea.

○   **What other endocrine disorder is associated with an increased frequency of sleep apnea?**

Acromegaly. Sleep apnea may be central or obstructive in origin.

○   **Define apnea, hypopnea and apnea/hypopnea index.**

1. Apnea: cessation of airflow for at least 10 sec.
2. Hypopnea: decrement of 50% or more in airflow with consequent 4% or more fall in O2 saturation or electroencephalographic arousal.
3. Apnea/hypopnea index: number of apneas and hypopneas per hour.

○   **When is obstructive sleep apnea present?**

When the apnea/hypopnea index exceeds 15, the patient has both daytime and nighttime symptoms that are due to obstruction of the airways.

○   **What are the risk factors for obstructive sleep apnea?**

Male gender, obesity, large neck size, tonsillar hypertrophy, nasal septal deviation, retrognathia, macroglossia, hypothyroidism, acromegaly, alcohol and sedatives

○   **Where is the site of obstruction?**

Retropalatal or retroglossal.

○   **What are the symptoms of obstructive sleep apnea?**

Excessive daytime sleepiness, intellectual impairment, memory loss, poor judgment, personality changes, snoring, morning headaches, decreased libido and restless sleep.

○   **How is obstructive sleep apnea diagnosed?**

Polysomnography – sleep study. This demonstrates lack of airflow from either nasal or oral leads while chest and abdominal motions continue. O2 saturation falls with apneic episodes.

○   **How is obstructive sleep apnea treated?**

Position (lateral decubitus), CPAP, intraoral appliances, weight loss and surgery.

○   **What surgical procedures can be performed for obstructive sleep apnea?**

Nasal surgery, tonsillectomy, adenoidectomy, uvulopalatopharyngoplasty and tracheostomy.

O   **What about protriptyline, acetazolamide, medroxyprogesterone and oxygen?**

Protriptyline decreases the amount of REM sleep and it is occasionally used in patients whose apnea mostly occurs during REM. Acetazolamide and medroxyprogesterone increase respiratory drive and are useful in central sleep apnea. Oxygen alone is discouraged as the use of oxygen with ongoing apneas could result in a more profound duration of obstruction.

O   **What are the side effects of nasal CPAP?**

Mask leaks, skin breakdown, claustrophobia, rhinitis and aerophagia.

O   **What is the obesity-hypoventilation (Pickwickian) syndrome?**

Obesity, hypoventilation and daytime hypercapnia with hypoxemia. Other findings include excessive sleepiness, pulmonary hypertension and right heart failure. These patients generally have obstructive sleep apnea as well.

O   **What are the treatment options for patients with Pickwickian syndrome?**

Weight loss is the optimal treatment. BiPAP and CPAP are used for the associated obstructive sleep apnea.

O   **What are the causes of central sleep apnea?**

Idiopathic, CNS disease, movement to high altitude and respiratory neuromuscular disease (as myasthenia gravis).

O   **How is central sleep apnea diagnosed on polysomnography?**

A lack of airflow coinciding with a lack of chest and abdominal movements.

O   **How is central sleep apnea treated?**

BiPAP ventilation and ventilatory stimulants.

O   **What is the upper airway resistance syndrome?**

Recurrent arousals occur due to airway resistance, which results in fragmented sleep. No oxygen desaturation occurs. Best diagnosed with nasal pressure tracings during polysomnography or with esophageal balloon tracings. Treatment is with CPAP.

O   **What is narcolepsy?**

This condition causes excessive daytime somnolence, cataplexy, sleep paralysis and hypnagogic hallucinations. Narcolepsy is diagnosed by the sleep latency test, in which patients with this condition will fall asleep in less than 5 minutes with early REM onset. Treatment is with stimulant drugs as dextroamphetamine.

O   **What is cataplexy?**

The sudden loss of muscle tone in which the patient falls asleep. It can be brought about by sudden emotions, as laughing.

O   **Compare REM (rapid eye movement) and NREM (non-rapid eye movement) sleep.**

During sleep, humans cycle between these two phases in intervals of 90 minutes. During REM the body occasionally twitches, respiration is irregular, and the EMG shows atonia. In NREM sleep, the body is still, respiration is regular and the muscle tone is stable. Vivid dreams occur in REM sleep. During NREM sleep, the parasympathetic tone increases, lowering the heart rate. During REM sleep marked fluctuations in the sympathetic outflow occur, which occasionally increases the heart rate.

○   **Why do animals sleep?**

No accepted answer. Theories include avoidance of predatory species and regeneration of cerebral metabolites.

○   **During which of the four phases of sleep are K waves seen on EEG?**

Second.

○   **What happens to the ventilatory response to pCO2 during sleep?**

It is less responsive.

○   **What is the differential diagnosis of persistent daytime sleepiness?**

Sleep apnea, narcolepsy, depression, insufficient sleep, medical problems limiting sleep (paroxysmal nocturnal dyspnea from CHF, prostatic enlargement), CNS disorders, drugs (benzodiazepines, narcotics, antihistamines) and idiopathic.

TRANSPLANTATION

"when I was at home, I was in a better place:
but travelers must be content."
As You Like It, Shakespeare

○ **Which drugs are used most often to prevent lung rejection?**

Cyclosporine, azathioprine and corticosteroids.

○ **What are the histopathological findings in acute rejection?**

Perivascular mononuclear cellular infiltrate and lymphocytic bronchitis or bronchiolitis.

○ **What are the clinical findings in acute rejection?**

Dyspnea, fever, hypoxemia and infiltrates on CXR.

○ **How is acute rejection diagnosed?**

Histologically, with transbronchial lung biopsy. BAL does not distinguish between infection and rejection.

○ **What is the treatment for acute rejection?**

High dose steroids. If this fails, OKT3 or ATL is used.

○ **What is the typical manifestation of chronic rejection?**

Progressive dyspnea with decline in FEV1 (at least 20% from baseline), usually after three months.

○ **Is tissue necessary to make the diagnosis of chronic rejection?**

No, not in the correct clinical scenario. Biopsy is useful to rule out concurrent acute rejection and infection.

○ **What is the histological hallmark of chronic rejection?**

Obliterative bronchiolitis and fibrointimal thickening of arteries and veins.

○ **What is the treatment for chronic rejection?**

Augmented steroids, OKT3 or ATL and FK506 have been used. The response is generally poor.

○ **What is the most common cause of infectious complications?**

Bacterial, which often occur early after the transplantation. Gram negative organisms are the most common.

○ **What is the most common viral infection?**

CMV, which occurs 1 to 3 months post-transplantation. Ganciclovir is the treatment and occasionally CMV hyperimmune globulin is added.

○ **Who is at risk for CMV pneumonitis?**

The seronegative recipient with a seropositive donor is at risk for primary disease. The seropositive recipient may develop reactivation disease. Ganciclovir is often given to patients at high risk for CMV disease.

○   **What other viral infections occur?**

RSV and herpes simplex. The latter has been less common since the use of prophylactic regimens containing acyclovir or ganciclovir.

○   **Which fungal infections are the most common in lung transplant patients?**

Candida and aspergillus.

○   **Which prophylactic drug has drastically reduced the incidence of PCP?**

Bactrim.

○   **What is post-transplant lymphoproliferative disorder?**

This is a proliferation of cells, either polyclonal or monoclonal, that usually occurs in the lung. The polyclonal variety is responsive to a reduction in immunosuppressive agents. The monoclonal variety is a lymphoma that requires chemotherapy. The response is poor, in general. These conditions are thought to be related to infection with EBV.

○   **What is the reimplantation response?**

This is a capillary leak syndrome thought to be due to ischemia and reperfusion of the grafted lung. It usually occurs in the first few days. The treatment is supportive care.

○   **What are the indications for single, double, or heart-lung transplantation?**

Single: COPD, primary pulmonary hypertension, IPF or other interstitial lung diseases
Double: cystic fibrosis, primary pulmonary hypertension, COPD
Heart-lung: Eisenmenger's syndrome (in congenital heart disease), primary pulmonary hypertension

○   **EBV infection is linked with what late complication (years)?**

Post transplant lymphoproliferative disorder.

○   **When is Pneumocystis carinii pneumonia most likely to be seen in a transplant patient?**

2 to 6 months post transplantation.

○   **What immunosuppressive agents have the highest risk of reactivating CMV infection?**

Azathioprine and OKT3/antilymphocyte globulin.

○   **What tests should be performed for rejection surveillance in a heart-lung transplant recipient?**

Pulmonary function tests
Systemic arterial oxygen tension
Chest roentgenogram
Transbronchial biopsy

○   **Fever, sternal tenderness, erythema and purulent drainage suggest what diagnosis 48 hours postoperative heart transplantation?**

Mediastinitis caused by S. aureus, S. epidermidis or gram negative bacilli.

○   **What is the most common site of bacterial infection in all types of transplant patients?**

Lung (35%).

○   **What is graft versus host disease (GVHD)?**

Engraftment of immunocompetent donor cells into an immunocompromised host, resulting in cell-mediated cytotoxic destruction of host cells if an immunologic incompatibility exists.

○   **What are the common factors which influence engraftment and graft rejection?**

1.   HLA disparity - most important
2.   Pretransplant alloimmunization by transfusions
3.   Conditioning regimen
4.   Transplanted marrow cell dose
5.   Marrow/stroma microenvironment
6.   Post-transplant immunosuppression
7.   Donor T cells
8.   Drug toxicity
9.   Viral infections

○   **When does acute GVHD present and what are the typical manifestations?**

Acute GVHD typically occurs around day 19 (median), just as the patient begins to engraft and is characterized by erythroderma, cholestatic hepatitis and enteritis.

○   **A 30 year-old female is 21 days status-post bone marrow transplant (BMT) and presents with a fever, maculopapular rash over 30% of her body, >1,000 ml diarrhea/day and rising LFTs, with a total bilirubin of 4 mg/100ml. What is the clinical stage of GVHD?**

Stage 2.

○   **The above patient, four days later, has evidence of generalized erythroderma with desquamation, severe abdominal pain with no bowel movements and a total bilirubin of 16mg/100ml. What is the clinical stage of GVHD?**

The patient has progressed to stage 4.

○   **What is the clinical definition of chronic GVHD (cGVHD)?**

As early as 60-70 days status-post engraftment, the patient exhibits signs of a systemic autoimmune process, manifesting as Sjogren's syndrome, systemic lupus erythematosus, scleroderma, primary biliary cirrhosis and commonly experiences recurrent infection with encapsulated bacteria, fungus, or viruses.

○   **What are the risk factors for development of cGVHD?**

1.   Advanced age
2.   Prior acute GVHD
3.   Buffy coat transfusions
4.   Parity of female donor
5.
○   **How long is immunosuppressive treatment required for BMT recipients?**

Usually 6-12 months or until a state of tolerance is attained.

O   **What agent may be a treatment alternative for patients with refractory chronic GVHD?**

Thalidomide.

O   **What is the mechanism of action of cyclosporine?**

It selectively inhibits the translation of IL-2 mRNA by helper T cells, thus attenuating the T cell activation pathways.

O   **What drugs <u>increase</u> blood levels of cyclosporine?**

1. Ketoconazole
2. Erythromycin
3. Methylprednisolone
4. Warfarin
5. Verapamil
6. Ethanol
7. Imipenem-cilastatin
8. Metaclopropamide
9. Fluconazole

O   **What drugs <u>decrease</u> blood levels of cyclosporine?**

1. Phenytoin
2. Phenobarbital
3. Carbamazepine
4. Valproate
5. Nafcillin
6. Rifampin

O   **What are significant toxic side effects of cyclosporine therapy?**

1. Neurotoxic: tremors, paraesthesia, headache, confusion, somnolence, seizures and coma.
2. Hepatotoxic: cholestasis, cholelithiasis and hemorrhagic necrosis.
3. Endocrine: ketosis, hyperprolactinemia, hypertestosteronemia, gynecomastia and impaired spermatogenesis.
4. Metabolic: hypomagnesemia, hyperuricemia, hyperglycemia, hyperkalemia and hypocholesterolemia.
5. Vascular: hypertension, vasculitic hemolytic-uremic syndrome and atherogenesis.
6. Nephrotoxic: oliguria, acute tubular damage, fluid retention, interstitial fibrosis and tubular atrophy.

O   **What drugs may exacerbate the nephrotoxicity of cyclosporine?**

Aminogylcosides, amphotericin B, acyclovir, digoxin, furosemide, indomethacin and trimethoprim.

O   **What are the long term effects of corticosteroid treatment?**

Growth failure, cushingoid appearance, hypertension, cataracts, GI bleeding, pancreatitis, psychosis, hyperglycemia, osteoporosis, aseptic necrosis of the femoral head and suppression of the pituitary-adrenal axis.

O   **What is the overall risk for developing a secondary malignancy, as compared to the general population?**

The risk is 6.7 times that of the general population.

O   **Common immunosuppressive drugs include:**

Cyclosporine, azathioprine, prednisone, OKT3 (monoclonal antilymphocyte antibody) and FK506.

O   **Child's Class C chronic liver disease is associated with what clinical manifestations?**

Serum bilirubin > 3, serum albumin < 3, PT of INR > 2, comatose neurologic state, difficult to control ascites and a wasting neurologic condition.

O   **Causes of encephalopathy in liver transplant candidates may include:**

Gastrointestinal bleeding or other protein loads, hepatic coma secondary to cerebral edema and elevated intracranial (ICP). Perioperative precautions to avoid increases in ICP are suggested (head up positioning, osmotic diuretics, consideration of ICP monitoring).

O   **What conditions predispose liver transplant patients to renal failure?**

1. Prerenal hypovolemia.
2. Ascites formation.
3. Hepatorenal syndrome.

O   **Why is adequate venous access so critical in liver transplantation anesthesia?**

Liver transplantation has been associated with major volume losses secondary to the coagulopathies associated with liver disease and massive transfusions are occasionally necessary.

O   **What are the major problems associated with reperfusion of the new liver?**

Retrograde flushing of the new liver via the portal vein can be associated with rapid blood loss and profound hypovolemia and hypotension, necessitating rapid transfusion. Flushing of the liver is also frequently associated with a dramatic rise in serum potassium. Serum potassium should be monitored during the anhepatic phase and be kept relatively low in anticipation of this dramatic rise.

O   **On induction for lung transplantation, patients with severe chronic obstructive pulmonary disease (COPD) are often hemodynamically unstable. Why?**

COPD patients are frequently very volume depleted. On induction and commencement of positive pressure ventilation, they have a tendency to auto-peep secondary to air trapping and "breath stacking," severely reducing venous return and cardiac output. These patients should be preloaded with approximately a liter of crystalloid and ventilated with shallow tidal volumes and a long expiratory time.

O   **T/F: Permissive hypercapnia is never utilized in lung transplantation.**

False. Ventilation is often marginal in lung transplantation patients, particularly during one lung ventilation. An elevated PCO2 is accepted so long as the pH is maintained above 7.2.

O   **What are the primary indications for heart-lung transplantation (HLTx)?**

Congenital heart disease with or without Eisenmenger's complex and primary pulmonary hypertension are the two main indications for HLTx, each accounting for about 28% of the total HLTxs performed in adults.

O   **Describe rate control for the heart transplanted patient.**

The transplanted heart frequently has two SA nodes. The native SA node is isolated from the myocardium by the suture line and does not influence the heart rate, although its p-wave may be visible on the EKG. The SA node from the donor heart controls the heart rate, but because of the resultant denervation it is isolated from sympathetic and parasympathetic modulation. Direct acting positive chronotropic agents are required to increase heart rate.

○   **In a patient undergoing renal transplantation, is succinylcholine contraindicated?**

Succinylcholine is only contraindicated if the patient has an elevated serum potassium level, risk factor for malignant hyperthermia or some other pre-existing medical condition that could cause the potassium level to become elevated (such as paralysis, muscular dystrophy, etc.) due to succinycholine administration.

○   **In a patient needing renal transplantation list some common preoperative problems that are often encountered?**

These problems include inadequate or excessive intravascular volume, electrolyte abnormalities, hypertension, anemia, concurrent drug therapy, or complications associated with DM (cardiac and vascular).

○   **In a patient needing renal transplantation why is the hemoglobin level low?**

Chronic anemia with hemoglobin levels of 5 to 7 results from decreased production of erythropoietin and diminished red cell survival time. Iron absorption from the gastrointestinal tract may also be decreased in patients with ESRD leading to iron deficiency.

○   **In a patient with ESRD needing renal transplantation are platelets affected?**

The platelet count is often low but the primary affect is on platelet function. Prolonged bleeding time and decreased platelet adhesiveness occur.

○   **In a patient with ESRD needing renal transplantation what other coagulation problems other than platelet dysfunction can be present?**

The vitamin K dependent coagulation factors (II, VII, IX, X) and factor V tend to be low.

○   **In a patient who has undergone renal transplantation what are some of the early postoperative complications?**

The early postoperative complications include renal artery occlusion, hyperacute rejection, acute renal failure, graft rupture, wound infection and urinary fistula.

○   **In a patient who has undergone renal transplantation what are the signs of rejection?**

Decreased urine output, fever and increased serum creatinine. The kidney is often enlarged and tender to palpation. A renal biopsy is necessary to verify the diagnosis.

○   **What is the primary indication for pancreas transplantation?**

Transplantation of the pancreas is the best method by which to establish a constant glycemic state in diabetic patients with permanent normalization of glycosylated hemoglobin.

○   **How does pancreatic islet transplantation differ from pancreas transplantation?**

Pancreatic islet transplantation is a form of selective transplantation since only the cells required by the recipient are transplanted. When only the islet cells are transplanted complications related to the exocrine portion of the pancreas are eliminated.

○   **What type of anesthesia is required for pancreatic islet cell transplantation?**

The transplantation of islet cells is performed by injecting purified islet suspension into the portal vein. Sedation combined with local anesthesia is usually all that is needed. This form of transplantation is often performed in the intensive care unit, not the operating room.

○   **What are some of the most common immunosuppressive agents used in patients status post pancreas transplantation?**

Cyclosporine, azathioprine, prednisone, OKT3 and antilymphocyte globulin.

TUMORS

"If I do grow great, I'll grow less"
King Henry IV, Shakespeare

○ **What intrathoracic neoplasms are associated with asbestos exposure?**

Malignant mesothelioma and lung cancer.

○ **T/F: Malignant mesothelioma usually presents with chest wall pain and dyspnea and has documented asbestos exposure in only 50% of patients.**

True.

○ **What is the most common intrathoracic neoplasm among cigarette smokers with a history of asbestos exposure?**

Bronchogenic lung carcinoma.

○ **What percentage of patients diagnosed with non-small cell lung cancer have the potential to undergo surgical resection for cure?**

Thirty percent.

○ **T/F: Paraneoplastic syndromes occur more frequently in association with non-small cell lung cancer than with small cell lung cancer.**

False.

○ **T/F: Small cell lung cancer is often widely disseminated at the time of diagnosis and is infrequently treated by surgical resection.**

True.

○ **T/F: Solitary pulmonary nodules found in patients over 50 years old are more likely to contain malignancy than those found in younger patients.**

True. The incidence of malignancy increases as patient age increases. By age 50, 50% of such nodules will harbor a malignancy.

○ **Following a history, physical examination and chest radiographs, what constitutes the minimum preoperative staging of patients with non-small cell lung cancer?**

Complete blood count, liver function test, electrolytes, computed tomography of the chest and upper abdomen and PFTs.

○ **What are the common sites for metastases of lung cancer?**

Brain, adrenal glands, bone, liver, contralateral lung and mediastinal and supraclavicular lymph nodes.

○   **T/F: Mediastinal lymph nodes that appear larger than 1.0 cm in size on CT scan confer N2 (stage IIIA) disease precluding curative resection of non-small cell lung cancer.**

False. 30% will show no evidence of malignancy when biopsied by mediastinoscopy or left parasternal incision (Chamberlain Procedure) and would not preclude curative resection.

○   **What is the best treatment for a patient with an isolated brain metastasis that otherwise appears to have stage I non-small cell lung cancer?**

Resection of the isolated brain metastasis followed by whole brain irradiation and resection of the primary lung tumor is associated with a 20% five-year survival in this subset of patients with stage IV disease.

○   **T/F: An ipsilateral pleural effusion is a contraindication to curative resection of a non-small cell lung cancer.**

False. Malignant pleural effusions (cytologically positive) confer T4 (stage IIIB) disease and preclude curative resection while non-malignant effusions do not change the tumor stage or resectability.

○   **What is the five-year survival of patients undergoing complete resection of a stage IA (T1N0M0) non-small cell lung cancer?**

70%.

○   **T/F: A solitary pulmonary nodule that has not changed in appearance on chest radiograph over six months can be assumed to be benign.**

False. Stability for two years is the classic duration for benignancy. Rarely, malignant lesions can appear stable over this period of time.

○   **Does postoperative radiation therapy for non-small cell lung cancer improve patient survival?**

No. It has, however, been shown to decrease the rate of local recurrence in patients with completely resected stage II and III squamous cell carcinoma of the lung.

○   **When is a pneumonectomy required for the resection of non-small cell lung cancer?**

When there is tumor invasion of the proximal mainstem bronchus or pulmonary arteries or veins in patients without other contraindications to resection.

○   **Horner's syndrome is most often associated with what intrathoracic malignancy?**

Superior sulcus (Pancoast) tumor.

○   **What is the advantage of lobectomy over segmentectomy and wedge resection in the treatment of a peripheral T1N0M0 (stage IA) non-small cell lung cancer?**

Lobectomy improves five-year survival and reduces the incidence of local recurrence from 15% to 5%.

○   **T/F: Non-small cell lung cancer that invades the parietal pleura or chest wall is not resectable for cure and should be treated with radiation.**

False. Complete resection by lobectomy and en-bloc chest wall resection is nearly always feasible. Adjunct radiation does not improve survival.

○   **What is the most common benign tumor of the lung?**

Hamartoma.

○   **What type of non-small cell lung cancer is often multicentric, metastasizes within the lung and requires extended follow-up?**

Bronchoalveolar carcinoma.

○   **What lung neoplasm in young to middle-aged patients is often centrally located, usually endobronchial and may present with obstructive symptoms or hemoptysis?**

Bronchopulmonary carcinoid.

○   **What three criteria must be obtained for a patient to benefit from the resection of metastases to the lung?**

Primary tumor controlled or controllable, metastatic disease confined to the lung and complete resection with adequate residual pulmonary function.

○   **What is the preferred technique for the resection of metastases to the lung?**

Wedge resection.

○   **Does the resection of metastases to the lung increase overall median survival in selected patients?**

Yes. 38 months versus 14 months in unresected patients. However, this is only in comparison to historical controls and has not been confirmed in randomized trials.

○   **What is the most common postoperative complication following pulmonary resection?**

Atelectasis.

○   **What is the most likely cause of severe head, neck and arm swelling in a patient with a centrally located mass on chest radiograph?**

Superior vena cava syndrome, the partial or complete mechanical obstruction of the superior vena cava by an intrathoracic tumor or nodal metastases.

○   **What is the preferred therapy for patients with superior vena cava syndrome caused by non-small cell lung cancer?**

Radiation therapy.

○   **What organs are frequently involved with metastases from primary lung cancer?**

Adrenal, brain, liver and bone.

○   **Hypercalcemia in the absence of bony metastases is associated with which lung cancer?**

Squamous cell carcinoma (a paraneoplastic syndrome associated with tumor elaboration of a PTH-like substance).

○   **The syndrome of inappropriate secretion of antidiuretic hormone is associated with which cell type of lung cancer?**

Small cell carcinoma.

○   **Bilateral periostitis, typically affecting the long bones and associated with lung cancer, is known as what other disease?**

Hypertrophic pulmonary osteoarthropathy (HPO).

○   **This finding is most frequently associated with which type of lung cancer?**

Adenocarcinoma.

○   **T/F: The presence of HPO alone contraindicate a surgical approach in the treatment of lung cancer.**

False.

○   **What myopathic syndrome is associated with lung cancer?**

Eaton-Lambert syndrome.

○   **What finding on physical examination can be used to differentiate Eaton-Lambert syndrome from myasthenia gravis?**

Muscle function improves with repeated activity in the former, but degrades in the latter.

○   **Tumor involvement in which lymph node location most clearly contraindicates a surgical approach to the therapy of non-small cell lung cancer? Hilar, contralateral mediastinal, infrapulmonary, or subcarinal?**

Contralateral mediastinal.

○   **T/F: Routine preoperative head CT scanning and nuclear scanning of liver and bone is advocated in patients with lung cancer.**

False.

○   **Of the following, which pattern of calcification of a solitary pulmonary nodule is most likely to be associated with a malignant lesion: lamellar (onion skin), popcorn, eccentric, or central?**

Eccentric.

○   **Radiographic stability for what period is assumed to indicate a benign origin of a solitary pulmonary nodule?**

Two years.

○   **Doubling of the volume of a solitary pulmonary nodule is associated with what percentage increase in its diameter?**

Twenty-six percent.

○   **What is the initial diagnostic test in a clinically stable patient suspected of having lung cancer?**

Sputum cytological examination.

○   **T/F: Patients who smoke >1 pack of cigarettes per day should be screened yearly with sputum cytology examinations.**

False.

O   T/F: Patients who smoke >2 packs of cigarettes per day should be screened annually with a PA radiograph of the chest.

False.

O   T/F: Local tumor invasion of the chest wall always contraindicates a surgical approach to lung cancer therapy.

No.

O   T/F: A malignant pleural effusion always contraindicates a surgical approach to lung cancer therapy.

True.

O   What are the components of Horner's Syndrome?

Ptosis, miosis and anhidrosis.

O   T/F: Pre-operative radiotherapy is indicated in the treatment of malignant tumors of the superior pulmonary sulcus.

True.

O   What finding indicates emergent radiation therapy for superior vena cava syndrome?

Cerebral edema.

O   What is the major indication for laser bronchoscopy in the treatment of bronchogenic carcinoma?

Tumor obstruction of large airways.

O   What predicted post-operative FEV1 contraindicates surgical therapy for lung cancer?

<800 cc.

O   Which of the following is the preferred method to predict post-operative FEV1 in patients whose pre-operative FEV1 is <2 liters: quantitative perfusion lung scanning, quantitative ventilation lung scanning, split lung function utilizing a Carlens tube, or the lateral position test?

Quantitative perfusion lung scanning.

O   Which of the following is an alternative method of assessing operability in patients with lung cancer: stress echocardiography, cardiopulmonary exercise testing, weighing the patient while submerged, or the helium mixing time?

Cardiopulmonary exercise testing.

O   Which method of mediastinal lymph node sampling is least likely to be useful in the pre-operative assessment of patients with lung cancer: mediastinoscopy, mediastinotomy (Chamberlain procedure), sternotomy, or transbronchial needle aspiration?

Sternotomy.

O   What is the 5 year survival in all patients diagnosed with primary lung cancer?

<15%.

O   **Which primary lung cancer is most likely to cavitate?**

Squamous cell carcinoma.

O   **Which primary lung cancer is least likely to present as a solitary pulmonary nodule?**

Small cell undifferentiated carcinoma.

O   **What is the 5 year survival of non-small cell carcinoma of the lung treated with combination chemotherapy?**

<10%.

O   **The best 5 year survival for non-small cell carcinoma of the lung is achieved by what therapy modality?**

Surgical resection.

O   **What is the surgical 5-year survival for stage 1 non-small cell carcinoma of the lung?**

50-60%.

O   **T/F: Curative doses of radiotherapy for inoperable lung cancer are effective in resultant long-term survival.**

False.

O   **In the absence of trauma, which of the following is most likely to be the etiology of a bloody pleural effusion: a leaking thoracic aortic aneurysm, pneumonia, tuberculosis, lung cancer or a pulmonary infarction?**

Lung cancer.

O   **What is the increase in death rate from lung cancer among smokers compared to non-smokers?**

8 to 20 fold.

O   **Bronchorrhea can be the presenting symptom in which subtype of adenocarcinoma of the lung?**

Bronchoalveolar cell carcinoma.

O   **T/F: Low tar cigarettes decrease the risk of lung cancer.**

False.

O   **The most common malignancy associated with asbestos exposure is which of the following: esophageal carcinoma, primary lung cancer, mesothelioma, or gastric carcinoma?**

Primary lung cancer.

O   **T/F: Alpha-1 antitrypsin deficiency is associated with an increased risk of lung cancer.**

False.

○   Which of the following physical findings is most specifically associated with lung cancer: cachexia, localized wheezing, acanthosis nigricans, or alopecia areata?

Localized wheezing.

○   T/F: A superior performance status has an association with improved survival among patients with non-small cell lung cancer.

True.

○   T/F: An ipsilateral pleural effusion in a patient with a malignant lung tumor is always assumed to represent tumor spread and contraindicates surgical therapeutic approach.

False.

○   T/F: A patient with lung cancer can be declared inoperable solely based on functional status.

True.

○   Which of the following can fill the vacated hemithorax following pneumonectomy: organized fluid, contralaterally shifted lung parenchyma, mediastinal contents, elevated hemi-diaphragm or intra-abdominal contents?

All of the above.

○   T/F: One should assume that two coexistent solitary pulmonary nodules always represent metastases.

False.

○   What percentage of solitary pulmonary nodules, in patients with a previous diagnosis of extrathoracic malignancy, represent metastatic disease?

50%.

○   T/F: The majority of solitary pulmonary nodules seen on routine chest x-ray are malignant.

False.

○   A solitary pulmonary nodule in an HIV-infected patient may represent which of the following: PCP, histoplasmosis, cryptococcosis, or bronchogenic carcinoma?

All of the above.

○   What are the major cell types of primary bronchogenic carcinoma?

Small cell, large cell, squamous cell and adenocarcinoma.

○   Differentiating which of these from the others is most important in planning the therapeutic approach?

Small cell.

○   Exposure to what mineral, used as insulation, greatly enhances the carcinogenic potential of exposure to cigarette smoke?

Asbestos.

○   **Second hand cigarette smoke exposure is a risk factor for the development of what two major lung diseases?**

Lung cancer and COPD.

○   **Which primary lung cancer is most frequently associated with paraneoplastic syndromes?**

Small cell undifferentiated carcinoma.

○   **What other exposures are also factors contributing to the development of bronchogenic carcinoma?**

Radon, uranium, nickel, arsenic, bis (chloromethyl) ether, ionizing radiation, vinyl chloride, mustard gas, polycyclic aromatic hydrocarbons and chromium.

○   **The incidence of lung cancer is increasing in the USA among members of which gender?**

Females.

○   **What accounts for this increase?**

Increased cigarette smoking prevalence.

○   **Which vitamin has been associated with a protective effect against the development of lung cancer?**

Vitamin A.

○   **What type of lung tumors can cause excessive ACTH production and Cushing's syndrome?**

Small cell carcinoma and carcinoid tumors.

○   **What is the most common cancer, excluding skin cancer, in the US?**

Lung cancer.

○   **What cancer is the leading cause of cancer death?**

Lung cancer.

○   **What cancers generally metastasize to the lungs?**

Breast, colon, prostate and cervical cancers.

○   **What routine program is recommended for screening lung cancer in the adult population?**

Screening programs for lung cancer have not demonstrated a decrease in morbidity or mortality. Practitioners must be aware of the signs and symptoms associated with lung cancer, including chronic non-productive cough, increased sputum production, hemoptysis, dyspnea, recurrent pneumonia, hoarseness, pleurisy, weight loss, shoulder pain, SVC syndrome, exercise fatigue and anemia. Incidental findings on chest x-ray should also be investigated.

○   **Where do the following cancers most commonly develop within the lung: adenocarcinoma, large cell, squamous cell and small cell?**

Adenocarcinoma and large cell carcinomas are usually located peripherally, while squamous and small cell carcinomas are located centrally.

❍ **Which form of lung cancer is the most common?**

Squamous cell carcinoma (40 to 50%), followed by adenocarcinoma (35%) and small-cell (oat cell) carcinoma (25%).

❍ **What is Pancoast syndrome?**

A tumor of the apex of the lung that gives rise to Horner's syndrome and shoulder pain. The tumor invades the bronchial plexus.

❍ **What cancer causes the most deaths in women?**

1. Lung cancer
2. Breast cancer
3. Colorectal cancer

❍ **What cancer causes the most deaths in men?**

1. Lung cancer
2. Colorectal cancer
3. Prostate cancer

❍ **What are the neuroendocrine tumors of the lung?**

Typical carcinoid, atypical carcinoid and small cell carcinoma.

❍ **Is carcinoid syndrome common with pulmonary carcinoid?**

No. It is rare, with incidence ranging from 2 to 7%.

❍ **How do metastatic malignant tumors spread in the lung?**

Hematogenously, via the lymphatics, direct invasion and via intrabronchial dissemination.

❍ **What is the differential diagnosis of multiple pulmonary nodules?**

Wegener's disease, sarcoidosis, AVM, histoplasmosis, coccidioidomycosis, tuberculosis, bacterial abscesses, paragonimiasis, nocardiosis, cryptococcosis and aspigillosis.

❍ **What are the radiological manifestations of metastatic malignant tumors?**

Nodules, masses, cavitation, lymphangitic spread, post-obstructive pneumonia, pleural effusions and atelectasis.

❍ **Which metastatic malignant tumors are amenable to chemotherapy?**

Hodgkin's disease, lymphomas, testicular and certain ovarian tumors and gestational trophoblastic neoplasms.

❍ **Which organ does osteosarcoma mostly metastasize to?**

Lung.

❍ **What is Castleman's disease (angiofollicular hyperplasia)?**

There are two types of presentation. The local variant presents as a middle mediastinal mass or as a pulmonary mass. The multicentric variant presents with systemic symptoms and involves the peripheral lymph nodes. The local variant is amenable to cure with surgery, while the multicentric variant is often responsive to chemotherapy.

○   **What are the pulmonary manifestations of Hodgkin's disease?**

Primary lung disease is uncommon. It may present with nodules, infiltration, or cavitation. Mediastinal nodal involvement is more typical. Local spread may occur into pleura, pericardium, chest wall and lungs. Radiation pneumonitis may occur, usually 3-4 months after treatment.

○   **What are the pulmonary manifestations of non-Hodgkin's lymphoma?**

Mediastinal disease, parenchymal masses, infiltrates and pleural involvement. Lesions may be single or multiple.

○   **What is a hamartoma?**

It is a benign neoplasm that contains connective tissue, fat, smooth muscle and cartilage. It occasionally has a popcorn calcification pattern. It usually presents as a coin lesion. Excision is performed usually to rule out carcinoma. Alternatively, if a lesion is a known hamartoma, it can be followed because it has a rare potential for malignant transformation.

○   **What is a carcinoid?**

A malignant tumor arising from the neuroendocrine cells of the lung. Patients present with incidental findings on CXR, hemoptysis, dyspnea, post-obstructive pneumonia and paraneoplastic syndrome. Associated paraneoplastic syndromes include carcinoid, Cushing's and acromegaly. Resection is the best available treatment.

○   **Which bronchogenic tumors are stage 0?**

Carcinoma in situ.

○   **What constitutes a stage 1 tumor?**

T1 or T2, N0 and M0. T1 is a tumor 3 cm or less without invasion proximal to a lobar bronchus. T2 is a tumor more than 3 cm or invades the visceral pleura, has obstructive atelectasis or pneumonitis that extends to the hilum.

○   **What constitutes a stage 2 tumor?**

N1, T1 or T2 and M0. N1 includes metastases to the peribronchial or ipsilateral hilar region.

○   **Stage 3a?**

T3 with N0 or N1, T1-T3 with N2 and all with M0. A T3 tumor extends into the chest wall, diaphragm, mediastinal pleura or pericardium without involving the heart, great vessels, trachea, esophagus, or vertebral bodies. A T3 tumor may also involve the mainstem bronchi within 2 cm of the carina but not involving the carina. An N2 tumor involves metastases to the ipsilateral mediastinum and the subcarinal lymph nodes.

○   **Stage 3b?**

Any T with N3 or T4 with any N. All with M0. A T4 tumor invades the mediastinum or involves the heart, great vessels, trachea, esophagus, vertebral bodies, or carina. A T4 tumor also may result in a malignant pleural effusion. An N3 tumor involves metastases to the contralateral mediastinum or hilum, scalene and supraclavicular lymph nodes.

○   **Stage 4?**

Any T, any N and M1. Distant metastases are present.

MULTIPLE CHOICE AND TRUE/FALSE REVIEW

I can see the light.

N Lorenzo

○ **What is a satisfactory initial tidal volume and rate setting for a patient with emphysema?**

A: 12 mL/kg of patient's estimated body weight at 12 breaths per minute
B: 12 mL/kg of patient's ideal body weight at 10 breaths per minute
C: 6 mL/kg of patient's ideal body weight at 18 breaths per minute
D: 10 mL/kg of patient's ideal body weight at 10 breaths per minute
E: 15 mL/kg of patient's ideal body weight at 6-8 breaths per minute

The correct answer is D: In a patient with chronic obstructive pulmonary disease, the initial selected tidal volume and rate are slightly reduced to avoid hyperinflation and hyperventilation.

○ **Which of the following is the proper amount of physiologic positive end-expiratory pressure (PEEP) to add on the initial ventilator setup when instituting mechanical ventilation?**

A: 3 cm water pressure
B: 5 cm water pressure
C: 1 cm water pressure
D: Difference between the peak and plateau pressure
E: 0 cm water pressure

The correct answer is E: Because PEEP is not a benign mode of therapy, most physicians believe that using the least amount of PEEP is better and that zero PEEP is best. Therefore, the initial ventilator setup involves the use of high fractions of inspired oxygen to oxygenate rather than immediately defaulting to PEEP. If the patient cannot be adequately oxygenated despite using a high fraction of inspired oxygen, then PEEP is appropriate.

○ **(T/F): When considering mechanical ventilation, a patient who requires 6 cm water of positive end-expiratory pressure (PEEP) for oxygenation should have 6 sighs per hour at a volume of 1.5 times the tidal volume delivered as a single sigh.**

The correct answer is False: Sighs used in combination with PEEP increase the risk of barotrauma; therefore, the use of sighs is not recommended.

○ **(T/F): The inspiratory-to-expiratory (I:E) ratio can be decreased by increasing the inspiratory flow rate.**

The correct answer is True: The I:E ratio can be adjusted by increasing the inspiratory flow rate, decreasing the tidal volume, and decreasing the ventilatory rate. Attention to the I:E ratio is important for avoiding barotrauma in patients with obstructive airway disease (eg, asthma, chronic obstructive pulmonary disease).

○ **(T/F): When starting mechanical ventilation, the fraction of inspired oxygen (FIO$_2$) should initially be set at 28%.**

The correct answer is False: When initiating mechanical ventilation, the highest priority is to provide effective oxygenation. After intubation, a 100% FIO_2 should always be used until adequate oxygenation has been documented based on postintubation and postmechanical ventilation arterial blood gas values. A short period on FIO_2 of 100% is not dangerous for patients on mechanical ventilation and offers the clinician several advantages. An FIO_2 of 100% protects the patient against hypoxemia if unrecognized problems develop from the intubation procedure. If the PaO_2 is measured while the patient is on an FIO_2 of 100%, the clinician can easily calculate the next desired FIO_2 and can quickly estimate the shunt fraction. Simply stated, until the patient is stabilized on mechanical ventilation, the initial FIO_2 should be 100%. Then, the FIO_2 can be decreased as the clinical situation allows.

○ **(T/F): Objective data have documented that the newer modes of mechanical ventilation are more successful for ventilating patients than conventional methods.**

The correct answer is False: No strong evidence supports the use of nonconventional modes of mechanical ventilation. Most physicians use alternative methods of ventilation in cases in which conventional methods have failed. However, this is rare.

○ **A 21-year-old man traveled from his home (near sea level) to Colorado to ski. He stayed at a lodge at nearly 10,000 feet in elevation. In the morning, after his second night at altitude, his friends reported that he had slurred speech, difficulty walking, and a mild headache. Which of the following conditions is most likely?**

A: High-altitude pulmonary edema (HAPE)
B: Acute mountain sickness (AMS)
C: High-altitude retinal hemorrhages
D: High-altitude cerebral edema (HACE)
E: Stroke

The correct answer is D: The CNS signs and symptoms, along with the recent gain in altitude, strongly suggest cerebral edema. Treatment, including descent to lower altitude, should be initiated immediately.

○ **A 25-year-old woman is planning a summer backpacking trip to Mount Whitney, California (>14,000 ft). She is concerned that she may develop acute mountain sickness (AMS) while on the trip. The incidence of AMS is highly variable among different people. Which of the following is the most reliable predictor of her chances for developing AMS?**

A: The amount of sleep she has during her first 2 nights at high altitude
B: Whether she has had AMS on previous trips to high altitude
C: Her sex because women are much less susceptible to AMS than men
D: Her body mass index (BMI) because individuals who are overweight are more likely to develop AMS than individuals who are not overweight
E: Geography because the region of the world to where she is going (ie, North America) suggests that she is more likely to develop AMS than if she were going to another region, for example, Nepal

The correct answer is B: Some individuals may be nearly incapacitated at altitudes encountered on a trip to Mount Whitney, whereas others may be only minimally affected or not affected at all. By far, the most reliable predictor is a person's response to past ascents to similar altitudes. While sleep at altitude is altered, the duration or quality of sleep is not useful in predicting whether someone will develop AMS. Similarly, AMS is not related to BMI or to the region of the world. Studies differ regarding the relative susceptibilities of men versus women; however, predicting the likelihood of subsequent episodes of AMS based on sex is not possible.

○ **(T/F): High-altitude pulmonary edema (HAPE) is a type of cardiogenic pulmonary edema.**

The correct answer is False: HAPE is a noncardiogenic form of pulmonary edema. Heart function in persons with HAPE is normal.

○   **(T/F): Sleep disruption at high altitude, along with hypoxia, contribute to impaired judgment and daytime performance.**

The correct answer is True: While hypoxia is the main cause of altered judgment and performance, sleep fragmentation also contributes to these changes. Frequent arousals (ie, a 2- to 5-s period of wakefulness within a 30-s epoch) cause sleep fragmentation, which, in turn, impairs daytime performance, even without concomitant hypoxia.

○   **(T/F): Use of acetazolamide (Diamox) ameliorates symptoms of acute mountain sickness (AMS) and improves nighttime arterial oxygenation.**

The correct answer is True: Acetazolamide (Diamox) is quite effective for both prevention and treatment of AMS. It also decreases nocturnal periodic breathing and improves arterial oxygen saturation, although the mechanism of action of acetazolamide in AMS is unclear.

○   **(T/F): Persons who have had a previous episode of high-altitude pulmonary edema (HAPE) should be cautioned to not go to high altitude again.**

The correct answer is False: A prior history of HAPE suggests that the individual probably is a susceptible person, but having had HAPE previously does not make someone more likely to have a second episode. A previous episode only serves to identify a susceptible individual. With proper acclimatization, many susceptible people have subsequently ascended to and above the altitude at which HAPE previously occurred.

○   **The American-European Consensus Conference (AECC) has defined acute respiratory distress syndrome (ARDS) by all but which one of the following criteria?**

A: A partial pressure of arterial oxygen (PaO_2)/fraction of inspired oxygen (FIO_2) ratio of less than 200
B: Pulmonary capillary wedge pressure of less than 18 mm Hg
C: A PaO_2/FIO_2 ratio of less than 100
D: Rapid development of bilateral pulmonary infiltrates
E: None of the above

The correct answer is C: The AECC developed a definition of ARDS to allow research on treatment and outcome. ARDS is defined by the rapid development of bilateral pulmonary infiltrates and severe hypoxemia (PaO_2/FIO_2 <200) in the absence of cardiogenic pulmonary edema (pulmonary capillary wedge pressure 18 mm Hg or compatible clinical picture).

○   **A patient with acute respiratory distress syndrome on mechanical ventilation with a tidal volume of 6 mL/kg, continuous positive airway pressure (CPAP) of 15 cm H_2O, and a fraction of inspired oxygen (FIO_2) of 70% develops hypotension and a fall in oxygen saturation to 40%. During the examination, jugular venous distention is present and absent breath sounds are noted on the left with tracheal deviation to the right. Which of the following actions should be taken?**

A: Increase FIO_2 to 100%, assess endotracheal tube position, suction the patient, obtain an emergent chest radiograph, and consider emergent chest tube placement.
B: Obtain an immediate chest radiograph and await results.
C: Pull the endotracheal tube back 1-2 cm.
D: Increase CPAP to 20.
E: Change the ventilator mode to pressure control.

The correct answer is A: The hypotension and acute decline in oxygenation are most likely caused by a tension pneumothorax. Other less likely possibilities include right mainstem intubation, a mucus plug in the left main bronchus, or the development of a left effusion or hemothorax. The patient may die unless quick action is taken. Unless rapid improvement ensues with increasing the FIO_2 or suctioning, a chest tube should be placed empirically.

○   **(T/F): Use the prone position in patients with acute respiratory distress syndrome (ARDS) only if all other means to improve oxygenation have failed.**

The correct answer is False: The prone position is effective in improving oxygenation in a high proportion of patients, especially if used early in the course of ARDS. Therefore, consider this positioning as a potential early therapeutic intervention.

○   **(T/F): High-dose intravenous corticosteroids are ineffective in preventing acute respiratory distress syndrome (ARDS) in patients with sepsis.**

The correct answer is True: Corticosteroids do not prevent the development of ARDS in patients with sepsis and are potentially detrimental. In selected patients with late ARDS (fibroproliferative phase) in whom infection has been carefully ruled out, corticosteroids are possibly beneficial, but further study is needed.

○   **(T/F): As in infants with neonatal respiratory distress syndrome, adults with acute respiratory distress syndrome (ARDS) benefit from the administration of inhaled surfactant.**

The correct answer is False: In 2 controlled trials of inhaled synthetic surfactant in adults with ARDS, no benefit was found.

○   **(T/F): Administration of inhaled nitric oxide improves survival in acute respiratory distress syndrome (ARDS).**

The correct answer is False: Although pulmonary hypertension is uniformly found in ARDS, the administration of nitrous oxide, a pulmonary vasodilator, may transiently improve oxygenation but does not change ultimate survival rates.

○   **A 62-year-old man underwent an uneventful elective cholecystectomy. After surgery, during extubation he vomited and developed severe shortness of breath. Examination showed that he had a temperature of 99.2°F, blood pressure of 108/68 mm Hg, pulse of 118 beats per minute, respiratory rate of 36 breaths per minute, and coarse breath sounds without wheezing. Arterial blood gases revealed Pa0$_2$ of 42, PaCO$_2$ of 28, and pH of 7.52. Which of the following is the next step?**

A: Start heparin administration intravenously and order a ventilation-perfusion lung scan.
B: Perform bronchoscopy.
C: Perform tracheal intubation and mechanical ventilation with positive end-expiratory pressure (PEEP) and oxygen supplementation.
D: Start administration of triple antibiotic therapy with clindamycin, an aminoglycoside, and a third-generation cephalosporin.
E: Start administration of intravenous aminophylline and nebulized albuterol.

The correct answer is C: The clinical presentation of this patient suggests acute aspiration and reveals acute respiratory failure. The appropriate first step is to provide oxygenation. In the context of severe oxygenation failure (ie, severe hypoxemia despite increased ventilation as indicated by hypocapnia) and the probability of ARDS, mechanical ventilation and institution of PEEP are appropriate management. The damage in this case is one of acute chemical pneumonia, and antibiotic therapy is not needed as the first step. The absence of known predisposing factors for venous thrombosis and the onset of symptoms soon after an elective cholecystectomy (an operation that takes about 1 h) oppose the diagnosis of acute pulmonary embolism; therefore, heparin is not indicated. Bronchoscopy is not indicated. No urgent indication for bronchodilators exists because bronchospasm and airway narrowing are not present.

○   **A 49-year-old man with a history of alcoholism presents with a 6-week history of malaise, low-grade fever, and a cough that produces greenish sputum tinged with blood. Examination showed periodontal disease with bad breath and clubbing of fingers. On chest radiograph, a 3-cm cavity with an air-fluid level**

was observed in the posterior segment of the right upper lobe. Sputum smear showed many neutrophils and a variety of microbes. Which of the following is the most appropriate treatment option?

A: Isolate the patient and initiate a 4-drug antituberculosis treatment.
B: Start intravenous administration of clindamycin.
C: Refer the patient to a dentist for periodontal care.
D: Schedule a bronchoscopy for the next day.
E: Start administration of methicillin and tobramycin.

The correct answer is B: The predisposing factors of alcoholism and periodontal disease, the duration of illness, the symptoms and signs, and the cavity in a dependent segment of the lung suggest the diagnosis of an anaerobic lung abscess caused by aspiration of bacteria from the mouth. Clindamycin is the drug of choice. Tuberculosis is not as likely a diagnosis as anaerobic lung abscess is, and empiric treatment without microscopic or culture evidence is not warranted in this chronically ill patient who is stable. Bronchoscopy prior to antibiotic treatment of a lung abscess carries a risk of dissemination and acute sepsis. Dental work without antibiotic coverage also carries a risk of sepsis. Staphylococcal and gram-negative antibiotics are not indicated.

○   **(T/F): The nature and volume of the aspirated material and the status of host defenses determine the manifestations, severity, and complications of aspiration pneumonia.**

The correct answer is True: The pH of the aspirate and volume aspirated are major factors in the type and severity of aspiration pneumonia. Large-volume acidic aspirate causes chemical pneumonia (CP) with high potential for the development of acute respiratory distress syndrome (ARDS). Periodontal disease and altered consciousness are major factors that predispose the patient to bacterial aspiration pneumonia.

○   **(T/F): Aspiration is the most common cause of community-acquired pneumonia (CAP).**

The correct answer is False: Although microaspiration of resident bacteria is thought to be part of the pathophysiology of CAP in general, aspiration pneumonia accounts for only 5-10% of CAP cases.

○   **(T/F): Acute respiratory distress syndrome (ARDS) is a complication of aspiration of gastric contents.**

The correct answer is True: Acidic gastric contents cause local inflammation and initiate cellular and cytokine reaction, causing ARDS.

○   **(T/F): Bronchoscopy is not indicated in all cases of aspiration pneumonia.**

The correct answer is True: Bronchoscopy is selectively indicated in aspiration pneumonia when bronchial obstruction due to a foreign body or neoplasm is suspected.

○   **A 36-year-old man has intermittent asthma exacerbations twice weekly that last approximately 2-3 hours. He denies any nocturnal symptoms. Which of the following is not appropriate therapy?**

A: Inhaled corticosteroids
B: Salmeterol
C: Theophylline
D: Albuterol prn
E: None of the above

The correct answer is C: Based on his twice-weekly symptoms, the patient has mild persistent asthma. Therapy should include a low-dose inhaled corticosteroid at baseline. Salmeterol, a long-acting beta-agonist, may be added if symptoms are not controlled with inhaled corticosteroids. Short-acting beta-agonists are always indicated for the acute relief of symptoms in any patient with asthma. Theophylline is not indicated for the treatment of mild persistent asthma unless the patient has nocturnal symptoms.

O   **A 26-year-old woman presents to the emergency department with severe shortness of breath after an argument with her spouse. She has a long history of asthma, with multiple hospitalizations despite maximal therapy. Examination reveals inspiratory and expiratory wheezes, normal saturations, and minimal response to nebulized beta-agonists based on peak expiratory flow measurements. Flow volume loops (FVLs) show truncation of the inspiratory limb. What is the most likely diagnosis for this patient?**

A: Aspirin sensitivity
B: Gastroesophageal reflux disease (GERD)
C: Foreign body aspiration
D: Vocal cord dysfunction (VCD)
E: None of the above

The correct answer is D: This is a typical presentation for a patient with VCD. This is a young woman with the diagnosis of asthma who has frequent exacerbations that do not respond to conventional asthma therapy. Key points are the stress-induced symptoms, the presence of inspiratory wheezes, and an FVL that shows variable extrathoracic obstruction or truncation of the inspiratory limb. Asthma resulting from aspirin sensitivity is difficult to treat unless aspirin is discontinued, but aspirin-induced asthma is not associated with a truncated inspiratory limb of the FVL. A patient with foreign body aspiration may not remember the event and may present with inspiratory and/or expiratory wheezing. If the upper airway is involved, the FVL would show either flattening of the expiratory limb because of a variable intrathoracic obstruction or truncation of both limbs if a fixed defect is present. GERD is an important consideration in patients with asthma that is difficult to control, but the symptoms may worsen at night while the patient is recumbent or in association with increasing heartburn symptoms. The FVLs would be normal.

O   **(T/F): Patients who have severe chronic obstructive pulmonary disease (COPD) and are current smokers do not benefit from smoking cessation.**

The correct answer is False: Even in patients with severe COPD smoking cessation slows decline in lung function.

O   **(T/F): Home oxygen therapy in a patient with hypoxemic chronic obstructive pulmonary disease (COPD) prolongs survival.**

The correct answer is True: Smoking cessation and oxygen therapy are the only interventions known to prolong survival in COPD.

O   **(T/F): Replacement of alpha1-antitrypsin in patients with emphysema who are deficient is a proven therapy.**

The correct answer is False: Replacement of alpha 1 antitrypsin is not established as beneficial, although large controlled studies are lacking.

O   **(T/F): A comprehensive pulmonary rehabilitation program improves lung function and survival in patients with chronic obstructive pulmonary disease (COPD).**

The correct answer is False: A comprehensive pulmonary rehabilitation improves quality of life and walking distance but not lung function or survival.

O   **Which of the following statements about pulmonary embolism (PE) is not accurate?**

A: PE is a common and lethal condition.
B: PE is not a disease but a complication of deep venous thrombosis (DVT).
C: The patients who die from PE do so within the first hour.
D: Further mortality occurs from recurrent embolism.
E: PE often resolves spontaneously.

The correct answer is E. PE does not resolve spontaneously; all of the other statements are accurate.

O **A 65-year-old man is seen for evaluation of progressive dyspnea. He has a 40-year smoking history. A spirometry is requested. Which of the following spirometric values is diagnostic of chronic obstructive pulmonary disease (COPD)?**

A: Forced vital capacity (FVC) 120% of predicted, forced expiratory volume in 1 second (FEV_1) 110% of predicted, and FEV_1/FVC 73%
B: FVC 90% of predicted, FEV_1 85% of predicted, and FEV_1/FVC 80%
C: FVC 75% of predicted, FEV_1/FVC 90%
D: FVC 85% of predicted, FEV_1/FVC 52%
E: FEV_1/FVC is 60% of predicted, improves to 75% post bronchodilator therapy

The correct answer is D. An obstructive spirometric pattern that does not normalize following bronchodilator administration is diagnostic of COPD (irreversible airflow obstruction).

O **(T/F): A comprehensive pulmonary rehabilitation program improves lung function and survival in patients with chronic obstructive pulmonary disease (COPD).**

The correct answer is False. A comprehensive pulmonary rehabilitation improves quality of life and walking distance but not lung function or survival.

O **(T/F): Pneumococcus is the most common cause of bacterial pneumonia.**

The correct answer is True. Streptococcus pneumoniae is the most common cause of bacterial pneumonia. Community-acquired pneumonia is caused most commonly by bacteria that traditionally have been divided into 2 groups, typical and atypical. Typical organisms include S pneumoniae (pneumococcus) and Haemophilus and Staphylococcus species. Atypical refers to pneumonia caused by Legionella, Mycoplasma, and Chlamydia species.

O **(T/F): A 62-year-old nonsmoking white male foundry worker presents with shortness of breath that has been gradually progressive over the past year. A chest radiograph (seen below) demonstrates multiple small (2-5 mm) nodules in all lung fields. Silicosis is the most likely pulmonary diagnosis.**

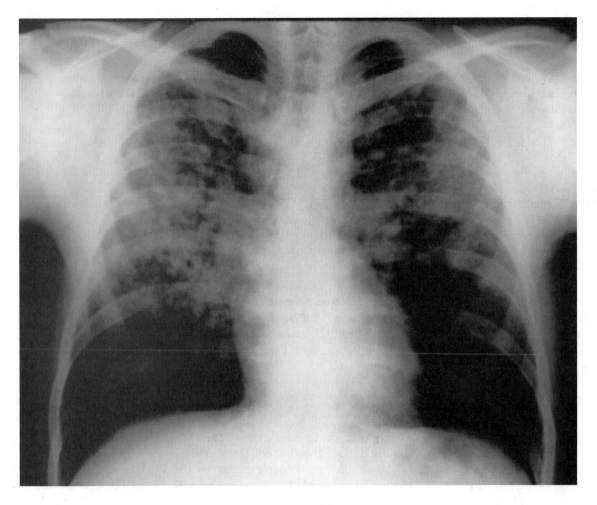

The correct answer is True. Foundry workers are at high risk to develop silicosis. Chest radiographs frequently demonstrate a diffuse pattern of small nodules.

○   **(T/F): Of the list of conditions that include foreign body aspiration, allergic bronchopulmonary aspergillosis, cystic fibrosis, primary ciliary dyskinesia, and human immunodeficiency virus (HIV) disease, HIV disease is most commonly associated with central bronchiectasis.**

The correct answer is False. Bronchiectasis as a result of infection generally involves the lower lobes, the right middle lobe, and the lingula. Right middle lobe involvement alone suggests right middle lobe syndrome or a neoplastic cause. Bronchiectasis caused by cystic fibrosis, Mycobacterium tuberculosis, or chronic fungal infections tends to affect the upper lobe. Allergic bronchopulmonary aspergillosis also affects the upper lobes but usually involves the central bronchi, whereas most other forms of bronchiectasis involve distal bronchial segments.

○   **A 71-year-old woman with a past medical history of myocardial infarction (MI) one year ago, diabetes, and congestive heart failure (CHF) requiring diuretics presents for elective cholecystectomy. What is her risk and what preoperative investigation is needed?**

A: Low-risk, proceed to surgery
B: Intermediate-risk; perform dobutamine methoxyisobutyl isonitrile testing, and, if results are negative, proceed to surgery
C: Intermediate-risk, proceed directly to surgery
D: High-risk, perform coronary angiography and possible revascularization prior to cholecystectomy
E: High-risk, cancel surgery

The correct answer is C: Based on the modified Detsky cardiac risk index, the patient`s age, MI, and CHF give her

15 points, thus categorizing her in class I. Her low-risk factors of diabetes and age categorizes her in the intermediate-risk. Because the patient is undergoing a nonvascular procedure, the patient may proceed directly to surgery. If the patient were undergoing a vascular procedure, then the correct answer would be B.

O   **Which of the following is not a reason to use preoperative pulmonary function tests?**

A: Help identify high-risk lung resection candidates
B: Help identify persons who smoke who have asymptomatic lung disease
C: Help optimize underlying chronic pulmonary obstructive disease or asthma
D: Help plan postoperative risk reduction strategies
E: Help reject and discourage high-risk patients

The correct answer is E: The objective of preoperative pulmonary function testing is not to reject patients for the surgery, but to identify high-risk patients, optimize their underlying disease, and plan postoperative risk reduction strategies.

O   **(T/F): Any level of lung function is considered safe enough to undergo lung resection for cancer.**

The correct answer is False: A minimum predicted postresection forced expiratory volume in one second of 0.8L/s, or 40% predicted, is associated with the least morbidity and mortality.

O   **(T/F): Preoperative interventions will not reduce postoperative pulmonary complications.**

The correct answer is False: Smoking cessation, optimization of an underlying chronic obstructive pulmonary disease or asthma, and patient education to emphasize lung expansion postoperatively are all known to reduce postoperative pulmonary complications.

O   **(T/F): An exercise stress test is a valuable diagnostic modality for preoperative evaluation.**

The correct answer is False: The sensitivity and specificity of exercise stress test results are only 65% and 85%, respectively.

O   **(T/F): The use of beta-blockers preoperatively is cardioprotective.**

The correct answer is True: In trials for nonvascular and vascular surgical procedures, atenolol and bisoprolol preoperatively showed a significant absolute reduction in long-term cardiac morbidity and mortality.

O   **Which of the following represents the most common presentation of acute disease in a person with hypersensitivity pneumonitis?**

A: Abdominal pain and diarrhea
B: Dyspnea, cough, fevers, and chills
C: Chest pain and wheezing
D: Loss of appetite and weight loss
E: None of the above

The correct answer is B: Acute exposure to an inciting agent in sensitized patients causes acute alveolitis, resulting in cough, sputum, and dyspnea. Systemic reactions manifest as fever, chills, and malaise.

O   **Which of the following is frequently found physical examination finding from a person with hypersensitivity pneumonitis (HP)?**

A: Splenomegaly
B: Peripheral lymphadenopathy
C: Crackles in the lower parts of the lungs
D: Skin changes
E: Clubbing

The correct answer is C: HP produces alveolitis, which causes atelectasis. During inspiration, these alveoli suddenly open, causing crackles.

○   (T/F): The presence of precipitating immunoglobulin G antibodies is a definitive finding for the diagnosis of hypersensitivity pneumonitis.

The correct answer is False: The presence of precipitating antibodies does not definitively indicate the diagnosis because 30-40% of farmers have these in the absence of clinical disease. Furthermore, testing precipitating antibodies carries a high rate of false-negative results.

○   (T/F): Histopathologic findings in hypersensitivity pneumonitis (HP) are frequently nonspecific and variable.

The correct answer is False: Poorly formed granulomas, mononuclear cell infiltration, and large histiocytes with foamy cytoplasm of alveolar walls are characteristic of HP.

○   (T/F): A micronodular interstitial pattern, particularly in the mid-to-upper lung zones, is characteristic of acute hypersensitivity pneumonitis (HP).

The correct answer is True: In acute and subacute HP, a micronodular interstitial pattern is most prominent in mid-to-upper lung zones. Chronic HP shows progressive fibrotic changes, with loss of lung volumes, particularly affecting the upper lobes.

○   (T/F): Bronchoalveolar lavage fluid from patients with hypersensitivity pneumonitis most frequently shows an increased percentage of lymphocytes.

The correct answer is True: Marked lymphocytosis (>20%) is common. The $CD4^+$-to-$CD8^+$ ratio is decreased to less than 1.

○   A 65-year-old man with no significant past medical history presents with a gradual onset of sore throat with hoarseness, which had subsided over 2 weeks and was followed by cough and nonpurulent sputum. His body temperature is normal, and physical examination reveals pharyngeal erythema without exudate and localized crackles on chest auscultation. His white blood cell count is within reference ranges, and chest radiography shows a single subsegmental infiltrate in the left lower lobe. Which of the following statements is least correct?

A: Chlamydia pneumoniae pneumonia is more common than mycoplasmal pneumonia in this age group.
B: Hoarseness is more common in mycoplasmal pneumonia than in C pneumoniae pneumonia.
C: Sinus tenderness to percussion is more likely to be observed with C pneumoniae pneumonia than with mycoplasmal pneumonia.
D: Outbreaks of C pneumoniae pneumonia have been reported in nursing homes and among military recruits.
E: Macrolides may be used in this patient.

The correct answer is B: Hoarseness is more common in C pneumoniae pneumonia than in mycoplasmal pneumonia.

○   Which of the following is considered disseminated coccidioidomycosis?

A: Hilar adenopathy
B: Pneumonia
C: Pulmonary nodule
D: Meningitis
E: Bronchopleural fistula

The correct answer is D: Only extrapulmonary disease is considered disseminated coccidioidomycosis. Dissemination usually occurs in hematopoietic tissues, skin, kidneys, bones, the CNS, and myocardium. Meningitis takes the form of granulomatous inflammation and presents as hydrocephalus.

O (T/F): Other than the lungs, the skin is the most common organ affected by blastomycosis.

The correct answer is True: When present, the characteristic skin lesion provides a strong clue to blastomycosis, and the diagnosis can be confirmed microscopically using a smear from drainage and small abscesses around the border of an ulcerating lesion.

O (T/F): Pneumococcus is the most common cause of bacterial pneumonia.

The correct answer is True: Streptococcus pneumoniae is the most common cause of bacterial pneumonia. Community-acquired pneumonia is caused most commonly by bacteria that traditionally have been divided into 2 groups, typical and atypical. Typical organisms include S pneumoniae (pneumococcus) and Haemophilus and Staphylococcus species. Atypical refers to pneumonia caused by Legionella, Mycoplasma, and Chlamydia species.

O (T/F): All patients with pneumonia should have a follow-up chest radiograph.

The correct answer is True: A follow-up chest radiograph at 6 weeks posttreatment is advised to rule out an underlying parenchymal abnormality (eg, tumor) as an etiology of pneumonia.

O (T/F): The prognosis for patients with Legionella pneumonia is poor despite adequate antibiotic therapy.

The correct answer is False: In most patients, the prognosis is good. However, if treatment is delayed or does not cover Legionella, then pneumonia due to this organism has a poor prognosis.

O A 72-year-old white man with a history of rheumatoid arthritis presents with the complaint of shortness of breath that has been worsening gradually over the past year. A chest radiograph demonstrates small lung volumes, a diffuse reticular-nodular infiltrate, and peripheral honeycombing. What are the likely pulmonary function abnormalities?

A: Increased total lung capacity, reduced forced expiratory volume in 1 second (FEV_1), reduced ratio of FEV_1 to FVC (forced vital capacity), and increased diffusing capacity of lung for carbon monoxide (DLCO).
B: Decreased total lung capacity, reduced FEV_1, increased ratio of FEV_1 to FVC, and decreased DLCO
C: Normal lung volumes, spirometry, and diffusing capacity
D: Decreased total lung capacity, increased FEV_1, reduced ratio of FEV_1 to FVC, and increased DLCO
E: Insufficient information is provided to predict the pulmonary function abnormality.

The correct answer is B: The patient presents with the typical clinical picture of fibrotic interstitial lung disease associated with rheumatoid arthritis. The chest radiograph demonstrates advanced findings that would suggest advanced disease. The usual pulmonary function pattern is restrictive, with decreased total lung capacity, reduced FEV_1, and an increased ratio of FEV_1 to FVC, which often is accompanied by a decreased DLCO.

O A 62-year-old nonsmoking white male foundry worker presents with shortness of breath that has been gradually progressive over the past year. A chest radiograph demonstrates multiple small (2-5 mm) nodules in all lung fields. What is the most likely pulmonary diagnosis?

A: Idiopathic pulmonary fibrosis
B: Hypersensitivity pneumonitis
C: Silicosis
D: Atypical pneumonia
E: Congestive heart failure

The correct answer is C: Foundry workers are at high risk to develop silicosis. Chest radiographs frequently demonstrate a diffuse pattern of small nodules.

○   (T/F): Incidence of diffuse parenchymal lung disease is higher in women than in men.

The correct answer is False: Incidence is 6 cases per 100,000 women and 31 cases per 100,000 men.

○   (T/F): Patients with pulmonary fibrosis who are tested for pulmonary function typically have findings of obstructive lung disease.

The correct answer is False: Pulmonary fibrosis is the prototypic restrictive lung disease. Most patients with pulmonary fibrosis manifest findings of restrictive lung disease. In some cases, this can be masked by coexistent obstructive lung disease, as in the case of some patients with long smoking histories.

○   (T/F): Congestive heart failure, lymphangitic carcinomatosis, and atypical pneumonia seldom are mistaken for chronic fibrotic lung disease.

The correct answer is False: Congestive heart failure, lymphangitic carcinomatosis, and atypical pneumonia are common disorders that most frequently are mistaken for chronic fibrotic lung disease.

○   (T/F): Routine blood analysis and serum chemistries are the most sensitive and specific tests for making the diagnosis of diffuse parenchymal lung disease.

The correct answer is False: Lung biopsy is the most sensitive and specific test for making the diagnosis of diffuse parenchymal lung disease. Routine blood analysis and serum chemistries are of limited value and generally are nonspecific.

○   A 65-year-old woman presents with the complaint of the onset of a cough and "squeaky" breathing, especially when she lies in a supine position. She notes that when she coughs, the cough is like a child with croup. Her symptoms have become worse in the past few days, even in an upright position. Her only medication is Synthroid, which she was put on 6 years ago for an underactive thyroid gland after she had part of her thyroid gland removed for a benign mass. Upon physical examination, a well-healed collar incision from the old surgery is seen and no masses or adenopathy can be felt in her neck or supraclavicular areas. Her chest radiograph shows a mass at the thoracic inlet and significant deviation of the tracheal shadow to the right. Which of the following should not be performed in this case?

A: CT scan of the neck, chest, and mediastinum
B: Radionuclide test with iodine I 131 or iodine I 123
C: Resection of the substernal mass
D: Hospital admission for a compromised airway
E: Doubling her dose of Synthroid because this will shrink the mass

The correct answer is E: This woman has a large mass at the thoracic inlet, which most likely is an intrathoracic goiter. The position of the mass in association with her sex, age, and history of thyroid disease and surgery make this the likeliest diagnosis, by far. She should be admitted to the hospital because the status of her airway is tenuous and acute obstruction may occur with these lesions. CT scan and/or radionuclide studies with tagged iodine may be performed for further workup. CT scan images will show the anatomic relationship of the mass and the mediastinal structures and will show the continuity between the intrathoracic mass and any cervical thyroid tissue.

Radionuclide scanning will help confirm that this mass is thyroid tissue. If both are desired, iodine-tagged studies must be performed before studies such as CT scan, for which iodinated contrast is administered. These tests may be somewhat difficult to perform in this woman because both require the patient to be in a supine position. These factors must be considered in light of her airway compromise.

Resection of an intrathoracic goiter should be undertaken. This can be performed through the cervical collar incision through which she had her previous surgery. Only occasionally is sternal splitting required for this resection. One important note is that of airway management. For safe management of the airway distorted or narrowed by a mediastinal mass, detailed preoperative assessment of the airway and adequate visualization and readily available supplementary equipment (eg, flexible bronchoscope) should be considered.

○   **A 26-year-old man presents with low-grade fever, malaise, 15-pound weight loss, and mild dyspnea. Chest radiograph reveals evidence of an anterior mediastinal mass and some lymphadenopathy in the hilar areas. Biopsy of the lymph nodes and a portion of the mass is performed using video-assisted thoracic surgery technique, and findings reveal the presence of Reed-Sternberg cells. In general, the lymph node tissue shows broad bands of collagenous material dividing the cellular components into nodular components. The cellular components include Reed-Sternberg cells, lymphocytes, neutrophils, plasma cells, eosinophils, and histiocytes. Which of the following is the most likely diagnosis for this patient?**

A: Sarcoidosis
B: Nodular sclerosing Hodgkin lymphoma
C: Tuberculosis
D: Seminoma
E: Thymoma

The correct answer is B: A characteristic feature of all forms of Hodgkin lymphoma is the presence of Reed-Sternberg cells. These are large cells with acidophilic cytoplasm that usually have binucleated or bilobed nuclei with large, prominent, deeply eosinophilic nucleoli. The nodular sclerosing variety is generally composed of broad bands of collagenous material, which appear to subdivide the tumor into nodular components. Cellular components include Reed-Sternberg cells, lymphocytes, neutrophils, plasma cells, eosinophils, and histiocytes. Some variants of the nodular sclerosing type have been described. None of the other pathologic entities described has Reed-Sternberg cells as a pathologic feature.

Note that in rare cases, Reed-Sternberg cells have been identified in benign lesions. However, in the case described, the patient has a fairly classic clinical presentation of Hodgkin lymphoma. The description of the lymph node histology including the presence of Reed-Sternberg cells is also quite typical for this disease.

○   **(T/F): The most common form of lymphoma found in the mediastinum is the nodular sclerosing type.**

The correct answer is True: Various lymphomas can be found in the mediastinum. They may be in the mediastinum as a primary process or as one of a number of involved locations in a systemic process. All forms of lymphoma originate from abnormalities of specific types of lymphocytes. They are generally divided into Hodgkin and non-Hodgkin lymphomas.

Many forms of non-Hodgkin lymphoma exist and are categorized by cell type. The most common types of lymphomas found in the mediastinum include immunoblastic T-cell, immunoblastic B-cell, follicular center cell, and lymphoblastic. The most common form of Hodgkin lymphoma found in the mediastinum is the nodular sclerosing type.

○   **(T/F): Substernal goiter is a condition in which all of the existing thyroid tissue is found in the anterior mediastinum instead of the neck.**

The correct answer is False: Substernal goiter is not true ectopic endocrine tissue but, rather, the direct extension of an abnormal cervical thyroid into the mediastinum. Surgical resection is indicated even in asymptomatic cases because of the risk of sudden airway obstruction and because of the somewhat increased chance of malignancy.

Resection can be performed via the standard cervical thyroidectomy incision in most cases. On rare occasions, sternotomy is required.

○   **(T/F): Surgical resection is indicated only for benign mesenchymal tumors of the mediastinum. Individuals with malignant mesenchymal tumors of the mediastinum undergo a combination of radiotherapy and chemotherapy.**

The correct answer is False: Surgical excision is indicated for most tumors of mesenchymal origin, both benign and malignant. One noted exception is that of rhabdomyosarcoma, for which a combination for radiation and chemotherapy offers the best survival results. Prognoses for specific tumors are as follows:

The prognosis for liposarcoma depends on several factors. Completely resected pseudoencapsulated tumors have a better prognosis compared to those that are nonencapsulated and invasive. Cell type and cell differentiation also play a role. Myxoid liposarcoma has a poorer prognosis. In one small series, approximately 30% of patients died of their disease after a mean period of less than 3 years.

Angiosarcomas of the mediastinum are rare but have a very poor prognosis, especially when they originate from the heart or great vessels.

Fibrosarcomas have a uniformly poor prognosis, and most patients die from their disease within a few years.

Primary leiomyosarcoma of the mediastinum has been described. In one reported series of 10 patients who underwent resection, 2 were alive and well at 4 and 6 years. Four of the others died of their disease or developed recurrence.

Rhabdomyosarcoma has the best long-term survival of all mesenchymal tumors because effective chemotherapeutic regimens have been identified. According to 1 report, 10-year actuarial survival rates range from 52-83% depending on the stage of disease at presentation and the existence of hematogenous metastases. Survival is much worse if the latter is present.

○   **(T/F): The technetium Tc 99m sestamibi scan, used for the identification of parathyroid tissue, may be particularly useful in finding a parathyroid gland located in the mediastinum.**

The correct answer is True: Approximately 1-3% of parathyroid tumors are located in the mediastinum and are approachable only via sternotomy. Accurate preoperative identification of these lesions is of paramount importance. Prior to the sestamibi scan, many patients underwent numerous unsuccessful explorations of the neck and mediastinum for parathyroid adenomas and treatment of hyperparathyroidism. Because of the accuracy with which this study can identify parathyroid tissue, it is a great asset in the treatment of these patients.

○   **Which of the following treatments is most appropriate for a patient who is HIV negative who has pulmonary tuberculosis (assuming directly observed therapy and a fully susceptible isolate)?**

A: Isoniazid and rifampin for 6 months
B: Isoniazid, rifampin, and pyrazinamide for 2 months followed by isoniazid and rifampin for 4 more months
C: Isoniazid and ethambutol for 12 months
D: Rifampin and ethambutol for 9 months
E: Isoniazid, rifampin, and ethambutol for 2 months followed by isoniazid and rifampin for 4 more months

The correct answer is B: Each of the drug combinations listed has shown good efficacy for the treatment of tuberculosis; however, the duration of therapy for isoniazid plus rifampin (without pyrazinamide) is 9 months. The duration of therapy for isoniazid plus ethambutol is 18 months. The duration of therapy for rifampin plus ethambutol is 12 months. Substitution of ethambutol for pyrazinamide results in lower efficacy of the short-course treatment.

○   32-year-old nurse presents for a preemployment physical examination. She reports having a positive purified protein derivative skin test in the past but denies taking any treatment. She currently is asymptomatic. What is the best course of action?

A: Obtain baseline and annual chest radiographs.
B: Administer bacille Calmette-Guérin vaccine.
C: Prescribe isoniazid at 300 mg PO qd for 6 months.
D: Perform a 2-step tuberculin skin test.
E: Document tuberculin skin test result as positive in patient's record without taking further action.

The correct answer is D: The history of a reaction to tuberculin skin testing is not a contraindication to future skin testing. Without documentation of the size of the reaction, whether the patient should truly be categorized as positive or administered preventive therapy remains unclear. In a health care worker or any individual who is likely to have annual skin testing, a 2-step test should be performed to eliminate the possibility of subsequent booster phenomenon.

○   (T/F): The risk of relapse after completing appropriate therapy (directly observed) for a fully susceptible isolate of *Mycobacterium tuberculosis* is 10%.

The correct answer is False: The risk for relapse is 0-4% with an optimal regimen and directly observed therapy. Other late complications of treated tuberculosis include aspergilloma, bronchiectasis, fibrothorax (trapped lung), broncholithiasis (manifested by hemoptysis, postobstructive pneumonia, or esophageal perforation), and possibly, an increased risk of lung cancer (controversial).

○   (T/F): Fever, sweats, weight loss, diarrhea, lymphadenopathy, and tender hepatosplenomegaly are symptoms of disseminated *Mycobacterium avium-intracellulare* (DMAC) infection in patients with AIDS.

The correct answer is True: Fever, sweats, weight loss, diarrhea, lymphadenopathy, and tender hepatosplenomegaly are symptoms of DMAC in patients with AIDS.

○   (T/F): Clarithromycin susceptibility should be requested in a patient with AIDS and disseminated *Mycobacterium avium-intracellulare* infection who does not respond to treatment with clarithromycin, ethambutol, and rifabutin.

The correct answer is True: Repeat blood cultures and do sensitivities to clarithromycin. If the isolate is sensitive to clarithromycin, add amikacin for 2-4 weeks. If the isolate is resistant to clarithromycin, consider changing clarithromycin to ciprofloxacin and add amikacin for 2-4 weeks.

○   (T/F): Isoniazid, pyrazinamide, and streptomycin, among others, have shown in vitro resistance to *Mycobacterium gordonae*.

The correct answer is True: *M gordonae* has proven resistant to isoniazid, pyrazinamide, and streptomycin. Clarithromycin and, possibly, azithromycin, quinolones (especially levofloxacin), and ethambutol are the recommended treatment options.

○   A 42-year-old man has right-sided chest pain and localized tenderness. His oxygen saturation is 98%, his chest x-ray findings are normal, and his CBC count is within normal limits. Which of the following is the next step for this patient?

A: Arterial blood gas determinations
B: Discharge patient
C: Ventilation-perfusion scan of the lungs
D: Heparinization
E: Compression ultrasound of legs

The correct answer is D: This patient most likely has pulmonary embolism. He should be heparinized immediately, before further investigations are carried out to confirm the diagnosis.

○   (T/F): The mortality rate of patients with pulmonary embolism (PE) could be reduced from 30% to less than 10% after adequate diagnosis and treatment.

The correct answer is True: If PE is undiagnosed and untreated, this condition has a high mortality rate.

○   (T/F): Any patient who has symptoms of thoracic disease but no alternate diagnosis should have investigations to rule out pulmonary embolism (PE).

The correct answer is True: Because symptoms and signs of PE are nonspecific, a high index of suspicion is required to aid in the diagnosis of this lethal condition.

○   (T/F): If a ventilation-perfusion scan reports a low probability in a patient suspected of having pulmonary embolism (PE), no further investigations are required.

The correct answer is False: As many as 12% of patients with a low-probability scan may have PE. Further investigations, such as a spiral CT scan, for pulmonary embolism are required in such patients.

○   (T/F): In a patient thought to have pulmonary embolism, echocardiography findings indicating right ventricular hypokinesis should prompt thrombolytic therapy.

The correct answer is True: The 2 indications for thrombolytic therapy are hemodynamic instability and right ventricular strain.

○   Which of the following statements about pulmonary embolism (PE) is not accurate?

A: PE is a common and lethal condition.
B: PE is not a disease but a complication of deep venous thrombosis (DVT).
C: The patients who die from PE do so within the first hour.
D: Further mortality occurs from recurrent embolism.
E: PE often resolves spontaneously.

The correct answer is E: PE does not resolve spontaneously; all of the other statements are accurate.

○   A 65-year-old man with a history of working as a sandblaster for 25 years presents with shortness of breath on minimal exertion (can walk only 1 city block without stopping to rest) and a productive cough. He has been retired for the past 10 years and is a smoker (1 pack daily for 50 y). His tuberculin skin status is unknown. He has lost approximately 15 pounds in the past 2 years. Prolonged expiration and wheeze are noted on examination. Chest radiograph (unchanged from one obtained 6 mo ago) shows bilateral upper zone densities without cavitation and bilateral upward retraction of the hila. Hyperinflation of the lower zones of the lungs also is noted. This clinical and radiographic presentation is most consistent with which of the following?

A: Silicoproteinosis
B: Asbestosis
C: Simple silicosis
D: Metastatic neoplasm
E: Complicated silicosis

The correct answer is E: The clinical and radiographic presentation is most consistent with complicated silicosis, as follows: (1) occupation and years of exposure to silica, (2) symptoms of marked shortness of breath and productive cough, and (3) upper zone densities with contraction. The clinical and radiographic appearance is not that of silicoproteinosis and simple silicosis. Asbestosis has lower zone predominance of infiltrates and often is accompanied by pleural changes. Densities only in the upper zones and hilar contractions are not expected in metastatic lung neoplasm.

○ **A 57-year-old man who has been a steam fitter for 25 years, who also worked in a shipyard many years ago, has a 2-cm noncalcified nodule in the right upper lobe of his lung. He has no symptoms. Previous chest radiographs are unavailable, but he states that his x-ray was normal 3 years ago. He has smoked 1-2 packages of cigarettes a day since he was in high school. A purified protein derivative (PPD) tuberculosis skin test showed 10-mm induration. He has traveled extensively in the United States and in Mexico. The findings during physical examination are normal. What is the most appropriate step?**

A: Start treatment with antituberculosis drugs.
B: Reassure the patient, and provide follow-up with chest radiographs every 3 months.
C: Administer chemoprophylaxis with isoniazid for 6 months.
D: Obtain a thoracic surgical consultation for resection of the nodule.
E: Perform bronchoscopy with transbronchoscopic biopsy.

The correct answer is D: In the absence of symptoms and without a confirmed diagnosis of tuberculosis, antituberculosis treatment is not indicated. PPD-positive status does not necessarily indicate active tuberculosis. A conservative approach to follow-up is risky and is not recommended for a patient with a solitary pulmonary nodule who has risk factors (eg, smoking, asbestos exposure) for bronchogenic carcinoma. Isoniazid chemoprophylaxis is a legitimate consideration, but the probability that the nodule may be a carcinoma demands priority consideration for treatment. The diagnostic yield from bronchoscopy and transbronchial lung biopsy of a 2-cm nodule is very low, and, therefore, a negative result does not exclude carcinoma. This patient's condition warrants an aggressive approach by resection of a solitary pulmonary nodule because it affords the best chance for cure in bronchogenic carcinoma.

○ **(T/F): During acute attacks of farmer's lung, an acute lymphocytic infiltration occurs with an increase in levels of interleukin-1 (IL-1) and tumor necrosis factor-alpha (TNF-alpha).**

The correct answer is True: During acute episodes, an acute neutrophilic infiltration is followed by a lymphocytic infiltration of the airways. Levels of IL-1 and TNF-alpha are increased. These cytokines have proinflammatory and chemotactic properties. They cause the recruitment of additional inflammatory mediators, resulting in direct cellular damage and changes in the complement pathway, which provide the necessary stimuli to increase vascular permeability and migration of leukocytes to the lung.

○ **(T/F): Shortness of breath, expiratory prolongation, and wheezing are features of asbestosis.**

The correct answer is False: While shortness of breath is a common symptom in asbestosis, expiratory prolongation and wheezing are not common features. The latter 2 features are associated with obstructive airway diseases.

○ **(T/F): A chemical worker who manufactures toluene diisocyanate (TDI) and has asthmalike symptoms with normal findings on chest radiographs describes a typical case of chemical worker's lung.**

The correct answer is True: Chemical worker's lung is an arbitrary, ill-defined, and confusing term because many chemicals are known to induce lung injury. For example, asbestosis could be considered a subclassification of chemical worker's lung, but in the real world, it is a separate disease entity and a subgroup of occupational lung disease and pneumoconiosis. By arbitrary definition, the implicated chemicals are restricted to the manufacture of polyurethane foam, moulding, insulation, synthetic rubber, and packaging materials and include TDI and trimellitic anhydride.

○ **(T/F): Avoidance of further exposure to the offending chemical is critical in the treatment of chemical worker's lung**

The correct answer is True: Providing health education, reducing exposures, and changing occupation are commonly used strategies.

○   **Which of the following indicates a complicated parapneumonic effusion that might need chest tube drainage?**

A: Loculated fluid identified by chest radiograph, ultrasound, or CT scanning
B: Pleural fluid pH greater than 7.2
C: Serosanguinous fluid
D: Cell count differential with greater than 95% lymphocytes
E: None of the above

The correct answer is A: Loculation indicates a fibrinopurulent parapneumonic effusion progressing to a closed space infection. Other indications for drainage of parapneumonic effusions are grossly purulent fluid, pleural fluid pH less than 7.0, and positive Gram stain result on the fluid. Parapneumonic effusions can be serosanguinous, but blood in the fluid does not necessarily indicate a need for drainage. Cell count differentials usually show a predominance of neutrophils; greater than 95% lymphocytes more commonly is found in malignant or tuberculous effusions.

○   **Which of the following tests should not be performed routinely on pleural fluid obtained at an initial thoracentesis?**

A: Cholesterol
B: Lactate dehydrogenase
C: Triglycerides
D: Protein
E: All of the above

The correct answer is C: Order cholesterol, lactate dehydrogenase, and protein measurements on pleural fluid to distinguish transudates from exudates on the initial evaluation. Triglyceride measurements on pleural fluid are indicated in the rare instance when a chylous effusion is suspected.

○   **(T/F): A shift in the trachea and heart toward the side of a large pleural effusion suggests obstruction of the bronchus.**

The correct answer is True: Endobronchial obstruction by malignancy or foreign body causes volume loss in the distal lung. The overlying effusion can obscure volume loss. The procedure of choice to evaluate such patients is bronchoscopy, not thoracentesis.

○   **(T/F): Elevated levels of pleural fluid adenosine deaminase (ADA) suggest tuberculous pleuritis as a cause of a lymphocytic exudative effusion.**

The correct answer is True: Tuberculosis is an important cause of lymphocytic exudative effusions and should be suspected clinically in high-risk populations. The absence of mesothelial cells (often counted as other cells) on the cell count differential further suggests the diagnosis. Pleural fluid ADA levels greater than 43 U support the diagnosis. Acid-fast stains on pleural fluid for tuberculosis rarely yield the diagnosis, but culture of pleural fluid and pleural biopsy tissue is positive in up to 90% of cases.

○   **(T/F): Herpes zoster virus is the etiology of pleurodynia.**

The correct answer is False: Coxsackievirus B is the etiology of pleurodynia.

○   **(T/F): Elevated levels of pleural fluid amylase support the diagnosis of pancreatitis as a cause of a left-sided exudative pleural effusion.**

The correct answer is True: Measure pleural fluid amylase in cases of suspected pancreatic disease producing pleural effusions.

○   **Spirometry shows the following results from an acceptable and reproducible test performed on a 45-year-old white man. He is 167 cm tall and weighs 80 kg. Forced vital capacity (FVC) is 3.03 L (69% of predicted and below the lower limit of normal [LLN]), forced expiratory volume in one second (FEV$_1$) is 2.28 L (63% of predicted and below the LLN), and FEV$_1$-to-FVC ratio is 75% (predicted ratio is 82%, LLN is 74%). These results can best be interpreted as which of the following?**

A: Mild airflow obstruction
B: Moderate airflow obstruction
C: Suggestive of restrictive lung disease
D: Normal
E: None of the above

The correct answer is C: The results are suggestive of restrictive lung disease, but the diagnosis of restrictive lung disease cannot be made by spirometry alone. The FVC can be reduced when obstruction is severe and commonly is reduced when patients are allowed to terminate their expiratory efforts early. The FEV$_1$ is reduced is this case, not because of airflow limitation caused by airway narrowing, but because the FVC is reduced and the FEV$_1$ is a component of the FVC. The FEV$_1$-to-FVC ratio is above the LLN. Lung volumes determination (by whole-body plethysmography or gas dilution) should be made to confirm the suspicion of restrictive lung disease. Measurement of the diffusing capacity of the lung for carbon monoxide also may be helpful if the residual volume and/or total lung capacity are reduced.

○   **Spirometry shows the following results from an acceptable and reproducible test performed on a 70-year-old white man. He is 183 cm tall and weighs 67 kg. The forced vital capacity (FVC) is 3.80 L (79% of predicted and above the lower limit of normal [LLN]), The forced expiratory volume in one second (FEV$_1$) is 1.23 L (33% of predicted), and the FEV$_1$-to-FVC ratio is 32% (predicted ratio is 76%, LLN is 68%). After administration of 2 puffs of a metered-dose inhaler of albuterol, the FVC is 3.84 L (1% increase) and the FEV$_1$ is 1.51 L (23% increase). These results are consistent with which of the following?**

A: Combined obstructive and restrictive ventilatory disorder with no significant response to bronchodilators
B: Combined obstructive and restrictive ventilatory disorder with significant response to bronchodilators
C: Severe obstructive ventilatory disorder with significant response to bronchodilators
D: Severe obstructive ventilatory disorder with no significant response to bronchodilators
E: None of the above

The correct answer is C: Although the FVC is less than 80% of predicted, it remains above the statistically defined LLN. The FEV$_1$ and FEV$_1$-to-FVC ratio are reduced severely. The FEV$_1$ shows a 23% increase after bronchodilators, and the absolute increase in the FEV$_1$ is 0.28 L. The threshold for a significant bronchodilator response is an increase in either the FVC or FEV$_1$ from a baseline of 12% and 0.2 L.

○   **(T/F): Pulse oximetry is an excellent test to evaluate operative risk.**

The correct answer is False: While useful as a means to monitor response to oxygen therapy postoperatively, pulse oximetry is a relatively insensitive index of gas exchange and should not be used to evaluate operative risk. Spirometry remains the best single test to evaluate risk for intraoperative and postoperative risk of pulmonary complications. For peripheral and abdominal surgery, when the forced expiratory volume in one second (FEV$_1$) is greater than 2 L and greater than 50% of predicted, complications are rare.

○   **(T/F): A reduced ratio of forced expiratory volume in one second (FEV$_1$) to forced vital capacity (FVC) is the hallmark of obstructive lung diseases.**

The correct answer is True: When obstructive lung disease is present, the ability of the airways to conduct airflow is reduced. The FEV$_1$ is reduced. In all but severe obstructive disease, the FVC generally is at or near normal. Thus, the FEV_1-to-FVC ratio always is reduced when obstructive lung disease is present. The ratio is considered to be reduced when it falls below the statistically defined lower limit of normal.

O   **(T/F): When obstructive lung disease is severe, the residual volume (RV) generally is reduced.**

The correct answer is False: The RV gradually increases when airflow obstruction is present, eventually reducing the vital capacity when obstruction is severe. A normal or reduced RV in the presence of moderate-to-severe airflow obstruction suggests a coexisting restrictive process.

O   **(T/F): When performing spirometry, the patient must exhale for only 6 seconds.**

The correct answer is False: While most patients with normal lung function are empty in 6 seconds, most patients with any degree of airflow obstruction are required to exhale for a full 15 seconds to obtain a valid estimate of their vital capacity. Having the patient exhale as forcefully as possible for the full 15 seconds is not necessary. The patient can be instructed to relax and push gently after just 3 seconds of forceful exhalation. Exhaling longer than 15 seconds is not recommended for safety reasons.

O   **A 65-year-old man with a history of chronic obstructive pulmonary disease (COPD) presents to the emergency department with a complaint of progressive dyspnea. He has an arterial blood gas analysis on room air with a pH of 7.28, a PCO_2 of 58 mm Hg, and a PO_2 of 50 mm Hg. An arterial blood gas analysis performed 6 months ago, when the patient was in stable condition, showed a pH of 7.39, PCO_2 of 44 mm Hg, and a PO_2 of 70 mm Hg. Oxygen is started at 4 L via face mask. A repeat arterial blood gas drawn 30 minutes later shows a pH of 7.22, a PCO_2 of 65 mm Hg, and a PO_2 of 70 mm Hg. Which of the following mechanisms is the most likely cause of this patient's worsening hypercapnia?**

A: Worsening shunt
B: Increased ventilation-perfusion mismatch
C: Anxiety
D: Worsening diffusion abnormality
E: Rebreathing of CO_2

The correct answer is B: Hypercapnia in COPD has multiple factors. These factors include decreased responsiveness to hypoxia and hypercapnia, increased ventilation-perfusion mismatch leading to increased dead space ventilation, and decreased diaphragm function secondary to fatigue and hyperinflation. In patients receiving oxygen therapy with a subsequent worsening of hypercapnia, increased ventilation-perfusion mismatch is the most likely cause of worsening hypercapnia.

O   **Which of the following drugs may not cause respiratory acidosis at toxic levels?**

A: Morphine
B: Aspirin
C: Lorazepam
D: Phenobarbital
E: Meperidine

The correct answer is B: All of these drugs except aspirin can cause respiratory depression with subsequent hypoventilation and respiratory acidosis. Aspirin is a salicylate, which initially can cause respiratory stimulation with subsequent hyperventilation and respiratory alkalosis. With continued toxicity, salicylates can cause metabolic acidosis.

O   **(T/F): A 65-year-old man with a history of chronic obstructive pulmonary disease (COPD) presents with a severe exacerbation complicated by respiratory acidosis. ABG analysis on a fraction of inspired oxygen (FiO_2) of 30% reveals the following: pH of 7.30, a $PaCO_2$ of 70 mm Hg, a PaO_2 of 65 mm Hg, and a bicarbonate (HCO_3^-) level of 32 mEq/L. The patient has been intubated and placed on mechanical ventilation.**

Now that the patient is on mechanical ventilation, the respiratory rate should be increased to obtain a PaCO₂ value of 45 mm Hg or less within several hours.

The correct answer is False: Respiratory acidosis should be corrected gradually over 2-3 days. Rapid overcorrection of hypercapnia in patients with chronic respiratory acidosis can result in metabolic alkalosis, hypokalemia, hypophosphatemia, and seizures.

○ **(T/F): Hypoxemia is a common finding in patients with hyperventilation syndrome.**

The correct answer is False: Hyperventilation syndrome is a diagnosis of exclusion, and symptoms may include dizziness, tetany, and paresthesia. Patients may benefit from treatment with rebreathing from a paper bag and reassurance. If hypoxemia is found in a patient with a diagnosis of hyperventilation syndrome, another diagnosis should be considered.

○ **(T/F): Respiratory alkalosis is an uncommon finding in critically ill patients.**

The correct answer is False: Respiratory alkalosis is one of the most common acid-base disturbances observed in critically ill patients. It is associated with many other metabolic derangements and is commonly observed in patients on mechanical ventilation.

○ **(T/F): Drugs that may cause respiratory alkalosis include methylxanthines such as theophylline and aminophylline.**

The correct answer is True: Respiratory alkalosis can be caused by several drugs. These drugs include salicylates, methylxanthines (eg, theophylline and aminophylline), progesterones, and catecholamines.

○ **A 22-year-old woman presents with a 3-day history of dyspnea, fatigue, and cough. Several months ago, while playing softball, she was hit by a ball in her right calf area. The patient denies use of diet suppressants. The area became swollen and painful; however, it improved slightly with cold compresses. Evaluation initially revealed a slightly dyspneic female with 2+ edema of the right-lower extremity, no cardiac murmurs, and normal findings after lung examination. Findings from a Doppler examination of the extremities were positive for deep venous thrombosis. The patient received warfarin anticoagulation for 3 months and her symptoms improved.**

She is now returning for a follow-up examination. She reports 2-block dyspnea upon exertion and a nonproductive cough. The swelling in her right leg, while improved, is worse, with some swelling of the left-lower extremity. Upon examination, her jugular venous pulsations are elevated, her second heart sound is accentuated, and a right ventricular heave is present. Laboratory evaluation reveals positive results for antinuclear antibody and anticardiolipin antibody. Ventilation-perfusion lung scan results show multiple segmental perfusion defects that are unmatched to ventilation. Which of the following is the most likely diagnosis?

A: Primary pulmonary hypertension
B: Mitral stenosis
C: Systemic lupus erythematosus
D: Chronic thromboembolic pulmonary hypertension
E: Anorexigen-associated pulmonary hypertension

The correct answer is D: This patient has chronic thromboembolic pulmonary hypertension, which may closely mimic primary pulmonary hypertension. Upon initial presentation, she was dyspneic and likely developed a pulmonary embolism related to her deep venous thrombosis. Despite anticoagulation, her symptoms persisted and she now presents with overt symptoms and signs of right ventricular failure. Chronic thromboembolic pulmonary hypertension can be associated with a hypercoagulable state, but often, findings from such a workup are negative. An antinuclear antibody test is a good screening tool for collagen vascular disease; however, results are nonspecific and often of little clinical significance.

O   **A 35-year-old man who has smoked all his life presents with worsening dyspnea and the presence of bilateral infiltrates on his chest radiograph. He has a hemoglobin of 9 g/dL and a serum creatinine of 3.8 mg/dL. Urinalysis reveals red blood cells and proteinuria. The serum anti–glomerular basement membrane (anti-GBM) is positive. Which of the following is a correct statement?**

A: The anemia is secondary to hemolysis.
B: Because hemoptysis is absent, pulmonary hemorrhage is not likely to be present.
C: Plasmapheresis will lead to recovery of renal function.
D: The disease activity correlates with the presence of anti-GBM antibodies.
E: This disease occurs predominantly in females.

The correct answer is D: This patient has a pulmonary-renal syndrome secondary to anti-GBM disease, or Goodpasture syndrome. A pulmonary-renal syndrome may be caused by Goodpasture syndrome, Wegener granulomatosis, systemic lupus erythematosus, or other vasculitides. The anti-GBM antibodies correlate with disease activity. A male predominance in the occurrence of Goodpasture disease exists. The pulmonary hemorrhage may occur without overt hemoptysis. Anemia is common and is due to chronic blood loss. Treatment includes plasmapheresis, corticosteroids, and immunosuppressive drugs. Renal function may be recovered; this is unlikely to occur once advanced renal dysfunction is present.

O   **(T/F): A 38-year-old woman with primary pulmonary hypertension currently being treated with epoprostenol is admitted for acute gastroenteritis. She is orthostatic and her standing blood pressure is 80/50 mm Hg. The nurse or doctor should immediately stop the epoprostenol drip to alleviate the hypotension.**

The correct answer is False: Do not stop the epoprostenol. It has a very short half-life, and its effect dissipates in a matter of minutes. Severe right-sided heart failure could ensue because of rebound pulmonary hypertension. More appropriate therapy would be gentle rehydration with intravenous fluids.

O   **(T/F): Patients taking combination therapy with prednisone and cyclophosphamide for Wegener granulomatosis should also be taking trimethoprim-sulfamethoxazole for *Pneumocystis carinii* pneumonia prophylaxis.**

The correct answer is True: The annual incidence of *Pneumocystis* pneumonia is approximately 1% in patients on combination therapy; therefore, these patients should be administered prophylactic therapy. Furthermore, this treatment has been shown to reduce the frequency of relapses in persons with Wegener granulomatosis.

O   **(T/F): The most common cause of mortality in patients with Churg-Strauss syndrome (CSS) is cardiovascular complications, including myocardial infarction secondary to coronary artery vasculitis.**

The correct answer is True: Cardiovascular complications, including myocardial infarction secondary to coronary artery vasculitis, are the most common causes of mortality in patients with CSS.

O   **(T/F): High-output congestive heart failure and bleeding following surgery are potential complications resulting from the hypervascularity of bone associated with Paget disease.**

The correct answer is True: High-output congestive heart failure and postoperative bleeding may occur from the hypervascularity of pagetic bone. Other complications of Paget disease include deafness, spinal stenosis, stroke, vascular steal syndrome, fractures, osteoarthritis, sarcomas, nephrocalcinosis, and the development of bone tumors (principally sarcomas).

O   **An individual presents with wheezing and eosinophilia. Which of the following is true?**

A: The patient most likely has Churg-Strauss syndrome (CSS).
B: The patient may need a stool examination.
C: The patient should receive systemic corticosteroids as soon as possible.

D: The patient should never receive corticosteroids.

E: The patient should be treated with thiabendazole if wheezing is refractory.

The correct answer is B: The patient may need a stool examination. None of the other answers is correct. Some patients with wheezing and eosinophilia may have a parasitic infection.

CSS is exceedingly rare. Patients with wheezing and eosinophilia are far more likely to have asthma than CSS; hence, answer A is incorrect. Systemic corticosteroids are indicated for persons with severe symptoms once the risks of administration have been excluded to a reasonable degree. No information regarding these issues exists, and no compelling reason is provided for immediate treatment; therefore, answers C and D are incorrect. Answer E is incorrect because patients with severe respiratory symptoms who are not at risk for dissemination of fungal or Strongyloides infection should not be denied the benefits of corticosteroids if they are indicated.

Empiric treatment with a medication associated with considerable adverse effects and a low probability of success is undesirable. Make reasonable and targeted diagnostic efforts. Administer bronchodilators and steroids, if indicated and justified, for persistent wheezing.

○   **When evaluating a patient with pulmonary infiltrates and eosinophilia, which of the following would provide the least helpful information?**

A: Bronchoalveolar lavage (BAL)

B: Computed tomography of the chest

C: Pulmonary function testing

D: Stool examination for ova and parasites

E: Tuberculin skin test

The correct answer is E: Tuberculin skin test is correct. The tuberculin skin test may help identify an individual who has latent tuberculous infection. A positive result from the skin test alone is not associated with eosinophilia. Active tuberculosis is an uncommon cause of eosinophilia.

Pulmonary function testing may be useful because a restrictive pattern suggests extensive or chronic inflammation, which is observed with tropical pulmonary eosinophilia, intrinsic eosinophilic syndromes, and interstitial lung diseases. An obstructive pattern may be observed with both extrinsic and intrinsic diseases.

Computed tomography of the chest is useful for helping define the extent and pattern of disease and provides a level of detail far beyond that offered by the plain radiograph.

Examination of the stool for ova and parasites may be helpful for diagnosing parasitic infection that may cause pulmonary infiltrates and eosinophilia. Examination of the stool is easily performed by experienced laboratory personnel.

BAL is often helpful for excluding infections and often improves diagnostic sensitivity over that provided by sputum specimens alone. BAL is commonly used to exclude infection when chronic eosinophilic pneumonia is high on the differential diagnosis list. Occasionally, BAL washings are positive for parasites such as Strongyloides.

○   **(T/F): Pulmonary hypertension is an infrequent complication of schistosomiasis.**

The correct answer is False: Pulmonary hypertension due to chronic embolization of ova is the most common pulmonary complication of schistosomiasis.

○   **(T/F): Allergic bronchopulmonary aspergillosis (ABPA) is largely a parenchymal lung disease requiring antifungal treatment.**

The correct answer is False: ABPA is an airway disease in which hypersensitivity to fungal elements creates chronic bronchospasm. Bronchiectasis develops from chronic inflammation and fungal proliferation. Antifungal treatment with itraconazole has been used as a steroid-sparing agent. If Aspergillus infection invades parenchymal tissue, antifungal treatment is indicated.

○   **(T/F): Antibiotics are a common cause of drug-induced pulmonary infiltrates and eosinophilia.**

The correct answer is True: Antibiotics are a common cause of drug-induced pulmonary infiltrates. Other common agents include nonsteroidal anti-inflammatory drugs.

○   **(T/F): Although the response to steroids in patients with chronic eosinophilic pneumonia (CEP) is dramatic and may occur in as few as 24 hours, the risk of relapse is high.**

The correct answer is True: The rapid (24-72 h) and dramatic response of CEP to steroids is actually a hallmark of CEP. The risk of relapse is high if steroids are discontinued within the first 6 months of therapy.

○   **A 45-year-old man presents with the chief symptom of excessive daytime sleepiness despite sleeping 8 hours every night. The findings of his physical examination are significant only for moderate obesity. Which of the following is the most likely diagnosis?**

A: Narcolepsy
B: Chronic insufficient sleep syndrome
C: Periodic limb movement disorder
D: Obstructive sleep apnea
E: Insomnia

The correct answer is D: In a 45-year-old man presenting with excessive daytime sleepiness and obesity, obstructive sleep apnea is clearly the most likely diagnosis. Narcolepsy generally develops in adolescents and young adults. Chronic insufficient sleep is unlikely in a patient sleeping 8 hours each night. Periodic limb movement disorder is a disorder of repetitive leg motions at night; it is much less common than obstructive sleep apnea. In insomnia, patients have difficulty sleeping at night.

○   **A 50-year-old woman has recently been diagnosed with obstructive sleep apnea (OSA), with an apnea-plus-hypopnea index (AHI) of 30 episodes per hour. Which of the following treatments should be recommended as first-line therapy for her OSA?**

A: Oral appliance
B: Conservative measures
C: Nasal continuous positive airway pressure (CPAP)
D: Uvulopalatopharyngoplasty (UPPP)
E: Protriptyline

The correct answer is C: Nasal CPAP should always be the first therapy for patients with OSA, especially those with moderate disease (AHI >20 episodes/h). Oral appliance usage is increasing, but this device should probably be considered second-line therapy if CPAP fails. Conservative measures should never be used alone for patients with moderate OSA. UPPP is second- or third-line therapy, given that it is effective in only 50% of patients.

○   **(T/F): The male-to-female ratio for obstructive sleep apnea is 8:1 in community-based studies.**

The correct answer is False: The male-to-female ratio, based on community studies, is 2-3:1. Evidence indicates that women underreport the symptoms of loud snoring and witnessed apneas, leading to underreferral to sleep centers. This may explain the marked male predominance (male-to-female ratio of approximately 8:1) in sleep center–based studies.

○   **(T/F): Adenotonsillar hypertrophy is the most common associated factor in both children and adults with obstructive sleep apnea.**

The correct answer is False: Obesity is the most common associated factor in adults, while adenotonsillar hypertrophy is the most common factor in children.

○ **(T/F): Obstructive sleep apnea (OSA) is an independent risk factor for the development of hypertension.**

The correct answer is True: The link between OSA and hypertension has been demonstrated in both cross-sectional and prospective studies.

○ **(T/F): Studies have shown a high rate of compliance with therapy in patients treated with nasal continuous positive airway pressure (CPAP) for obstructive sleep apnea.**

The correct answer is False: Most studies show that most patients use CPAP 4-5 hours at night only 4-5 times/wk. The rate of compliance at 1 year is only 68%.

○ **Which of the following is not an acceptable donor criterion related to lung transplantation?**

A: Age younger than 55 years
B: Minimal smoking history
C: PaO_2 of greater than 300 mm Hg, fraction of inspired oxygen equal to 1, and peak end-expiratory pressure of 5 cm H_2O
D: No significant chest trauma
E: Diffuse erythema present but purulent secretions absent upon bronchoscopic examination

The correct answer is E: Individuals with lower respiratory infections are not donor candidates. A bronchoscopy is the preferred evaluation used to decide this issue. If purulent secretions are present but erythema is not, lungs may be harvested. The presence of diffuse erythema is a contraindication.

○ **When considering lung transplantation, which of the following requirements does not need to be met when matching a recipient to a donor?**

A: ABO compatibility
B: Lung size, ie, a total lung capacity within 500 mL of each other
C: Human leukocyte antigen (HLA) matching
D: Matching cytomegalovirus (CMV) serological status
E: All of the above

The correct answer is C: HLA compatibility of donors and recipients does not correlate with subsequent rejection or mortality.

○ **(T/F): Lung transplant should not be offered to patients with poorly controlled collagen vascular diseases.**

The correct answer is True: Patients with systemic collagen vascular diseases other than scleroderma, if active or poorly controlled, are at risk of disease recurrence after the transplant.

○ **(T/F): When considering patients who have undergone lung transplants, diagnosing cytomegalovirus (CMV) infection requires bronchoscopy and bronchoalveolar lavage.**

The correct answer is True: Because of the high morbidity and mortality associated with CMV pneumonitis, patients with a positive result on "shell-vial" accelerated centrifugation culture from bronchoalveolar lavage fluid in the appropriate setting require therapy.

○   **(T/F): A patient developed clinical and radiologic evidence of pulmonary edema 3 days after lung transplantation. This patient very likely has a pulmonary reimplantation response.**

The correct answer is True: Pulmonary reimplantation response is pulmonary edema following transplant, which develops secondary to ischemic injury to the donor lung and peaks by the fourth day after the transplant.

○   **(T/F): Bronchiolitis obliterans is a form of chronic rejection and is observed in 50% of patients who undergo lung transplantation.**

The correct answer is True: Obliterative bronchiolitis is an inflammatory disorder of the airways that leads to disease of the respiratory bronchioles. Presently, bronchiolitis obliterans is believed to be a manifestation of chronic rejection.

○   **A 65-year-old white man reports progressively worsening dyspnea and cough. In the last few weeks, he has observed blood-tinged sputum. The patient does not report any weight loss. He is a mechanic and is still working full time. He has smoked 1 pack of cigarettes per day since age 20 years.**

Physical examination reveals a well-built, otherwise healthy-looking man in no distress. Vital signs are stable. Except for finger clubbing, no other positive findings are noted. His chest radiograph reveals a right hilar mass. His CT scan reveals a 5 X 4-cm mass at the right hilum and enlarged nodes in the right hilum and the subcarinal region. Additionally, a 2.5-cm lymph node is observed in the left paratracheal region. The rest of the lung parenchyma, liver, and adrenals appear normal. Bronchoscopy is performed and reveals a normal trachea and mainstem bronchi. The right upper lobe bronchus appears abnormal, with extrinsic compression. Biopsy specimens taken during bronchoscopy reveal an adenocarcinoma.

The patient undergoes mediastinal lymph node sampling because the surgeon considers his tumor resectable, provided the cancer does not involve the contralateral mediastinal lymph node. The results of the biopsy of a lymph node from the left paratracheal region indicate malignancy. Therefore, the final pathologic stage is IIIB. What is the optimum management strategy?

A: Radiation therapy alone
B: Chemotherapy alone
C: Combined chemotherapy and radiation given in sequence
D: Combined chemotherapy and radiation therapy given concurrently
E: Palliative care

The correct answer is D: The standard of care for patients with unresectable stage III non–small cell lung cancer and a good performance status has been combined-modality therapy with chemotherapy and radiation. This has been proven in several studies. The Cancer and Leukemia Group B and Radiation Therapy Oncology Group (RTOG) both showed improvements in 3- and 5-year survival rates with a combined-modality approach. A recent phase 3 randomized trial (RTOG 9410) compared the value of combined-modality therapy administered concurrently versus sequentially and found further survival benefit with the concurrent approach.

○   **(T/F): Adenocarcinoma is the lung tumor most commonly associated with hypercalcemia.**

The correct answer is False: Hypercalcemia is a paraneoplastic manifestation most commonly associated with squamous cell carcinoma of the lung.

○   **(T/F): All patients with small cell lung cancer (SCLC) should be offered chemotherapy and thoracic radiotherapy.**

The correct answer is False: The benefit of thoracic radiation therapy has been proven only in limited-stage SCLC. The addition of thoracic radiotherapy results in a modest survival improvement of 5% in this situation. No evidence currently exists to support routine use of thoracic radiotherapy in extensive-stage SCLC.

○ **(T/F): A patient with small cell carcinoma with a pulmonary mass, ipsilateral mediastinal and supraclavicular adenopathy, and a malignant pleural effusion has limited-stage disease.**

The correct answer is False: Presence of a malignant pleural effusion in a patient with small cell carcinoma of the lung makes it extensive-stage disease.

○ **(T/F): The most common paraneoplastic syndrome associated with small cell lung cancer (SCLC) is syndrome of inappropriate secretion of antidiuretic hormone (SIADH).**

The correct answer is True: The primary management of low serum sodium level associated with SCLC is treatment of the underlying illness; however, those with very low sodium level or with symptoms can be treated with fluid restriction. Demeclocycline is a tetracycline antibiotic that decreases the sensitivity of distal renal tubules to the effect of antidiuretic hormone and has been used successfully to correct serum sodium in SIADH.

○ **Which condition is most commonly associated with central bronchiectasis?**

A: Foreign body aspiration
B: Allergic bronchopulmonary aspergillosis
C: Cystic fibrosis
D: Primary ciliary dyskinesia
E: Human immunodeficiency virus (HIV) disease

The correct answer is B: Bronchiectasis as a result of infection generally involves the lower lobes, the right middle lobe, and the lingula. Right middle lobe involvement alone suggests right middle lobe syndrome or a neoplastic cause. Bronchiectasis caused by cystic fibrosis, Mycobacterium tuberculosis, or chronic fungal infections tends to affect the upper lobe. Allergic bronchopulmonary aspergillosis also affects the upper lobes but usually involves the central bronchi, whereas most other forms of bronchiectasis involve distal bronchial segments.

○ **Which diagnostic study is not generally helpful in the evaluation of bronchiectasis?**

A: High-resolution computed tomography (HRCT) scanning
B: Pilocarpine iontophoresis (sweat test)
C: Chest radiography
D: Bronchoscopy
E: Sputum analysis

The correct answer is D: In general, bronchoscopy is not useful in diagnosing bronchiectasis and subsequently is of use only when foreign body or neoplastic obstruction is suspected. The diagnosis of bronchiectasis is generally made by the use of an HRCT scan, although in the appropriate clinical setting, suggestive chest radiograph findings may be enough to aid in making the diagnosis. Once the diagnosis of bronchiectasis is made, further workup should be pursued to identify contributing causes. A pilocarpine iontophoresis (sweat test) for cystic fibrosis and a sputum analysis are 2 useful tests in this evaluation.

○ **(T/F): A chronic cough and daily mucopurulent sputum production are the 2 most common presenting clinical complaints in bronchiectasis.**

The correct answer is True: A chronic cough and daily mucopurulent sputum production lasting months to years are the most common presenting complaints in bronchiectasis.

○ **(T/F): Pseudomonas aeruginosa is the most common organism recovered from sputum cultures in patients with cystic fibrosis.**

The correct answer is True: Patients with cystic fibrosis have a predilection for colonization with P aeruginosa. Once colonized, P aeruginosa tends to persist.

○   **(T/F): Recurrent otitis media is one of the presentations of cystic fibrosis.**

The correct answer is False: Otitis media is not one of the typical features of cystic fibrosis.

○   **(T/F): Pulmonary function testing in a patient with cystic fibrosis typically shows restrictive lung disease.**

The correct answer is False: Obstructive pulmonary defect, as demonstrated on pulmonary function testing, is the typical finding in a patient with cystic fibrosis.

○   **A 65-year-old white man reports progressively worsening dyspnea and cough. In the last few weeks, he has observed blood-tinged sputum. The patient does not report any weight loss. He is a mechanic and is still working full time. He has smoked 1 pack of cigarettes per day since age 20 years.**

Physical examination reveals a well-built, otherwise healthy-looking man in no distress. Vital signs are stable. Except for finger clubbing, no other positive findings are noted. His chest radiograph reveals a right hilar mass. His CT scan reveals a 5 X 4-cm mass at the right hilum and enlarged nodes in the right hilum and the subcarinal region. Additionally, a 2.5-cm lymph node is observed in the left paratracheal region. The rest of the lung parenchyma, liver, and adrenals appear normal. Bronchoscopy is performed and reveals a normal trachea and mainstem bronchus. The right upper lobe bronchus appears abnormal, with extrinsic compression. Biopsy specimens taken during bronchoscopy reveal an adenocarcinoma. What is the clinical and radiologic stage?

A: Stage IIA
B: Stage IIIA
C: Stage IIIB
D: Stage IV
E: Stage IB

The correct answer is C: Involvement of contralateral mediastinal nodes is nodal stage N3. Even though the patient does not have a malignant pleural effusion or involvement of major mediastinal structures, his cancer is staged as N3. His final tumor stage is T2 N3 M0 (ie, stage IIIB).

○   **(T/F): Pulmonary function tests (PFTs), high-resolution CT scan, and manometry or esophagogastroduodenoscopy (EGD) are used to determine a baseline value and evaluate function on patients with scleroderma.**

The correct answer is True: All of these tests help evaluate the patient's baseline function.

○   **(T/F): Rheumatoid arthritis rarely affects the lungs of patients with active, long-standing rheumatoid arthritis.**

The correct answer is False: RA involvement of the lungs may take several forms, including pleural effusions, interstitial fibrosis, nodules (Caplan syndrome), and bronchiolitis obliterans-organizing pneumonia

○   **(T/F): Restrictive lung disease may occur in patients with late-stage AS, with costovertebral and costosternal involvement causing limited chest expansion**

The correct answer is False: Restrictive lung disease may occur in patients with late-stage AS, with costovertebral and costosternal involvement causing limited chest expansion.

○   **(T/F): Pulmonary hypertension is not a feature of mixed connective tissue disease.**

The correct answer is False: Pulmonary hypertension, particularly in the setting of myocardial ischemia and myocarditis, must be suspected when cardiopulmonary symptoms occur in these patients.

O   **Which of the following is a major American College of Rheumatology (ACR) criterion for the classification of scleroderma?**

A: Proximal scleroderma - Symmetric thickening, tightening, and induration of the skin of the fingers and skin proximal to the metacarpophalangeal or metatarsophalangeal joints (These changes may affect the entire extremity, face, neck, and trunk [thorax and abdomen].)
B: Sclerodactyly - Changes limited to the fingers
C: Digital pitting scars or loss of substance from the finger pad - Depressed areas of finger tips or loss of digital pad tissue as a result of ischemia
D: Bibasilar pulmonary fibrosis - Bilateral reticular pattern of linear or lineonodular densities most pronounced in basilar portions of the lungs on standard chest roentgenograms, which may assume the appearance of diffuse mottling or a honeycomb lung (Changes likely are not attributable to primary lung disease,)
E: A positive test result for Scl-70 or a positive result for centromere pattern antinuclear antibody (ANA)

The correct answer is A: Proximal scleroderma is the only major criterion and is enough to classify a patient as having scleroderma. The others criteria are minor, and the presence of 2 is required to classify a patient as having scleroderma. A positive result for Scl-70 or a positive result for centromere pattern ANA is not part of the classification system.

O   **A 36-year-old African-American woman presents with complaints of dyspnea and cough. Approximately 2 weeks ago she noted the onset of a red rash on her lower extremities. She also reports bilateral arthralgias. She has had no recent purified protein derivative (PPD) tuberculin test, reports no ill contacts, and is otherwise healthy. A chest radiograph reveals bilateral hilar adenopathy. Which of the following is not included in the differential diagnosis of this presentation?**

A: Lymphoma
B: Sarcoidosis
C: Systemic lupus erythematosus (SLE)
D: Tuberculosis
E: Histoplasmosis

The correct answer is C: All of the above but lupus may be associated with erythema nodosum and bilateral hilar adenopathy. Lupus, although associated with joint complaints, rarely causes bilateral hilar adenopathy. When SLE does cause adenopathy in the chest, it is more often mediastinal. This patient has Löfgren syndrome.

O   **A 36-year-old African-American woman presents with complaints of dyspnea and cough. Approximately 2 weeks ago, she noted the onset of a red rash on her lower extremities. She also reports bilateral arthralgias. She has had no recent purified protein derivative (PPD) tuberculin test, reports no ill contacts, and is otherwise healthy. A chest radiograph reveals bilateral hilar adenopathy. What is the most appropriate medical therapy?**

A: Prednisone, 30 mg PO qd
B: Motrin, 800 mg PO tid
C: Methotrexate, 10 mg PO q wk
D: No therapy indicated
E: Azathioprine, 50mg PO qd

The correct answer is B: This patient has Löfgren syndrome, which has an excellent prognosis. She only requires symptomatic therapy with Motrin.

O   **(T/F): Infection is the most common cause of acute bronchiolitis.**

The correct answer is True: Infectious bronchiolitis are most common in children, the offending organisms include adenovirus (types 3, 7, 21), respiratory syncytial virus, measles, mycoplasma, influenza A and pertussis.

○   **(T/F): All patients with hereditary angioedema or acquired angioedema who are undergoing procedures involving the oropharyngeal region should receive prophylaxis for angioedema.**

The correct answer is True: Short-term prophylaxis with androgens and fresh frozen plasma is required for patients with hereditary angioedema or acquired angioedema who have minor trauma or are undergoing procedures involving the oropharyngeal region, including dental procedures, secondary to the association of these procedures with inciting angioedema.

○   **(T/F): C1q levels are low in persons hereditary angioedema (HAE) and acquired angioedema (AAE).**

The correct answer is False: While C1-esterase inhibitor levels may be low in patients with either HAE and AAE, the C1q level is usually normal or only slightly decreased in persons with HAE.

○   **(T/F): Measurement of C1 esterase inhibitor (C1-INH) functional and quantitative levels can be used to confirm a diagnosis of hereditary angioedema (HAE).**

The correct answer is True: The definitive diagnosis of HAE is made by measurement of C1-INH levels. This can be performed by either a quantitative or a functional assay.

BIBLIOGRAPHY

ACCP Critical Care Board Review, 2004.

Advanced Cardiac Life Support. Dallas: American Heart Association; 2000.

Advanced Trauma Life Support. Chicago: American College of Surgeons; 1995.

Albert, DM. *Clinical Practice Principles and Practice of Ophthalmology,* Vol. 2. Philadelphia: W.B. Saunders Co.; 1994.

Anderson, JE. *Grant's Atlas of Anatomy,* 8th ed. Baltimore: Williams & Wilkins; 1983.

Arieff, A. & Defronzo, R. *Fluid, Electrolyte and Acid Base Disorders*, 2nd ed. New York: Churchill Livingstone; 1995.

Auerbach, PS. *Management of Wilderness and Environmental Emergencies,* 4th ed. St. Louis: CV Mosby Company; 2001.

Bakerman, S. *ABCs of Interpretive Laboratory Data,* 2nd ed. Greenville: Interpretive Laboratory Data, Inc; 1984.

Baum's Textbook of Pulmonary Diseases, Lippincott, 2003.

Barash PG, Cullen BF, Stoelting RK (eds): *Clinical Anesthesia*, 4th ed. Philadelphia: Lippincott-Raven; 2000.

Barie PS, Shires GT (eds): *Surgical Intensive Care.* Boston: Little, Brown and Co.; 1993.

Berkow, R. *The Merck Manual,* 15th ed. Rahway: Merck Sharp & Dohme Research Laboratories; 1987.

Blomquist, IK & Bayer, AS. Life-threatening deep fascial space infections of the head and neck. *Infect Dis Clin N America.* 1988; 2 (1):237.

Bone LB, Johnson KD, Weigelt J, et al: Early versus delayed stabilization of femoral fractures: a prospective randomized study. *J Bone Joint Surg.* 1989; 71;336.

Bone, RC (ed): *Pulmonary and Critical Care Medicine.* 1993.

Bouachour G, Tirot P, Varache N, Gouello JP, Harr P, Alquier P. Hemodynamic changes in acute adrenal insufficiency. *Intensive Care Med.* 1994; 20:138-41.

Bracken MB, Shepard MJ, Collins WF, et al: A randomized, controlled trial of methylprednisolone or naloxone in the treatment of acute spinal cord injury: results of the Second National Acute Spinal Cord Injury Study. *N Engl J Med.* 1990; 322:1405-11.

Bradley, WG. *Neurology in Clinical Practice,* 4th ed. Newtown: Butterworth-Heineman; 2003.

Braverman LE & Utiger RD, eds: *The Thyroid*, 7th ed. Philadelphia: Lippincott-Raven; 1996:286-296.

Cahill, BC & Ingbar, DH. Massive hemoptysis. *Clinics in Chest Medicine.* 1994; 15:147.

Calleja, GA & Barkin, JS. Acute Pancreatitis. *Med Clin North Am.* 1993; 77:1037-1056.

Civetta JM, Taylor RW, Kirby RR. *Critical Care,* 3rd ed. New York: Lippincott-Raven Publishers; 1997.

Claussen MS, Landercasper J, Cogbill THE. Acute adrenal insufficiency presenting as shock after trauma and surgery: Three cases and review of the literature. *J Trauma.* 1992; 32:94-100.

Current Diagnosis & Treatment in Pulmonary Medicine, McGraw-Hill/Appleton & Lange; 1 edition (October 17, 2003)

Chronic Obstructive Pulmonary Disease, Oxford University Press, 2003.

Critical Care Transport, Jones & Bartlett, 2003.

Cynober, L, *Nutrition and Critical Care*, Ag Med & Sci, 2003.

DeGowin, EL. *Bedside Diagnostic Examination,* 4th ed. New York: Macmillan Publishing Co. Inc; 1981.

Diepenbrock, Nancy, *Quick Reference to Critical Care*, Lippincott Williams and Wilkins, 2003.

Doods, Chris, *Anaesthesia and Critical Care*, Churchill Livingstone, 2003.

Edelstein, PH. Legionnaire's disease. *Clin Infect Dis.* 1993; 16:741.

Ellenhorn, MJ. *Ellenhorn's Medical Toxicology: Diagnosis and Treatment of Human Poisoning,* 2nd ed. Baltimore: Williams & Wilkins; 1997.

Farb, Daniel, *Basic Critical Care,* Atlasbooks, 2004.

Farwell, AP. Sick euthyroid syndrome. *J Intens Care Med.* vol. 12: 5:249-260.

Fauci, AS & Braunwald, E. *Harrison's Principles of Internal Medicine*, 14th ed. New York: McGraw-Hill; 1998.

Feliciano DV, Moore EE, Mattox KL (eds): *Trauma*, 3rd ed. Stamford: Appleton & Lange; 1996.

Fishman, AP. *Fishman's Pulmonary Diseases and Disorders*, 3rd ed. New York: McGraw-Hill; 1998.

Forrester JS, Diamond G, Chatterjee K, Swan JC. Medical therapy of acute myocardial infarction by application of hemodynamic subsets (parts 1 and 2). *N Engl J Med.* 1976; 295, 1356-1362 & 1204-1213.

Flomenbaum, N. *Emergency Diagnostic Testing,* 2nd ed. St. Louis: Mosby-Year Book, Inc.; 1995.

Goldfrank, LR, et al: *Goldfrank's Toxicologic Emergencies*, 6th ed. Stamford: Appleton & Lange; 1998.

Greenfield, LJ. *Surgery Scientific Principles and Practice.* Philadelphia: J.B. Lippincott Company; 1993.

Guyton, AC. *Textbook of Medical Physiology.* 10th ed. Philadelphia: W.B. Saunders Co.; 2000.

Hall JB, Schmidt GA, Wood LDH. *Principles of Critical Care*, 3rd ed. New York: McGraw Hill; 2005.

Harris, JH. *The Radiology of Emergency Medicine,* 2nd ed. Baltimore: Williams and Wilkins; 1981.

Harrison, TR. *Principles of Internal Medicine,* 16th ed. New York: McGraw-Hill Book Company; 2004.

Harwood-Nuss, A. *The Clinical Practice of Emergency Medicine,* 3rd ed. Philadelphia: JB Lippincott Company; 2001.

Holland, JF. *Cancer Medicine,* 6th ed. Baltimore: Williams & Wilkins; 2003.

Hoppenfeld, S. *Physical Examination of the Spine and Extremities.* Norwalk: Appleton-Century-Crofts; 1976.

International Consensus Conference: Clinical Investigation of Ventilator-Associated Pneumonia. *Chest.* Nov 1992; vol. 102; 5: 1.

International Study Group, The. In-hospital mortality and clinical course of 20,891 patients with suspected acute myocardial infarction randomized between alteplase and streptokinase with and without heparin. *Lancet.* 1990; 336: 71-75.

International Consensus Conference: Clinical Investigation of Ventilator-Associated Pneumonia. *Chest.* Nov 1992; vol. 102; 5: 1.

Ivatury, RR & Cayten, CG (eds): *The Textbook of Penetrating Trauma.* Philadelphia: Williams & Wilkins; 1996: 319-332.

Jenison, S & Hejelle, B. Hantavirus pulmonary syndrome; clinical, diagnostic and virologic aspects. *Seminars in Respiratory Infections.* December 1995; vol. 10; 4: 259 – 269.

Johnson D & Cunha, B. Drug Fever. *Infectious Disease Clinics of North America.* March 1996; vol 10; 1: 85-91.

Kelley, WN. *Textbook of Internal Medicine*, 3rd ed. Lippincott-Raven; 1997.

Kelly C, Pothoulakis C, LaMont J. Clostridium difficile colitis. *NEJM.* January 1994; vol. 330; 4: 257-261.

Koenig, K. *Clinical Emergency Medicine.* New York: McGraw-Hill; 1996.

Leach, Richard, *Critical Care Medicine at a Glance,* Blackwell, 2004.

Levin, DL & Morris, FC. *Essentials of Pediatric Intensive Care.* Quality Medical Publishing, Inc.; 1990.

Linden, BE & Aguilar, EA. Sinusitis in the nasotracheally intubated patient. *Arch Otolaryngol Head Neck Surg.* August 1988; vol. 114: 860-861.

Mandell, D & B. *Principles and Practice of Infectious Diseases*, 5th ed. WB Saunders; 2000.

Marino, P. *The ICU Book*, 2nd ed. Baltimore: Williams and Wilkins; 1998.

Marrie, TJ. Community-acquired pneumonia. *Clin Infect Dis.* 1994; 18:501.

Marriott, HJL. *Practical Electrocardiography,* 10th ed. Baltimore: Williams and Wilkins; 2001.

Marshall JB. Acute Pancreatitis. A review with an emphasis on new developments. *Arch Int Med.* 1993;153:1185-1198.

MayoSmith MF, Hirsch PJ, Wodzinski SF, Schiffman FP: Acute epiglottitis in adults. An eight-year experience in the state of Rhode Island. *N Engl J Med.* 1986; 314(18): 1133.

Meduri, GU. Diagnosis of ventilator-associated pneumonia. *Infect Dis clin North Am.* 1993; 7:295.

Miller, RD (ed): *Anesthesia*, 5th ed. New York: Churchill Livingstone; 2000.

Mittman, Bradley, *Frontrunner's Internal Medicine Board Revew*, Frontrunners, 2004.

Mirvis, Stuart, *Imaging in Trauma and Critical Care*, Elsevier Science Health, 2003.

Molitoris, Bruce, *Critical Care Nephrology,* Remedica, 2003.

Montaner JS, Lawson LM, Levitt N, Belzber A, Schechrer,MT, Ruedy J. Corticosteroids prevent early deterioration in patients with moderately sever Pneumocystitis carinii pneumonia and the acquired immunodeficiency syndrome. *Ann Intern Med.* 1990; 113:14-20.

Moore, KL. *Clinically Oriented Anatomy.* 4th ed. Baltimore: Williams & Wilkins; 1999.

Murray, JF and Nadel, JA (ed): *Textbook of Respiratory Medicine*, 3rd ed. Philadelphia: WB Saunders; 2004.

Musher, DM: Infections caused by Streptococcus pneumoniae: Clinical spectrum, pathogenesis, immunity and treatment. *Clin Infect Dis.* 1992;14:801.

Nelson, W.E. *Textbook of Pediatrics.* 17th ed. Philadelphia: W.B. Saunders Company; 2004.

Niederman MS et al.: Guidelines for the initial management of adults with community-acquired pneumonia: Diagnosis, assessment of severity and initial antimicrobial therapy. *Am Rev Respir Dis.* 1993; 148:1418.

Oelkers, W. Adrenal Insufficiency. *N Engl J Med.* 1996; 335:1206-1212.

Owings JT, Kennedy JP, Blaisdell. FW. *Injuries to the Extremities.* Surgery, Scientific American; 1997.

Peitzman AB, Rhodes M, Schwab CW, Yealy DM (eds): *The Trauma Manual.* 2nd ed. Philadelphia: Lippincott-Raven; 2002.

Physicians' Desk Reference, 50th ed. Oradell: Medical Economics Company Inc; 1996.

Plantz, SH. *Emergency Medicine PreTest, Self-Assessment and Review.* McGraw-Hill; 1990.

Plantz, SH. *Emergency Medicine.* Baltimore: Williams & Wilkins; 1998.

Plantz, SH. *Emergency Medicine Pearls of Wisdom,* 6th ed. McGraw-Hill, 2005.

Practical Pulmonary Pathology: A Diagnostic Approach, Churchill Livingstone, 2004.

Principles of Pulmonary Medicine, W.B. Saunders Company, 4th Edition, 2003.

Reddy PS, Curtiss EL, O'Toole JD, Shaver JA. Cardiac tamponade: hemodynamic observations in man. *Circulation.* 1978; 58: 265-272.

Reese, RE & Betts, RF (eds): *A Practical Approach to Infectious Diseases*, 4th ed. Boston: Little, Brown and Company.

Robbins, SL. *Pathologic Basis of Disease,* 3rd ed. Philadelphia: WB Saunders Company; 1984.

Roland, L. *Merritt's Textbook of Neurology.* Williams & Wilkins; 1995.

Rosen, P. *Emergency Medicine Concepts and Clinical Practice,* 4th ed. St. Louis: Mosby Year Book; 1998.

Rosenow EC, Myers JL, Swenson SJ & Pisani RJ: Drug-Induced Pulmonary Disease. *Chest.* 1992; 102:239-250.

Rowe, RC. *The Harriet Lane Handbook: A Manual for Pediatric House Officers,* 16th ed. C.V Mosby; 2002.

Sabiston, DC. *Textbook of Surgery; The Biologic Basis of Modern Surgical Practice.* 17th ed, Philadelphia: W.B. Saunders Co.; 2004.

Salit, IE. Diagnostic approaches to head and neck infections. *Infect Dis Clin N America.* 1988; 2 (1):35.

Savage EB. *Essentials of Basic Science in Surgery.* Philadelphia: J.B. Lippincott Company; 1993.

Schrier, RW & Gottschalk, CW. *Diseases of the Kidney and Urinary Tract,* 7th ed. Williams & Wilkins; 2001.

Shapiro BA, Kacmarek RM, Cane RD, et al: *Clinical Application of Respiratory Care,* 4th.ed. St. Louis: Mosby-Year Book, Inc.; 1991.

Shapiro BA, Peruzzi WT, Templin R. *Clinical Application of Blood Gases,* 5th ed. St. Louis: Mosby-Year Book, Inc.; 1994.

Simon, RR. *Orthopedics in Emergency Medicine: The Extremities,* 2nd ed. Norwalk: Appleton & Lange; 1992.

Simon, RR. *Emergency Procedures and Techniques,* 2nd ed. Baltimore: Williams and Wilkins; 1987.

Squire, LF. *Fundamentals of Radiology,* 6th ed. Cambridge: Harvard University Press; 2004.

Stedman, TL. *Illustrated Stedman's Medical Dictionary,* 24th ed. Baltimore: Williams & Wilkins; 1982.

Stewart, CE. *Environmental Emergencies.* Baltimore: Williams and Wilkins; 1990.

Suarez, Jose, *Crtical Care Neurology and Neurosurgery,* Humana Press, 2003.

Tietjen PA, Kaner, RJ and Quinn CE: Aspiration Emergencies. *Clinics in Chest Medicine* 1994;15:117-135.

Tintinalli, JE. *Emergency Medicine A Comprehensive Study Guide,* 6th ed. New York: McGraw-Hill, Inc; 2003.

Urokinase Pulmonary Embolization Trial Study Group. Urokinase Pulmonary embolism trial- Phase I results. *JAMA.* 1970; 214: 2163-2172.

Vance, ML. Hypopituitarism. *N Engl J Med.* 1994; 330:1651-62 (Erratum, *N Engl J Med.* 1994; 331:487.)

Weigelt, JA & Lewis, FR (eds): *Surgical Critical Care.* Philadelphia: WB Saunders Co.; 1996.

Weiner, HL. *Neurology for the House Officer,* 7th ed. Baltimore: Williams & Wilkins; 2004.

Werber, SS & Ober, KP. Acute adrenal insufficiency. *Endocrinol Metab Clin North Am.* 1993; 22:303-28.

West, JB. *Respiratory Physiology: The Essentials,* 6th ed. Baltimore: Williams & Wilkins; 2000.

Whitley, RJ. Viral Encephalitis. *NEJM.* July 1990; 242 – 248.

Williams, RD & Larsen, PR. *Williams Textbook of Endocrinology,* 10th ed. Philadelphia: W.B. Saunders; 2002.

Wilson, R & Walt, A. *Management of Trauma: Pitfalls and Practice,* 2nd ed. Philadelphia: Williams & Wilkins; 1996.

Yoshikawa, TT & Quinn, W. The aching head: intracranial suppuration due to head and neck infections. *Infect Dis Clin N America.* 1988; 2 (1):265,

Youmans, JR. *Neurological Surgery,* 5th ed. Philadelphia: W.B. Saunders; 2003.

Zevitz, M. *Cardiovascular Pearls of Wisdom.* McGraw-Hill, 2005.

Zevitz, M. *Internal Medicine Pearls of Wisdom.* McGraw-Hill, 2005.

NOTES

NOTES

NOTES

NOTES

NOTES

NOTES